T0137425

Regenerative Medicine for Spine and Joint Pain

Grant Cooper • Joseph Herrera
Jason Kirkbride • Zachary Perlman
Editors

Regenerative Medicine for Spine and Joint Pain

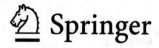 Springer

Editors
Grant Cooper
Princeton Spine and Joint Center
Princeton, NJ
USA

Jason Kirkbride
Princeton Spine and Joint Center
Princeton, NJ
USA

Joseph Herrera
Department of Rehabilitation Medicine
Mount Sinai Hospital
New York, NY
USA

Zachary Perlman
Princeton Spine and Joint Center
Princeton, NJ
USA

ISBN 978-3-030-42773-3   ISBN 978-3-030-42771-9   (eBook)
https://doi.org/10.1007/978-3-030-42771-9

This Springer imprint is published by the registered company Springer Nature Switzerland AG
The registered company address is: Gewerbestrasse 11, 6330 Cham, Switzerland

Contents

Contributors

Walter Alomar-Jimenez, MD, JD Department of Rehabilitation and Human Performance, Icahn School of Medicine at Mount Sinai, New York, NY, USA

Allison C. Bean, MD, PhD Department of Physical Medicine and Rehabilitation, University of Pittsburgh Medical Center, Pittsburgh, PA, USA

Tina Bijlani, DO Rehabilitation Medicine, The Mount Sinai Hospital, Mount Sinai, New York, NY, USA

Eliana Cardozo, DO Sports Medicine and Interventional Spine, Department of Rehabilitation Medicine and Human Performance, Icahn School of Medicine at Mount Sinai, New York, NY, USA

Richard G. Chang, MD, MPH Department of Rehabilitation & Human Performance, Icahn School of Medicine at Mount Sinai, New York, NY, USA

Grant Cooper, MD Princeton Spine and Joint Center, Princeton, NJ, USA

Andrew Creighton, DO Physiatry, Hospital for Special Surgery, Rehabilitation Medicine, Weill Cornell Medicine, New York, NY, USA

Emily N. Fatakhov, MD Rehabilitation Medicine, The Mount Sinai Hospital, Mount Sinai, New York, NY, USA

Alfred C. Gellhorn, MD Department of Rehabilitation Medicine, Weill Cornell Medicine, New York, NY, USA

Michael Guthrie, MD University of Pittsburgh Medical Center, Department of PM&R, Pittsburgh, PA, USA

Behnum Habibi, MD NewYork-Presbyterian University Hospital, Columbia University Medical Center and Weill Cornell Medical Center, New York, NY, USA

Joseph Herrera, DO Department of Rehabilitation Medicine, Mount Sinai Hospital, New York, NY, USA

Jason Kirkbride, MD Princeton Spine and Joint Center, Princeton, NJ, USA

Jonathan S. Kirschner, MD Physiatry, Hospital for Special Surgery, Rehabilitation Medicine, Weill Cornell Medicine, New York, NY, USA

Anthony J. Mazzola, MD Department of Rehabilitation and Human Performance, Icahn School of Medicine at Mount Sinai, New York, NY, USA

Dayna McCarthy, DO Sports Medicine and Interventional Spine, Department of Rehabilitation and Human Performance, Icahn School of Medicine at Mount Sinai, New York, NY, USA

Anokhi Mehta, MD Department of Rehabilitation and Human Performance, Icahn School of Medicine at Mount Sinai, New York, NY, USA

Gerardo Miranda-Comas, MD Department of Rehabilitation and Human Performance, Icahn School of Medicine at Mount Sinai, New York, NY, USA

Kentaro Onishi, DO University of Pittsburgh School of Medicine, Department of PM&R, Department of Orthopaedic Surgery, Pittsburgh, PA, USA

Zachary Perlman, DO Princeton Spine and Joint Center, Princeton, NJ, USA

Jonathan Ramin, DO Sports Medicine and Interventional Spine, Department of Rehabilitation Medicine and Human Performance, Icahn School of Medicine at Mount Sinai, New York, NY, USA

Krutika Parasar Raulkar, MD Department of Physical Medicine and Rehabilitation, NewYork-Presbyterian Hospital – The University Hospital of Columbia and Cornell, New York, NY, USA

Stephen Schaaf, MD University of Pittsburgh Medical Center, Department of PM&R, Pittsburgh, PA, USA

Caroline Schepker, DO NewYork-Presbyterian University Hospital, Columbia University Medical Center and Weill Cornell Medical Center, New York, NY, USA

Allison N. Schroeder, MD University of Pittsburgh Medical Center, Department of PM&R, Pittsburgh, PA, USA

David A. Spinner, DO, RMSK, CIPS, FAAPMR Department of Rehabilitation and Human Performance, Icahn School of Medicine at Mount Sinai, New York, NY, USA

Katherine V. Yao, MD Weill Cornell Medical College, New York, NY, USA

Xiaoning (Jenny) Yuan, MD, PhD Department of Rehabilitation Medicine, NewYork-Presbyterian Hospital, New York, NY, USA

Mariam Zakhary, DO Department of Rehabilitation and Human Performance, Icahn School of Medicine at Mount Sinai, New York, NY, USA

Nadia N. Zaman, DO Sports Medicine and Interventional Spine, Department of Rehabilitation and Human Performance, Icahn School of Medicine at Mount Sinai, New York, NY, USA

Chapter 1
Introduction to Regenerative Medicine

Grant Cooper, Joseph Herrera, Jason Kirkbride, and Zachary Perlman

Regenerative Medicine Intro Combined

Patients suffering from musculoskeletal ailments frequently seek additional treatment options after more traditional methods have failed. Though eager for alternative methods, they may have reservations over the safety and efficacy of the broad range of regenerative medicine techniques, which can make regenerative medicine a somewhat controversial topic [1, 2]. A large pool of anecdotal evidence exists, but there is no standardization of techniques, and evidence-based research has strained to catch up (Table 1.1). As is the case with cutting-edge treatments, research is continually emerging. By reviewing, evaluating, and exploring the current state of regenerative medicine research, we hope to provide a foundation upon which the practitioner can converse with the patient. Organizing the book based on the anatomic site of injury will allow the medical practitioner to easily reference evidence-based regenerative medicine treatment options and help guide open discussion with their patients about additional treatments that may be appropriate to offer.

In the broad sense of the term, "regenerative medicine" is delivering cells or products to diseased tissues or organs in the attempt to restore tissue or organ function. What we are interested in is connective tissue and bone regeneration [3]. The rationale for using these therapies is that the injected product will stimulate repair of these damaged structures as opposed to only treating the patient's symptoms. To understand these regenerative options, it is important to look back at the history of platelet-rich plasma (PRP) and stem cell therapy.

G. Cooper (✉) · J. Kirkbride · Z. Perlman
Princeton Spine and Joint Center, Princeton, NJ, USA
e-mail: drcooper@princetonsjc.com

J. Herrera
Department of Rehabilitation Medicine, Mount Sinai Hospital, New York, NY, USA

© Springer Nature Switzerland AG 2020
G. Cooper et al. (eds.), *Regenerative Medicine for Spine and Joint Pain*,
https://doi.org/10.1007/978-3-030-42771-9_1

Table 1.1 Regenerative Medicine Questions

What is the particular "injectate"?
Are we using leukocyte-reduced or leukocyte-enriched PRP?
How are you harvesting your stem cells?
Bone marrow aspirate, bone marrow concentrate, or mesenchymal from adipose tissue?
What about embryonic products?
Which therapy is the most powerful "regenerator"?
How do we price them?
How much volume is just right for your patient?
Do they need a single or series of multiple injections?
If we are treating an arthritic condition, then what stage of arthritis responds best?
How active is the patient?/What level of competition?
Gender?
What is the post-injection rehabilitation protocol?
As you can see, there are many possible combinations of answers to the above questions, which makes this field very intimidating to patients and practitioners because of the many variables.

Platelet-rich plasma was developed in the field of hematology in the 1970s [4]. PRP releases growth factors, which are also known as bioactive proteins. These proteins aid in stimulating the body's natural ability to heal. Hematologists were treating thrombocytopenia with a product that was plasma with a platelet count higher than peripheral blood. In the late 1980s, it was used during open heart surgery. Then, in the 1990s, maxillofacial surgeons were using PRP to aid in healing skin flaps. Next, it was used in musculoskeletal medicine. The first documented case in *Sports Medicine* was in 1999, when Dr. Allan Mishra used PRP to treat San Francisco 49ers quarterback Steve Bono's Achilles tendon injury. In 2006, PRP use for elbow tendonitis was published in the *American Journal of Sports Medicine*. That study showed 60% improvement in pain levels immediately, 81% improvement in 6 months, and 93% improvement at 2 years. This is when PRP gained significant popularity and many well-known professional athletes began using PRP therapy including Kobe Bryant and Tiger Woods [5]. It then gained popularity among orthopedic surgeons for treating fracture nonunion, arthritis, tendonitis, muscle strains, cartilage injuries, and more [6]. Today, PRP is being used in pediatric surgery, gynecology, urology, plastic surgery, dermatology, and ophthalmology.

Stem cells are cells that have the ability to differentiate or change into a particular cell. A specific type of stem cell known as a mesenchymal stem cell can transform into a bone, cartilage, muscle, or fat cell. The first scientists who defined the key properties of stem cells were Ernest McCulloch and James Till in the 1960s. They discovered that the cells can divide and differentiate into mature cell types [7]. Then, in 1996, scientists were crossing ethical boundaries when attempting to clone "Dolly the sheep" by using stem cells. In the early 2000s, Dr. Shinya Yamanaka discovered skin cells can be converted into stem cells by altering gene expression. This was the birth of induced pluripotent stem cells, or iPS. Since then, stem cells have been used in musculoskeletal medicine and many other areas including gene therapy for inheritable disorders.

As you will find, the research is not unambiguous. Patients who have been failed by more traditional treatment options are frequently desperate for additional potential treatments. Demand for regenerative medicine is growing as the amount of evidence increases. Oftentimes, patients are initiating the conversation about regenerative medicine and it is important for the physician to be well prepared for such a discussion. Practitioners must be ready to acknowledge the lack of clear-cut evidence at times and be open to frank discussions regarding the risks of treatment and potential benefits [8]. Informed consent is paramount and cannot be stressed enough. The ability to counsel on the risks and benefits of different regenerative medicine techniques based on the current literature is the first step to offering regenerative medicine treatment options. Though it is important to remain hopeful that regenerative treatment will allow for improvements when more conservative measures have failed, it is essential to develop realistic goals with the patient.

As the number of degenerative and chronic conditions continues to climb among the population, demand for regenerative medicine is increasing. Regenerative medicine and tissue engineering have been identified as top research priorities by the Medical Research Council in the United Kingdom and the National Research Council of the United States [9]. With increased interest and research into regenerative medicine, the ambition to transition healthcare from a focus on symptomatic treatment to a more curative treatment approach grows [10]. Because of this growing expectation, significant controversies exist. Concerns include research misconduct and tumor development [11, 12], while unproven therapies are creating an entire stem cell tourism industry with little safety oversight for patients desperate for therapeutic treatment [13]. In addition, there are multiple manufacturers of the systems that isolate the injectate, so not every physician offering regenerative medicine is using the same concentration of growth factors. Another major barrier to administering regenerative medicine to patients is that insurance companies generally do not cover these injections. It is difficult to say if the Food and Drug Administration (FDA) could administer an approval since "the injectate" is not a product of a pharmaceutical laboratory, but it stems from the patient themselves. Despite these obstacles, regenerative medicine continues to make progress with regard to safety and its use of evidence-based treatment options. As the number of clinical trials continue to increase, regenerative medicine is at the cutting edge of translational research and will require a collaborative effort among a vast array of interdisciplinary researchers and clinicians [14]. This further cements the need for an evidence-based, practitioner-friendly guide to regenerative treatments.

References

1. Matthews KR, Iltis AS. Unproven stem cell-based interventions and achieving a compromise policy among the multiple stakeholders. BMC Med Ethics. 2015;16:75. https://doi.org/10.1186/s12910-015-0069-x.
2. Alta CR. On the road (to a cure?) — stem-cell tourism and lessons for gene editing. N Engl J Med. 2016;374:901–3. https://doi.org/10.1056/NEJMp1600891.

3. https://www.mayo.edu/research/centers-programs/center-regenerative-medicine/patient-care/about-regenerative-medicine.
4. Andia I, Abate M. Platelet rich plasma: underlying biology and clinical correlates. Regen Med. 2013;8:645–58.
5. Mishra A, Pavelko T. Treatment of chronic elbow tendinosis with buffered platelet-rich plasma. Am J Sports Med. 2006;34(11):1774–8.
6. https://www.movementortho.com/2017/11/03/the-history-of-prp-therapy/.
7. http://sitn.hms.harvard.edu/flash/2014/stem-cells-a-brief-history-and-outlook-2/.
8. Bubela T, Li MD, Hafez M, Bieber M, Atkins H. Is belief larger than fact: expectations, optimism and reality for translational stem cell research. BMC Med. 2012;10:133. https://doi.org/10.1186/1741-7015-10-133.
9. O'Dowd A. Peers call for UK to harness "enormous" potential of regenerative medicine. BMJ. 2013;347:f4248. https://doi.org/10.1136/bmj.f4248.
10. Nelson TJ, Behfar A, Terzic A. Strategies for therapeutic repair: the "R3" regenerative medicine paradigm. Clin Transl Sci. 2008;1:168–71.
11. Berkowitz AL, Miller MB, et al. Glioproliferative lesion of the spinal cord as a complication of "stem-cell tourism". N Engl J Med. 2016;375:196–8. https://doi.org/10.1056/NEJMc1600188.
12. Wang Y, Han Z-B, Song Y-P, Han ZC. Safety of mesenchymal stem cells for clinical application. Stem Cells Int. 2012;2012:4. https://doi.org/10.1155/2012/652034.652034.
13. Brown C. Stem cell tourism poses risks. CMAJ. 2012;184(2):E121–2. https://doi.org/10.1503/cmaj.109-4073.
14. Jessop ZM, et al. Transforming healthcare through regenerative medicine. BMC Med. 2016;14(1):115. https://doi.org/10.1186/s12916-016-0669-4.

Chapter 2
Basic Science Concepts in Musculoskeletal Regenerative Medicine

Allison C. Bean

Introduction

Injury and degeneration of musculoskeletal tissues of the spine and joints are common causes of pain and disability, creating a significant worldwide health and economic burden. These tissues are particularly at risk due to their limited intrinsic healing capacity in conjunction with repetitive exposure to high mechanical loads over a lifetime. Following injury, many musculoskeletal tissues are unable to fully recover, leading to persistent alterations in mechanical properties that may initiate a cascade of progressively worsening tissue degradation and functional impairment.

Regenerative medicine has been studied as a method to repair or replace damaged cells, tissues, and organs. Numerous strategies have been investigated, including but not limited to tissue engineering, autologous cell therapy, gene therapy, and administration of growth factors (Fig. 2.1) [1]. Tissue engineering strategies typically focus on combining cells, scaffolds, and biochemical factors to create a functional tissue in vitro that may subsequently be implanted. Other regenerative approaches may rely on altering the in vivo environment via injection or implantation of cells and biochemical factors in order to stimulate the body's innate healing mechanisms to repair or regenerate the damaged tissue.

Regardless of the approach, thorough knowledge of the biological structure and function of the tissue niche is essential to develop effective regenerative therapies. This chapter will focus on the basic science concepts that guide the development and application of regenerative medicine for treatment of spine and joint dysfunction. An overview of the developmental biology of the joints, spine, and associated

A. C. Bean (✉)
Department of Physical Medicine and Rehabilitation,
University of Pittsburgh Medical Center, Pittsburgh, PA, USA
e-mail: beanac2@upmc.edu

© Springer Nature Switzerland AG 2020
G. Cooper et al. (eds.), *Regenerative Medicine for Spine and Joint Pain*,
https://doi.org/10.1007/978-3-030-42771-9_2

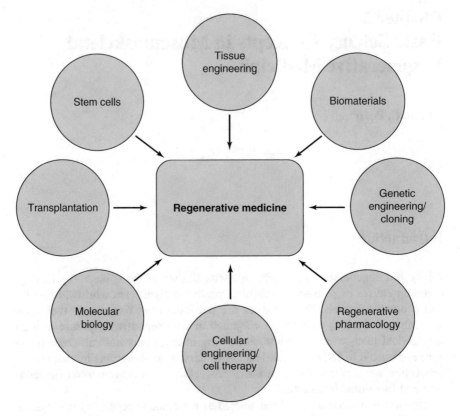

Fig. 2.1 Schematic representation of the various components of regenerative medicine. (Reprinted from Yalcinkaya et al. [1], with permission from Elsevier)

tissues from fertilization to maturity will be presented, followed by a summary of the current scientific understanding of the pathophysiology underlying degeneration of skeletal tissues.

Musculoskeletal Development

Developmental biology focuses on understanding the physical and chemical cues that lead to tissue and organ formation. Regenerative medicine seeks to create or heal tissues through manipulation of cells and the diseased tissue environment. Applying knowledge of developmental processes to regenerative medicine strategies can allow for improved control over cell behavior and potentially result in more effective therapies.

Early Musculoskeletal Embryogenesis

Most scientific knowledge of musculoskeletal development is derived from experiments performed in chick and mouse embryos. The majority of musculoskeletal tissues, except for craniofacial tissues that arise from the neural crest, are derived from the mesodermal layer of the embryo. The axial skeleton arises from the paraxial mesoderm while the limbs are derived from the lateral plate mesoderm [2]. Skeletogenesis is regulated through several signaling pathways. In particular, members of the transforming growth factor-beta (TGF-β) superfamily, which include TGF-β as well as bone morphogenic proteins (BMPs), fibroblast growth factors (FGFs), and growth differentiation factors (GDFs) play important roles throughout bone and cartilage development and in maintaining tissue homeostasis during adulthood [3].

Bone Embryogenesis

Bone formation occurs through two different mechanisms. The flat bones of the skull form through a process known as intramembranous ossification, during which mesenchymal cells directly differentiate into osteoblasts, laying down osteoid matrix that is then mineralized. The process of intramembranous ossification will not be covered in this chapter, but has been described in detail elsewhere [4, 5]. In contrast, long bones and vertebrae develop through a process known as endochondral ossification, where tissues proceed through a cartilaginous phase prior to mineralization (Fig. 2.2).

The initial step in limb bone and joint formation begins with clustering of mesenchymal cells within the limb bud in a process known as mesenchymal condensation. Following condensation, under regulation by the transcription factor Sox9, the mesenchymal cells begin to differentiate into two separate populations of cells – an avascular core containing rounded chondrocytes and an outer layer of flattened perichondrial cells closely associated with the surrounding vasculature [7, 8]. The chondrocytes proliferate, producing an initial cartilaginous extracellular matrix template, or anlage, which segments to form early the individual skeletal elements. Chondrocytes at the center of the anlage eventually stop proliferating and undergo hypertrophy, shifting from secretion of type II to X collagen and inducing matrix mineralization. Hypertrophic chondrocytes also secrete paracrine factors including Indian hedgehog (IHH), signaling perichondrial cells to undergo differentiation, and vascular endothelial growth factor (VEGF), triggering blood vessel invasion.

Hypertrophic chondrocytes eventually undergo apoptosis as mineralization limits nutrient delivery to the interior of the tissue [9–12]. Perichondrial cells adjacent to the hypertrophic zone differentiate into osteoblasts, which create a mineralized

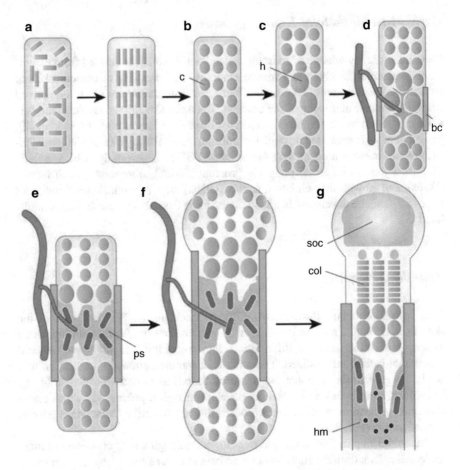

Fig. 2.2 Endochondral bone formation. (**a**) Mesenchymal cells condense. (**b**) Cells of condensations become chondrocytes (c). (**c**) Chondrocytes at the center of condensation stop proliferating and become hypertrophic (h). (**d**) Perichondrial cells adjacent to hypertrophic chondrocytes become osteoblasts, forming the bone collar (bc). Hypertrophic chondrocytes direct the formation of mineralized matrix, attract blood vessels, and undergo apoptosis. (**e**) Osteoblasts of primary spongiosa accompany vascular invasion, forming the primary spongiosa (ps). (**f**) Chondrocytes continue to proliferate, lengthening the bone. Osteoblasts of primary spongiosa are precursors of eventual trabecular bone; osteoblasts of the bone collar become the cortical bone. (**g**) At the end of the bone, the secondary ossification center (soc) forms through cycles of chondrocyte hypertrophy, vascular invasion, and osteoblast activity. The growth plate below the secondary center of ossification forms orderly columns of proliferating chondrocytes (col). Hematopoietic marrow (hm) expands in the marrow space along with stromal cells. (Reprinted from Kronenberg [6] with permission from Springer Nature)

bone collar, forming early the cortical bone, and endothelial cells, which initiate vascular invasion into the tissue [7]. As blood vessels invade, they bring chondroclasts and hemopoietic stem cells. The chondroclasts resorb the cartilaginous matrix and osteoblast precursors use the remnants as a scaffold for bone matrix deposition. This tissue is known as the primary spongiosa and is later remodeled into a mature trabecular bone. Hemopoietic stem cells migrate to the center of the eventual diaphysis, where they reside within the bone marrow postnatally [13]. This region is called the primary ossification center (POC). Chondrocytes at the epiphyseal ends continue to proliferate, elongating the bone, while progressive chondrocyte hypertrophy and subsequent ossification continue from the POC toward the epiphysis. Postnatally, a secondary ossification center (SOC) forms at the epiphysis in a process similar to the POC. Chondrocyte proliferation is then limited to the epiphyseal or growth plate, which closes at the end of puberty [9–12, 14, 15].

Synovial Joint Development

Development of synovial joints begins at the time of cartilage anlagen segmentation as mentioned previously. The first step is condensation of cells into a densely packed region called the interzone. The interzone layer gradually thickens and then separates to form early the joint space. Cells in the interzone express Gdf5 and eventually give rise to the articular cartilage covering the joint surface, as well as other joint tissues including the joint capsule, synovium, ligaments, and menisci. They also contribute to chondrocyte proliferation and bone maturation at the SOC [16–18].

Articular cartilage maturation continues postnatally, with chondrocytes continuing to proliferate and produce matrix proteins. Eventually, the tissue is organized into four zones: superficial, middle, deep, and calcified. Articular cartilage ECM is primarily composed of type II collagen and proteoglycans, the most prevalent being aggrecan. The superficial zone contains flattened chondrocytes expressing lubricin and hyaluronic acid, creating a smooth, low-friction surface and preventing overgrowth of synovial cells [19]. The collagen matrix in the superficial zone runs parallel to the tissue surface. In the middle/intermediate zone, chondrocytes have a more rounded morphology while collagen fibers are thicker and loosely organized into radial bundles. Chondrocytes in the deep zone are organized into columns and secrete less collagen and more aggrecan. Lastly, chondrocytes in the deep calcified zone located adjacent to the subchondral bone are hypertrophic and terminally differentiated, expressing type X collagen and alkaline phosphatase [20]. This tissue organization enables cartilage to effectively absorb and dissipate the forces generated during loading.

Spine Joint Development

At each spinal level, three joints link adjacent vertebrae and stabilize the spine. Zygapophysial or facet joints are located posteriorly on each side of the vertebral column and are articular joints that form between superior and inferior processes of adjacent vertebrae [21]. Between each bony vertebra lies an intervertebral disc (IVD) which functions to stabilize the spine, acts as a shock absorber during loading, and allows for multidirectional movement of the spinal column [22]. The IVD is bound rostrally and caudally by the endplate (EP), a thin layer of articular cartilage less than 1 mm thick, that separates the IVD from the vertebral bodies and aids in mechanical load distribution [23]. During embryogenesis, blood vessels transverse through the EP and into the IVD, supplying nutrients to the AF and NP. As development progresses, the vessels regress, and the IVD becomes avascular by adulthood, relying on diffusion of nutrients through the endplate from vessels terminating within the subchondral bone [23, 24].

The NP is derived from cells originating from the embryonic notochord [25, 26]. The notochord initially begins as a rod-like structure oriented along the rostro-caudal access of the embryo and acts as a signaling center, directing patterning of the neural tube and other tissues. The mechanisms driving the transformation of the notochord into the NP are not fully understood; however, notochordal cells eventually differentiate into chondrocytic NP cells and secrete a gelatinous ECM composed primarily of aggrecan along with sparse, randomly oriented type II collagen fibers. The glycosaminoglycan (GAG) chains of aggrecan proteoglycans are negatively charged and hydrophilic, creating high osmotic pressures within the NP and giving it the ability to withstand and distribute compressive loads [22].

The AF is composed of fibrochondrocytes that secrete an ECM predominately composed of aligned collagen with small amounts of proteoglycans organized into 15–25 lamellar sheets. The collagen fibers of consecutive layers are obliquely oriented and alternate in direction with each layer, creating an angle-ply structure. This arrangement gives the AF the ability to withstand the high tensile forces during compressive loading [22, 27]. The outer AF has a more fibrous structure containing more type I collagen, while the inner zone is more cartilaginous with higher aggrecan and type II collagen content [28].

Tendon and Ligament Development

While not part of the joint proper, tendons play an important role in joint motion, since they couple muscle to bone across joints. Ligaments also play an important role in joint stabilization as they form bone-to-bone connections. Research focused on ligament development is limited; however, there appears to be significant overlap with tendon, as these tissues have comparable composition and properties [29]. Given these similarities and lack of scientific literature specific to ligament development, this text will focus predominately on the formation of tendons.

Cells that will differentiate into mature tendon cells are known as tenocytes. Axial tenocytes originate from a dorsolateral strip of the sclerotome in a region known as the syndetome. Syndetome formation is dependent on FGF signaling from the myotome, which induces expression of the transcription factor scleraxis (Scx), a key regulator of tendon development. Tendon progenitors are initially loosely organized between the developing bone and muscle. Then, under regulation by TGF-β secreted by the bone and muscle, additional tendon precursors are recruited and the cells become organized, begin to differentiate, and integrate with bone and muscle at the enthesis and myotendinous junction [30, 31].

Limb tenocytes arise from the lateral plate mesoderm and in the early limb bud consist of ventral and dorsal blastema, from which the flexor and extensor tendons arise, respectively. Unlike the axial skeleton, muscle is not required for initial induction of tendon progenitors in the limbs, though it does appear to be required in later stages of differentiation. Instead, the blastemas are located under the ectodermal layer, from which they receive signals required for induction of Scx expression, which mediates expression of BMP4 [32]. As the limb bud lengthens, the tendon progenitor cells of the proximal limb realign between the differentiating muscle and bone, while distal tendon cells are already near their eventual position prior to induction.

Mature tendon ECM is predominately composed of aligned type I collagen fibers assembled in a hierarchical pattern, with small amounts of other collagens and proteoglycans. Initial tendon matrix synthesis begins with formation of thin collagen fibrils, which assemble together, gradually increasing in length and width, eventually forming collagen fibers. Fibers are bundled together into fascicles, which are separated by loose connective tissue composed of small collagen fibers and elastin called the endotenon, which is contiguous with the surrounding epitenon. Some tendons also have an outer sheath known as the paratenon, which allows tendons, such as at the Achilles, to slide more easily over bony protuberances [33].

The underlying mechanisms of the juncture of tendon with bone at the enthesis and tendon with muscle at the myotendinous junction (MTJ) are incompletely understood. Muscle cells, or myocytes, originate from the somite myotome. Cells in the dorsomedial portion of the myotome give rise to the axial muscles while those in the ventrolateral portion migrate toward the lateral plate mesoderm to eventually form the limb muscles [34]. As tendon and muscle precursors become closely approximated, a disorganized ECM including integrin ligands and thrombospondin 4 (Tsp4) is secreted by myoblasts, forming early the basement membrane. These proteins facilitate integrin binding, stabilizing myofibers and tendon collagen fibers at the MTJ. As myotubes begin to contract, the tension generated at the MTJ interface stimulates increased production and alignment of tendon collagen and parallel assembly of sarcomeres. Persistent mechanical forces promote maturation of collagen fibers and formation of the finger-like processes characteristic of the MTJ as noted above [35–37]. Unlike much of the musculoskeletal system, MTJ formation is complete by the time of birth [36].

Mature fibrocartilaginous entheses, which typically occur near joints, consist of four zones, gradually transitioning from tendinous to cartilaginous to mineralized tissue [38, 39]. After establishment of the primary cartilage anlagen, eminences appear at the site of the future enthesis and are composed of a separate pool of progenitor cells that initially co-express Scx and Sox9, as well as Gdf5 and later Gli1 [40, 41]. Gli1 is a downstream target of Hedgehog, and its expression is essential for enthesis development, where it may play a role in mineralization and widening of the enthesis [42, 43]. Mechanical loading of the enthesis during early post-natal development has been shown to be essential for enthesis maturation, likely through modulation of Hedgehog expression, as reduction of loading results in impaired mineralization [42, 44].

Musculoskeletal Tissue Homeostasis and Response to Injury

Osteoarthritis (OA) is estimated to affect 10–15% of the population and is a leading cause of disability worldwide, particularly among older individuals [45]. OA most commonly affects the hips, knees, fingers, and spine but can occur in any joint. Development of OA is often multifactorial and is associated with systemic and biomechanical risk factors including but not limited to age, sex, genetics, weight, occupation, joint shape, joint alignment, and comorbid medical conditions [46]. OA is primarily characterized by cartilage deterioration, but surrounding joint tissues including the synovium, meniscus, ligaments, and subchondral bone are often involved [47]. In this section, we provide a brief summary of the pathophysiology of degenerative disease of joints, spine, and tendons, identifying potential mechanisms through which regenerative therapies may prevent or manage pain and disease progression. Proposed mechanisms of repair in currently used regenerative therapies such as platelet-rich plasma and stem cells will be covered in later chapters.

Osteoarthritis of Articular Cartilage

The normal cartilaginous tissues of articular joints are avascular and hypoxic, relying on diffusion for delivery of nutrients from the joint capsule, synovium, and underlying subchondral bone. As a result, chondrocyte metabolism and ECM turnover are limited under normal physiologic conditions, with the half-life of type II collagen and aggrecan estimated to be 120 years and 120 days, respectively [48]. Tissue homeostasis is maintained through a balance of anabolic and catabolic factors released by chondrocytes in response to environmental cues, carefully modulating the slow ECM turnover. Disruption of this balance leads to the complex cascade of changes seen in OA. Below, we briefly highlight some of the mechanisms that drive the development of OA. Additional comprehensive discussions of the important molecular pathways are found in other reviews [49–54]. It is important to note that much of the knowledge regarding these pathways has been obtained from animal studies and may not be completely translatable to the general human population.

The primary driver in development of osteoarthritis is thought to be abnormal mechanical loading of the joint. Chondrocytes are mechanoresponsive cells, altering their phenotype based on changing mechanical cues. Cyclic physiologic loading is important for maintaining cartilage health, and it has been suggested that in the absence of altered biomechanics or biology of the tissue, the cartilage becomes conditioned to the physiologic loads generated during locomotion, maintaining homeostasis [55]. Previous studies have demonstrated that reduced loading due to immobilization has been shown to lead to decreased cartilage thickness [56, 57]. In several experiments using canine models, immobilization resulted in loss of proteoglycans in the cartilage superficial zone and reduced mechanical properties [58–60]. Mechanical overloading either through strenuous repetition or single high-magnitude loads can lead to increased catabolic activity and cartilage degradation. In in vitro and canine models, supramaximal repetitive loading causes tissue swelling, chondrocyte apoptosis, increased oxidative stress, reduced matrix protein production (including GAGs), increased matrix protein breakdown, and reduced mechanical properties, with the severity of findings often proportional to the magnitude of loading [61–68]. Furthermore, injuries to other joint tissues such as menisci or ligaments can lead to increased risk of developing post-traumatic osteoarthritis, which likely occurs secondary to long-term changes in joint kinematics as a result of the previous injuries [69]. Re-establishing healthy joint kinematics should be part of any OA treatment plan; however, this is a difficult task as small variations are difficult to detect.

The earliest change typically seen in OA is disruption of the collagen fibers in the superficial layer [70, 71]. In response to injury, chondrocytes proliferate and form clusters around the damaged area, releasing both anabolic and catabolic factors in an attempt to remodel the injured tissue [72]. However, the overall anabolic capabilities of chondrocytes are limited, and unless there is a full thickness injury penetrating the subchondral bone, progenitor cells with increased reparative abilities cannot be recruited due to the lack of vasculature. Even in full thickness injuries, the repair response is limited, with the repaired tissue lacking the organization and mechanical strength of the native tissue [73, 74]. In contrast, the catabolic processes initiated by chondrocytes following injury are robust and self-sustaining, shifting the balance toward progressive tissue degeneration and OA.

In a process akin to endochondral ossification that occurs normally during development of long bones, following initial clustering and proliferation, chondrocytes in injured cartilage become hypertrophic, eventually initiating mineral deposition and thickening of the deep calcified zone. VEGF expression in the underlying subchondral bone increases concomitantly, inducing bone remodeling and vascular invasion into the cartilage layers, leading to impaired mechanical properties and progressive cartilage degradation and chondrocyte apoptosis. In later stages of OA, persistent activation of catabolic pathways may also stimulate other pathologic changes throughout the joint including meniscus and ligament degeneration, osteophyte formation, subchondral bone sclerosis, joint capsule hypertrophy, and synovial inflammation and fibrosis [75, 76]. Blood vessel ingrowth occurs with many of these changes and is typically accompanied by sensory nerves containing substance P and calcitonin gene-related peptide. These small unmyelinated nerves are thought to contribute to the development of pain typically seen in OA [77, 78].

Cartilage homeostasis is maintained by transcriptional control of the chondrocyte phenotype through several different interconnecting pathways. Following injury, activation of these pathways shift, driving chondrocytes toward a hypertrophic

phenotype and terminal differentiation, similar to that seen in endochondral ossification. Each of these pathways induces downregulation of Sox9 and upregulation of
Runx2, and the cells begin to synthesize type X collagen while reducing production
of type II collagen and aggrecan. Hypertrophic chondrocytes in injured articular
cartilage also express high levels of proteases including metalloproteinases (MMPs)
and a disintegrin and metalloproteinase with thrombospondin motifs (ADAMTS),
which degrade collagen and aggrecan, respectively. MMP-1, MMP-3, and MMP
-13 and ADAMTS-4 and ADAMTS-5 have been shown to be particularly important
in tissue degeneration in OA. Conversely, tissue inhibitors of metalloproteinases
(TIMPs) are downregulated. Thus, inhibition of MMP and ADAMTS activity has
been seen as a potential therapeutic target. While most of the specific inhibitors
of these enzymes have not yet made it past pre-clinical testing [79, 80], an oral
ADAMTS-5 inhibitor is currently being tested in a phase II clinical trial [81].

Inflammation plays an integral role in the progression of OA (Fig. 2.3). Molecules
known as damage-associated breakdown products (DAMPs) are released by chondrocytes following injury and serve as ligands for pattern recognition receptors
(PRRs) including toll-like receptors (TLRs) and receptor for advanced glycation
end products (RAGE) expressed by chondrocytes and synovial cells. Interaction
between DAMPs and PRRs induces release of pro-inflammatory cytokines including pro-inflammatory interleukins, IL-1β and IL-6, and tissue necrosis factor-
alpha (TNF-α) from chondrocytes and macrophages. This signals chondrocytes to
undergo hypertrophy and terminal differentiation and promotes tissue degradation
through nuclear factor-kappaB (NF-κB) and MAPK pathways, resulting in upregulation of MMPs and ADAMTS, as well as other pro-inflammatory mediators including nitric oxide (NO), cyclooxygenase-2 (COX-2), and prostaglandin E2 (PGE2)
[50, 52]. Activation of the complement system and infiltration of cell mediators of
the adaptive immune system including T-cells, B-cells, and macrophages have also
been found to be increased in the synovium of osteoarthritic joints [82–84]. In sum,
the pro-inflammatory environment induced by cartilage injury leads to progressive
synovitis and chondrocyte activation, promoting a cycle of inflammation and cell
damage that results in progressive cartilage breakdown and changes in the other
joint tissues as described above.

Medications commonly used in OA including corticosteroids, nonsteroidal anti-
inflammatory drugs (NSAIDs), COX inhibitors, and hyaluronic acid are directed
toward inhibition of inflammatory pathways; however, long-term use can result
in significant side effects, including adverse gastrointestinal and cardiovascular
events, and may even accelerate OA progression [85–87]. Anti-cytokine therapies
have been demonstrated to be effective in the treatment of rheumatoid arthritis;
however, their efficacy in OA thus far appears to be limited [88].

TGF-β is essential for chondrocyte maturation and differentiation during development and is present in low concentrations in young, healthy articular cartilage.
TGF-β signaling through the Alk5-SMAD2/3 pathway has been shown to be essential for inhibiting chondrocyte hypertrophy and terminal differentiation [89, 90].
Following injury, TGF-β downstream signaling appears to shift from signaling
through the Alk5-SMAD2/3 pathway to the Alk1-SMAD1/5/8 pathway, inducing

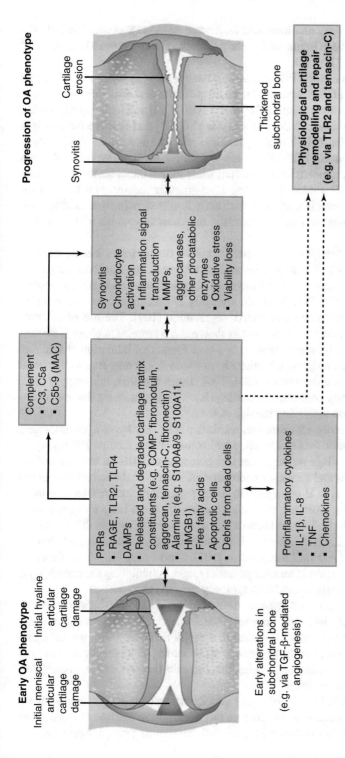

Fig. 2.3 Several of the different classes of inflammatory mediators, including PRRs and their DAMP ligands, conventional inflammatory cytokines, and activated complement proteins C5a and C5b-9 network to augment meniscal fibrocartilage and articular cartilage damage in early and progressive OA. These mediators promote macroscopic inflammation, including synovitis, and can drive cartilage matrix catabolism, but some also promote cartilage remodeling and repair. The number and diversity of inflammatory mediators in OA joints, the paradoxical roles of some of these mediators in tissue damage and repair, and the physiological roles of some mediators in host defense mean targeting individual mediators for OA therapy is difficult. Abbreviations: COMP, cartilage oligomeric matrix protein; DAMP, danger-associated molecular pattern; HMGB1, high mobility group box protein 1; MAC, membrane attack complex; MMP, matrix metalloproteinase; OA, osteoarthritis; PRR, pattern recognition receptor; RAGE, receptor for advanced glycation end products; TGF-β, transforming growth factor β; TLR, toll-like receptor. (Reprinted from Liu-Bryan and Terkeltaub [82], with permission from Springer Nature)

chondrocyte hypertrophy and increased MMP and ADAMTS expression [89, 91–95]. TGF-β has also been implicated in early osteophyte formation and subchondral bone sclerosis [96, 97].

Fibroblast growth factors (FGFs) have also been shown to play an important role in OA. In particular, FGF-2 is released from the pericellular matrix following injury, inhibiting anabolic growth factors BMP-7 and IGF-1 [98] and inducing expression of matrix degrading factors MMP-13 and ADAMTS-5, and reactive oxygen species. This suggests that FGF-2 plays a dual anti-anabolic and pro-catabolic role in OA [99–102]. In contrast, FGF-18 appears to promote cartilage synthesis through inhibition of noggin, a known BMP inhibitor, while FGF-2 increases noggin expression [102]. A phase II clinical trial using intra-articular recombinant FGF-18 for treatment of OA is currently underway, with early results showing that the drug may increase or at least help to maintain cartilage thickness in patients with moderate knee OA [103].

Wnt signaling pathways are important in skeletal development, health, and disease, modulating both chondrogenesis and osteogenesis through both canonical Wnt/β-catenin or non-canonical pathways. As described in a recent review, several studies have shown that Wnt/β-catenin signaling is upregulated in OA, promoting chondrocyte hypertrophy and matrix degradation [104]. The use of a small-molecule inhibitor of the Wnt pathway has shown some promise in phase II clinical trials [105]. Importantly, while some studies have found that inhibition of Wnt signaling can reduce OA progression, others have found that it may lead to increased cell death and cartilage destruction [104, 106]. Taken together, this suggests that Wnt signaling is tightly controlled in cartilage homeostasis, with significant disruption in either direction increasing the risk of OA.

Due to its avascularity, chondrocytes reside in a relatively hypoxic environment. A group of transcription factors known as hypoxia-inducible factors (HIFs) play an important role in cartilage development and homeostasis. HIF-1α is expressed by healthy chondrocytes and promotes expression of several anabolic cartilage genes including Sox9 and type II collagen. However, under abnormal mechanical loading or inflammatory conditions, pro-inflammatory cytokines induce expression of HIF-2α through NF-κB. HIF-2α induces chondrocyte hypertrophic differentiation by increasing Runx2, IHH, and VEGF expression and cartilage degradation by increasing MMP and ADAMTS expression [107]. Suppressing HIF-2α while maintaining HIF-1α expression is another potential target in inhibiting the chondrocyte hypertrophy and cartilage degradation typically seen in OA.

Finally, it is important to discuss the role of aging in OA. The incidence of OA increases dramatically with age; however, recent research has suggested that aging in and of itself does not cause OA. Instead, changes that occur with normal aging increase cartilage susceptibility to damage in the setting of trauma or altered joint kinematics. Changes secondary to aging that increase this risk can be seen at cellular, tissue, and systemic level.

One of the main hallmarks of aging is cell senescence, an irreversible arrest in the cell cycle. Senescence can occur either through replicative senescence via telomere shortening that occurs with each cell division or through stress-induced senescence triggered by oxidative stress. Since mature chondrocytes rarely divide, stress-induced senescence has been hypothesized to be the main driver of chondrocyte senescence or "chondrosenescence" and likely contributes to development of OA [108]. Oxidative stress can be induced through intracellular processes as described below or by external dysfunction such as abnormal mechanical loading or inflammatory cytokines released from surrounding tissues. Chondrosenescence increases susceptibility to OA due to decreased responsiveness to anabolic growth factors and increased production of catabolic factors [108].

Inflammation has also been implicated in aging. As cells age, their anti-inflammatory responses gradually become less robust and are eventually unable to neutralize the pro-inflammatory processes, resulting in a chronic low-grade inflammation known as "inflammaging" [109, 110]. Increased longevity has been associated with reduced inflammatory and more robust anti-inflammatory responses. The intrinsic effects of aging on cells contributes to the development of inflammaging and OA. Aging cells have been shown to progressively lose their ability to remove dysfunctional proteins and organelles through lysosomal degradation in a process known as autophagy. Loss of autophagic capacity results in protein aggregation, mitochondrial dysfunction, and accumulation of oxygen species (ROS) such as NO. ROS activate the NF-κB signaling pathway, increasing production of pro-inflammatory cytokines including IL-1β and TNF-α. Autophagy may be further suppressed in OA through inhibition of the HIF-2α pathway described previously [109].

These changes in the cellular environment due to aging eventually lead to development of fibrillations on the cartilage surface, decreased size of proteoglycan aggregates due to reduced length of glycosaminoglycan side chains, increased cross-linking of collagen, and decreased total water content, all of which contribute to decreased stiffness and strength that may make the tissue more susceptible to injury [111, 112]. Regenerative therapies that increase cellular resilience to oxidative stress through inhibition of premature chondrosenescence and loss of autophagy could potentially prevent or delay the onset of OA.

Intervertebral Disc Degeneration

Most individuals will experience back pain at some point in their lives. As the leading cause of disability globally, back pain carries a high social and economic burden [113]. In the United States alone, healthcare costs for treatment of low back and neck pain are estimated to exceed $85 billion per year [114]. The most common underlying etiology in the development of low back pain is IVD degeneration [115]. While less is known about the mechanisms underlying IVD degeneration compared to articular cartilage, many similarities are apparent. First, the primary driver of progressive IVD degeneration is biomechanical stress; however, aging, genetics, and other systemic factors also play an important secondary role. Additionally, loss of the delicate balance between anabolic and catabolic processes triggers a degenerative cascade, leading to upregulation of the same inflammatory mediators and tissue degrading enzymes that are active in articular cartilage degeneration. Lastly, aging and cellular senescence also appear to play an important role in IVD degeneration [116–118]. Despite this overlap, the structure of the IVD is significantly different than that of articular cartilage; thus, regenerative therapies targeting the IVD will likely require a unique approach. Below, we will briefly discuss the pathophysiology of IVD degeneration, focusing on cellular and ECM structure and function in the diseased state.

The first pathologic change noted in IVD degeneration is dysfunction of the NP. Over time, aggrecan content in the NP decreases, leading to a loss of hydrophilicity and compressive resistance. This causes shifting of mechanical loads onto surrounding structures including the AF and EP, increasing mechanical stresses on these tissues. As described above for articular cartilage, persistent mechanical stress disrupts the balance between anabolic and catabolic processes, including upregulation of pro-inflammatory cytokines and matrix degrading enzymes. Under stress, aggrecan and type II collagen within the NP are progressively replaced with fibrous type I collagen leading to worsening dehydration and loss of disc height. The lamellae composed of predominately type I collagen in the outer AF also become increasingly disorganized, increasing susceptibility to disc bulging or AF rupture leading to NP herniation [116, 119].

Nutrients are delivered to the NP and AF primarily by diffusion from the vertebral bodies through the avascular, cartilaginous EP. With degeneration and aging, the EP becomes increasingly thin and calcified. Decreased nutrient perfusion and altered mechanical properties can lead to increased apoptosis and progressive IVD degeneration [118]. NP herniation through the EP into the adjacent vertebral body due to EP mechanical failure results in development of a calcification called a "Schmorl's node" [119].

Development of regenerative therapies for treatment of IVD degeneration require considerations of the different cell types and tissue structure within the IVD. Targeting replacement or preventing loss of aggrecan in the NP may be the most beneficial, as it is the earliest change that is seen with IVD degeneration and is the workhorse in dissipating mechanical forces on the spine. Similar to articular cartilage, regenerative therapies that effectively disrupt the pro-catabolic cycle that occurs in IVD degeneration may also slow progression of the disease and ease symptoms. Finally, restoration of appropriate mechanical loading will need to accompany any regenerative therapy in order to prevent reignition of the pathological processes following treatment.

Tendon and Ligament Degeneration

Tendon and ligament injuries are estimated to account for nearly 50% of musculoskeletal injuries and are common among athletes as well as the general population [120]. While tears or ruptures may occur acutely due to trauma or sudden mechanical overload, injuries of these tissues occur more frequently as a result of progressive degenerative changes secondary to repetitive mechanical overloading in combination with other factors including aging, genetics, and systemic disorders. In this chapter, we will focus on the pathogenesis of tendinopathy as this is the most frequently encountered and commonly investigated. Similar concepts to those discussed with tendinopathy may also be applied to ligamentous injuries.

Tendinopathy is characterized by several changes including tenocyte proliferation, disruption and disorganization of collagen fibers, increase in the ratio of type III to type I collagen, and increase in non-collagenous matrix proteins including GAGs [121]. The water content of the tissue increases, leading to increased cross-sectional area. Vascular ingrowth, often accompanied by sensory nerves, has also been noted [122].

Much remains to be understood regarding pathophysiology of tendinopathy, and key components continue to be debated. Like other degenerative joint diseases, tendinopathy is considered to be the result of a failed healing response, with a loss of balance between anabolic and catabolic factors. Mechanical loading is a central regulator, with appropriate physiologic loading resulting in an increase in anabolic activity, particularly in the periphery, while underloading or overloading can induce factors that promote tissue degeneration [123]. One of the most popular models proposed to describe the pathophysiology of tendinopathy is the continuum model. Initially published in 2009 [124] and updated in 2016 [125], this model suggests that tendon pathology occurs as a potentially reversible continuum across three stages in the setting of abnormal mechanical loading: reactive tendinopathy, tendon disrepair, and degenerative tendinopathy (Fig. 2.4). As the tendon moves toward the degenerative tendinopathy stage, it becomes more difficult to reverse the pathologic process. A fourth stage, reactive-on-degenerative, was added in the 2016 model to highlight the potential for only a portion of a tendon to have progressed to the degenerative stage, while another area may be in a reactive stage.

The role of inflammation in tendinopathy has remained controversial. In the 1970s, histological studies on degenerated tendons demonstrated an absence of acute inflammatory cells, leading to a shift away from an inflammatory etiology for chronic tendon pain and toward a degenerative model [127, 128]. However, recent studies using more advanced techniques have confirmed the presence of macrophages, lymphocytes, and mast cells in acutely injured and chronically degenerated tendons [129–132]. Interestingly, macrophages found in chronic tendinopathy typically express the M2 phenotype, which produces immunosuppressive cytokines to reduce inflammatory responses, unlike the M1 phenotype, which is pro-inflammatory. Similar to OA pathogenesis, inflammatory mediators appear to play an important role in modulating matrix composition and tenocyte phenotype. By binding to cell surface receptors and inducing downstream pathways, pro-inflammatory cytokines including interleukins and TNF-α, as well as PGE2 and NO among others, can enhance inflammation, induce collagen remodeling, increase tenocyte proliferation, and promote angiogenesis [133–135].

Fig. 2.4 Continuum
model of tendinopathy.
(Reprinted from Rudavsky
and Cook [126] with
permission from Elsevier)

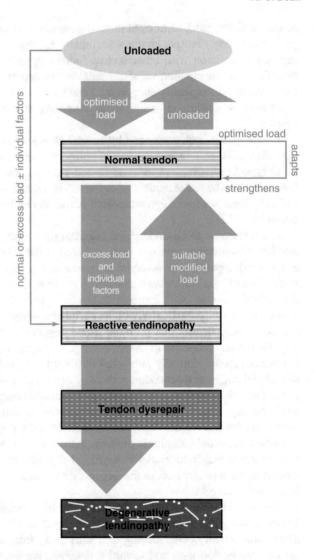

Studies investigating the changes that occur in otherwise healthy tendons with aging, particularly in humans, are somewhat limited. Results from in vitro studies suggest that aging may cause a decline in tenocyte migration and proliferation capacity. However, there is no clear evidence that aging leads to impairment in the ability of tenocytes to synthesize collagen, consistent with findings that aging does not independently lead to reduced cross-sectional area. Whether aging affects mechanical properties of the tendon remains uncertain, though physical activity appears to increase tissue stiffness independent of aging [123].

Conclusion

Unlike many current therapies that focus primarily on reducing physical symptoms, regenerative medicine has the potential to either halt or even reverse tissue disease and degeneration. The high prevalence of pathology and disability related to degeneration of skeletal tissues including articular cartilage, IVD, and ligaments/tendons makes them an important focus for regenerative therapies. As the field advances, understanding the biology of tissue development and disease can provide invaluable insight into potential therapeutic targets. Potential targets for regenerative therapies include inhibition of catabolic pathways including the inflammatory cascade, matrix degrading enzymes and their upstream effectors, vascular and neural ingrowth, and cellular senescence, as well as enhancing anabolic pathways by increasing cell proliferation and the availability of anabolic growth factors and antioxidants. Finally, as altered mechanical loading is often the sentinel change that leads to progressive degeneration, it is imperative that normal kinematics and mechanical stress on the tissue are restored and that appropriate cyclic loading through exercise is continued in conjunction with the use of regenerative therapies.

References

1. Yalcinkaya TM, Sittadjody S, Opara EC. Scientific principles of regenerative medicine and their application in the female reproductive system. Maturitas. 2014;77:12–9.
2. Ono N, Kronenberg HM. Developmental biology of musculoskeletal tissues for tissue engineers. In: Developmental biology and musculoskeletal tissue engineering. Elsevier Academic Press; 2018. p. 1–24.
3. Wu M, Chen G, Li Y-P. TGF-β and BMP signaling in osteoblast, skeletal development, and bone formation, homeostasis and disease. Bone Res. 2016;4:16009.
4. Berendsen AD, Olsen BR. Bone development. Bone. 2015;80:14–8.
5. Teti A. Bone development: overview of bone cells and signaling. Curr Osteoporos Rep. 2011;9:264–73.
6. Kronenberg HM. Developmental regulation of the growth plate. Nature. 2003;423:332–6.
7. Colnot C, Lu C, Hu D, Helms JA. Distinguishing the contributions of the perichondrium, cartilage, and vascular endothelium to skeletal development. Dev Biol. 2004;269:55–69.
8. Bi W, Deng JM, Zhang Z, Behringer RR, de Crombrugghe B. Sox9 is required for cartilage formation. Nat Genet. 1999;22:85–9.
9. Long F, Chung U, Ohba S, McMahon J, Kronenberg HM, McMahon AP. Ihh signaling is directly required for the osteoblast lineage in the endochondral skeleton. Development. 2004;131:1309–18.
10. Hu H, Hilton MJ, Tu X, Yu K, Ornitz DM, Long F. Sequential roles of Hedgehog and Wnt signaling in osteoblast development. Development. 2005;132:49–60.
11. Chung UI, Lanske B, Lee K, Li E, Kronenberg H. The parathyroid hormone/parathyroid hormone-related peptide receptor coordinates endochondral bone development by directly controlling chondrocyte differentiation. Proc Natl Acad Sci U S A. 1998;95:13030–5.

12. Duan X, Murata Y, Liu Y, Nicolae C, Olsen BR, Berendsen AD. Vegfa regulates perichondrial vascularity and osteoblast differentiation in bone development. Development. 2015;142:1984–91.
13. Coskun S, Hirschi KK. Establishment and regulation of the HSC niche: roles of osteoblastic and vascular compartments. Birth Defects Res C Embryo Today. 2010;90:229–42.
14. Shen G. The role of type X collagen in facilitating and regulating endochondral ossification of articular cartilage. Orthod Craniofac Res. 2005;8:11–7.
15. Kobayashi T, Kronenberg HM. Overview of skeletal development. Methods Mol Biol. 2014;1130:3–12.
16. Decker RS. Articular cartilage and joint development from embryogenesis to adulthood. Semin Cell Dev Biol. 2017;62:50–6.
17. Shwartz Y, Viukov S, Krief S, Zelzer E. Joint development involves a continuous influx of Gdf5-positive cells. Cell Rep. 2016;15:2577–87.
18. Pacifici M, Koyama E, Shibukawa Y, Wu C, Tamamura Y, Enomoto-Iwamoto M, Iwamoto M. Cellular and molecular mechanisms of synovial joint and articular cartilage formation. Ann N Y Acad Sci. 2006;1068:74–86.
19. Greene GW, Banquy X, Lee DW, Lowrey DD, Yu J, Israelachvili JN. Adaptive mechanically controlled lubrication mechanism found in articular joints. Proc Natl Acad Sci U S A. 2011;108:5255–9.
20. Poole AR, Kojima T, Yasuda T, Mwale F, Kobayashi M, Laverty S. Composition and structure of articular cartilage: a template for tissue repair. Clin Orthop Relat Res. 2001;391:S26–33.
21. Bowles RD, Setton LA. Biomaterials for intervertebral disc regeneration and repair. Biomaterials. 2017;129:54–67.
22. Whatley BR, Wen X. Intervertebral disc (IVD): structure, degeneration, repair and regeneration. Mater Sci Eng C. 2012;32:61–77.
23. Sivakamasundari V, Lufkin T. Bridging the gap: understanding embryonic intervertebral disc development. Cell Dev Biol. 2012;1(2):103.
24. Raj PP. Intervertebral disc: anatomy-physiology-pathophysiology-treatment. Pain Pract. 2008;8:18–44.
25. McCann MR, Tamplin OJ, Rossant J, Séguin CA. Tracing notochord-derived cells using a Noto-cre mouse: implications for intervertebral disc development. Dis Model Mech. 2012;5:73–82.
26. Choi K-S, Cohn MJ, Harfe BD. Identification of nucleus pulposus precursor cells and notochordal remnants in the mouse: implications for disk degeneration and chordoma formation. Dev Dyn. 2008;237:3953–8.
27. Cox MK, Serra R. Development of the intervertebral disc. In: Shapiro IM, Risbud MV, editors. The intervertebral disc. Vienna: Springer Vienna; 2014. p. 33–51.
28. Chu G, Shi C, Wang H, Zhang W, Yang H, Li B. Strategies for annulus fibrosus regeneration: from biological therapies to tissue engineering. Front Bioeng Biotechnol. 2018;6:90.
29. Tozer S, Duprez D. Tendon and ligament: development, repair and disease. Birth Defects Res C Embryo Today. 2005;75:226–36.
30. Schweitzer R, Zelzer E, Volk T. Connecting muscles to tendons: tendons and musculoskeletal development in flies and vertebrates. Development. 2010;137:2807–17.
31. Rothrauff BB, Yang G, Tuan RS. Tendon resident cells—functions and features in section I—developmental biology and physiology of tendons. In: Tendon regeneration. Elsevier Academic Press; 2015. p. 41–76.
32. Blitz E, Viukov S, Sharir A, Shwartz Y, Galloway JL, Pryce BA, Johnson RL, Tabin CJ, Schweitzer R, Zelzer E. Bone ridge patterning during musculoskeletal assembly is mediated through SCX regulation of Bmp4 at the tendon-skeleton junction. Dev Cell. 2009;17:861–73.
33. Benjamin M, Kaiser E, Milz S. Structure-function relationships in tendons: a review. J Anat. 2008;212:211–28.
34. Chal J, Pourquié O. Making muscle: skeletal myogenesis in vivo and in vitro. Development. 2017;144:2104–22.

35. Valdivia M, Vega-Macaya F, Olguín P. Mechanical control of myotendinous junction formation and tendon differentiation during development. Front Cell Dev Biol. 2017;5:26.
36. Charvet B, Ruggiero F, Le Guellec D. The development of the myotendinous junction. A review. Muscles Ligaments Tendons J. 2012;2:53–63.
37. Asahara H, Inui M, Lotz MK. Tendons and ligaments: connecting developmental biology to musculoskeletal disease pathogenesis. J Bone Miner Res. 2017;32:1773–82.
38. Jensen PT, Lambertsen KL, Frich LH. Assembly, maturation, and degradation of the supraspinatus enthesis. J Shoulder Elb Surg. 2018;27:739–50.
39. Apostolakos J, Durant TJ, Dwyer CR, Russell RP, Weinreb JH, Alaee F, Beitzel K, McCarthy MB, Cote MP, Mazzocca AD. The enthesis: a review of the tendon-to-bone insertion. Muscles Ligaments Tendons J. 2014;4:333–42.
40. Sugimoto Y, Takimoto A, Akiyama H, Kist R, Scherer G, Nakamura T, Hiraki Y, Shukunami C. Scx+/Sox9+ progenitors contribute to the establishment of the junction between cartilage and tendon/ligament. Development. 2013;140:2280–8.
41. Blitz E, Sharir A, Akiyama H, Zelzer E. Tendon-bone attachment unit is formed modularly by a distinct pool of Scx- and Sox9-positive progenitors. Development. 2013;140:2680–90.
42. Schwartz AG, Long F, Thomopoulos S. Enthesis fibrocartilage cells originate from a population of Hedgehog-responsive cells modulated by the loading environment. Development. 2015;142:196–206.
43. Dyment NA, Breidenbach AP, Schwartz AG, et al. Gdf5 progenitors give rise to fibrocartilage cells that mineralize via hedgehog signaling to form the zonal enthesis. Dev Biol. 2015;405:96–107.
44. Thomopoulos S, Kim H-M, Rothermich SY, Biederstadt C, Das R, Galatz LM. Decreased muscle loading delays maturation of the tendon enthesis during postnatal development. J Orthop Res. 2007;25:1154–63.
45. WHO|Chronic rheumatic conditions 2019. https://www.who.int/chp/topics/rheumatic/en/. Accessed 14 June 2019.
46. Barbour KE, Helmick CG, Boring M, Brady TJ. Vital signs: prevalence of doctor-diagnosed arthritis and arthritis-attributable activity limitation – United States, 2013–2015. MMWR Morb Mortal Wkly Rep. 2017;66:246–53.
47. Mobasheri A, Batt M. An update on the pathophysiology of osteoarthritis. Ann Phys Rehabil Med. 2016;59:333–9.
48. Houard X, Goldring MB, Berenbaum F. Homeostatic mechanisms in articular cartilage and role of inflammation in osteoarthritis. Curr Rheumatol Rep. 2013;15:375.
49. Ripmeester EGJ, Timur UT, Caron MMJ, Welting TJM. Recent insights into the contribution of the changing hypertrophic chondrocyte phenotype in the development and progression of osteoarthritis. Front Bioeng Biotechnol. 2018;6:18.
50. Rigoglou S, Papavassiliou AG. The NF-κB signalling pathway in osteoarthritis. Int J Biochem Cell Biol. 2013;45:2580–4.
51. Xia B, Chen D, Zhang J, Hu S, Jin H, Tong P. Osteoarthritis pathogenesis: a review of molecular mechanisms. Calcif Tissue Int. 2014;95:495–505.
52. Marcu KB, Otero M, Olivotto E, Borzi RM, Goldring MB. NF-kappaB signaling: multiple angles to target OA. Curr Drug Targets. 2010;11:599–613.
53. Haseeb A, Haqqi TM. Immunopathogenesis of osteoarthritis. Clin Immunol. 2013;146:185–96.
54. Mariani E, Pulsatelli L, Facchini A. Signaling pathways in cartilage repair. Int J Mol Sci. 2014;15:8667–98.
55. Andriacchi TP, Koo S, Scanlan SF. Gait mechanics influence healthy cartilage morphology and osteoarthritis of the knee. J Bone Joint Surg Am. 2009;91(Suppl 1):95–101.
56. Hinterwimmer S, Krammer M, Krötz M, Glaser C, Baumgart R, Reiser M, Eckstein F. Cartilage atrophy in the knees of patients after seven weeks of partial load bearing. Arthritis Rheum. 2004;50:2516–20.
57. Vanwanseele B, Eckstein F, Knecht H, Spaepen A, Stüssi E. Longitudinal analysis of cartilage atrophy in the knees of patients with spinal cord injury. Arthritis Rheum. 2003;48:3377–81.

58. Haapala J, Arokoski J, Pirttimäki J, Lyyra T, Jurvelin J, Tammi M, Helminen HJ, Kiviranta I. Incomplete restoration of immobilization induced softening of young beagle knee articular cartilage after 50-week remobilization. Int J Sports Med. 2000;21:76–81.

59. Palmoski M, Perricone E, Brandt KD. Development and reversal of a proteoglycan aggregation defect in normal canine knee cartilage after immobilization. Arthritis Rheum. 1979;22:508–17.

60. Jurvelin J, Kiviranta I, Tammi M, Helminen JH. Softening of canine articular cartilage after immobilization of the knee joint. Clin Orthop Relat Res. 1986;207:246–52.

61. Alexander PG, Song Y, Taboas JM, Chen FH, Melvin GM, Manner PA, Tuan RS. Development of a spring-loaded impact device to deliver injurious mechanical impacts to the articular cartilage surface. Cartilage. 2013;4:52–62.

62. Bonnevie ED, Delco ML, Fortier LA, Alexander PG, Tuan RS, Bonassar LJ. Characterization of tissue response to impact loads delivered using a hand-held instrument for studying articular cartilage injury. Cartilage. 2015;6:226–32.

63. Jeffrey JE, Gregory DW, Aspden RM. Matrix damage and chondrocyte viability following a single impact load on articular cartilage. Arch Biochem Biophys. 1995;322:87–96.

64. Kurz B, Jin M, Patwari P, Cheng DM, Lark MW, Grodzinsky AJ. Biosynthetic response and mechanical properties of articular cartilage after injurious compression. J Orthop Res. 2001;19:1140–6.

65. Loening AM, James IE, Levenston ME, et al. Injurious mechanical compression of bovine articular cartilage induces chondrocyte apoptosis. Arch Biochem Biophys. 2000;381:205–12.

66. Torzilli PA, Grigiene R, Borrelli J, Helfet DL. Effect of impact load on articular cartilage: cell metabolism and viability, and matrix water content. J Biomech Eng. 1999;121:433–41.

67. Kiviranta I, Tammi M, Jurvelin J, Arokoski J, Säämänen AM, Helminen HJ. Articular cartilage thickness and glycosaminoglycan distribution in the canine knee joint after strenuous running exercise. Clin Orthop Relat Res. 1992;283:302–8.

68. Arokoski J, Kiviranta I, Jurvelin J, Tammi M, Helminen HJ. Long-distance running causes site-dependent decrease of cartilage glycosaminoglycan content in the knee joints of beagle dogs. Arthritis Rheum. 1993;36:1451–9.

69. Carbone A, Rodeo S. Review of current understanding of post-traumatic osteoarthritis resulting from sports injuries. J Orthop Res. 2017;35:397–405.

70. Andriacchi TP, Mündermann A, Smith RL, Alexander EJ, Dyrby CO, Koo S. A framework for the in vivo pathomechanics of osteoarthritis at the knee. Ann Biomed Eng. 2004;32:447–57.

71. Brandt KD, Dieppe P, Radin E. Etiopathogenesis of osteoarthritis. Med Clin North Am. 2009;93(1–24):xv.

72. Lotz MK, Otsuki S, Grogan SP, Sah R, Terkeltaub R, D'Lima D. Cartilage cell clusters. Arthritis Rheum. 2010;62:2206–18.

73. Temenoff JS, Mikos AG. Review: tissue engineering for regeneration of articular cartilage. Biomaterials. 2000;21:431–40.

74. Buckwalter JA. Articular cartilage: injuries and potential for healing. J Orthop Sports Phys Ther. 1998;28:192–202.

75. van der Kraan PM. The changing role of TGFβ in healthy, ageing and osteoarthritic joints. Nat Rev Rheumatol. 2017;13:155–63.

76. Lories RJ, Luyten FP. The bone-cartilage unit in osteoarthritis. Nat Rev Rheumatol. 2011;7:43–9.

77. Ashraf S, Wibberley H, Mapp PI, Hill R, Wilson D, Walsh DA. Increased vascular penetration and nerve growth in the meniscus: a potential source of pain in osteoarthritis. Ann Rheum Dis. 2011;70:523–9.

78. Mapp PI, Walsh DA. Mechanisms and targets of angiogenesis and nerve growth in osteoarthritis. Nat Rev Rheumatol. 2012;8:390–8.

79. Malemud CJ. Inhibition of mmps and ADAM/ADAMTS. Biochem Pharmacol. 2019;165:33–40.

80. Clouet J, Vinatier C, Merceron C, Pot-vaucel M, Maugars Y, Weiss P, Grimandi G, Guicheux J. From osteoarthritis treatments to future regenerative therapies for cartilage. Drug Discov Today. 2009;14:913–25.
81. Identifier NCT03595618, a study to assess efficacy and safety of GLPG1972/S201086 in patients with knee osteoarthritis (Roccella). In: ClinicalTrials.gov 2018. https://clinicaltrials.gov/ct2/show/NCT03595618?term=GLPG1972&recrs=d&rank=1. Accessed 30 Apr 2019.
82. Liu-Bryan R, Terkeltaub R. Emerging regulators of the inflammatory process in osteoarthritis. Nat Rev Rheumatol. 2015;11:35–44.
83. Loeser RF, Goldring SR, Scanzello CR, Goldring MB. Osteoarthritis: a disease of the joint as an organ. Arthritis Rheum. 2012;64:1697–707.
84. Kandahari AM, Yang X, Dighe AS, Pan D, Cui Q. Recognition of immune response for the early diagnosis and treatment of osteoarthritis. J Immunol Res. 2015;2015:192415.
85. Zeng C, Lane NE, Hunter DJ, Wei J, Choi HK, McAlindon TE, Li H, Lu N, Lei G, Zhang Y. Intra-articular corticosteroids and the risk of knee osteoarthritis progression: results from the osteoarthritis initiative. Osteoarthr Cartil. 2019;27:855–62.
86. McAlindon TE, LaValley MP, Harvey WF, Price LL, Driban JB, Zhang M, Ward RJ. Effect of intra-articular triamcinolone vs saline on knee cartilage volume and pain in patients with knee osteoarthritis: a randomized clinical trial. JAMA. 2017;317:1967–75.
87. Malemud CJ. Anticytokine therapy for osteoarthritis: evidence to date. Drugs Aging. 2010;27:95–115.
88. Kim J-R, Yoo JJ, Kim HA. Therapeutics in osteoarthritis based on an understanding of its molecular pathogenesis. Int J Mol Sci. 2018;19(3):674. https://doi.org/10.3390/ijms19030674.
89. Furumatsu T, Matsumoto E, Kanazawa T, Fujii M, Lu Z, Kajiki R, Ozaki T. Tensile strain increases expression of CCN2 and COL2A1 by activating TGF-β-Smad2/3 pathway in chondrocytic cells. J Biomech. 2013;46:1508–15.
90. Bougault C, Aubert-Foucher E, Paumier A, Perrier-Groult E, Huot L, Hot D, Duterque-Coquillaud M, Mallein-Gerin F. Dynamic compression of chondrocyte-agarose constructs reveals new candidate mechanosensitive genes. PLoS One. 2012;7:e36964.
91. Yang X, Chen L, Xu X, Li C, Huang C, Deng CX. TGF-beta/Smad3 signals repress chondrocyte hypertrophic differentiation and are required for maintaining articular cartilage. J Cell Biol. 2001;153:35–46.
92. Ballock RT, Heydemann A, Wakefield LM, Flanders KC, Roberts AB, Sporn MB. TGF-beta 1 prevents hypertrophy of epiphyseal chondrocytes: regulation of gene expression for cartilage matrix proteins and metalloproteases. Dev Biol. 1993;158:414–29.
93. van de Laar IMBH, Oldenburg RA, Pals G, et al. Mutations in SMAD3 cause a syndromic form of aortic aneurysms and dissections with early-onset osteoarthritis. Nat Genet. 2011;43:121–6.
94. Yao J-Y, Wang Y, An J, Mao C-M, Hou N, Lv Y-X, Wang Y-L, Cui F, Huang M, Yang X. Mutation analysis of the Smad3 gene in human osteoarthritis. Eur J Hum Genet. 2003;11:714–7.
95. Patwari P, Cook MN, DiMicco MA, Blake SM, James IE, Kumar S, Cole AA, Lark MW, Grodzinsky AJ. Proteoglycan degradation after injurious compression of bovine and human articular cartilage in vitro: interaction with exogenous cytokines. Arthritis Rheum. 2003;48:1292–301.
96. Zhen G, Wen C, Jia X, et al. Inhibition of TGF-β signaling in mesenchymal stem cells of subchondral bone attenuates osteoarthritis. Nat Med. 2013;19:704–12.
97. Blaney Davidson EN, Vitters EL, van der Kraan PM, van den Berg WB. Expression of transforming growth factor-beta (TGFbeta) and the TGFbeta signalling molecule SMAD-2P in spontaneous and instability-induced osteoarthritis: role in cartilage degradation, chondrogenesis and osteophyte formation. Ann Rheum Dis. 2006;65:1414–21.
98. Loeser RF, Chubinskaya S, Pacione C, Im H-J. Basic fibroblast growth factor inhibits the anabolic activity of insulin-like growth factor 1 and osteogenic protein 1 in adult human articular chondrocytes. Arthritis Rheum. 2005;52:3910–7.

99. Im H-J, Li X, Muddasani P, Kim G-H, Davis F, Rangan J, Forsyth CB, Ellman M, Thonar EJ. Basic fibroblast growth factor accelerates matrix degradation via a neuro-endocrine pathway in human adult articular chondrocytes. J Cell Physiol. 2008;215:452–63.

100. Im H-J, Muddasani P, Natarajan V, Schmid TM, Block JA, Davis F, van Wijnen AJ, Loeser RF. Basic fibroblast growth factor stimulates matrix metalloproteinase-13 via the molecular cross-talk between the mitogen-activated protein kinases and protein kinase Cdelta pathways in human adult articular chondrocytes. J Biol Chem. 2007;282:11110–21.

101. Wang X, Manner PA, Horner A, Shum L, Tuan RS, Nuckolls GH. Regulation of MMP-13 expression by RUNX2 and FGF2 in osteoarthritic cartilage. Osteoarthr Cartil. 2004;12:963–73.

102. Ellman MB, Yan D, Ahmadinia K, Chen D, An HS, Im HJ. Fibroblast growth factor control of cartilage homeostasis. J Cell Biochem. 2013;114:735–42.

103. Hochberg M, Guermazi A, Guehring H, Aydemir A, Wax S, Fleuranceau-Morel P, Reinstrup Bihlet A, Byrjalsen I, Ragnar Andersen J, Eckstein F. OP0059 efficacy and safety of intra-articular sprifermin in symptomatic radiographic knee osteoarthritis: pre-specified analysis of 3-year data from a 5-year randomised, placebo-controlled, phase II study. Wednesday 13 June 2018. BMJ Publishing Group Ltd and European League Against Rheumatism. 2018;80–1.

104. Teufel S, Hartmann C. Wnt-signaling in skeletal development. Curr Top Dev Biol. 2018;133:235–79. https://doi.org/10.1016/bs.ctdb.2018.11.010.

105. Yazici Y, McAlindon TE, Gibofsky A, et al. Results from a 52-week randomized, double-blind, placebo-controlled, phase 2 study of a novel, intra-articular wnt pathway inhibitor (SM04690) for the treatment of knee osteoarthritis. Osteoarthr Cartil. 2018;26:S293–4.

106. Zhu M, Chen M, Zuscik M, Wu Q, Wang Y-J, Rosier RN, O'Keefe RJ, Chen D. Inhibition of beta-catenin signaling in articular chondrocytes results in articular cartilage destruction. Arthritis Rheum. 2008;58:2053–64.

107. Saito T, Kawaguchi H. HIF-2α as a possible therapeutic target of osteoarthritis. Osteoarthr Cartil. 2010;18:1552–6.

108. Loeser RF. Aging and osteoarthritis: the role of chondrocyte senescence and aging changes in the cartilage matrix. Osteoarthr Cartil. 2009;17:971–9.

109. Salminen A, Kaarniranta K, Kauppinen A. Inflammaging: disturbed interplay between autophagy and inflammasomes. Aging (Albany, NY). 2012;4:166–75.

110. Franceschi C, Capri M, Monti D, et al. Inflammaging and anti-inflammaging: a systemic perspective on aging and longevity emerged from studies in humans. Mech Ageing Dev. 2007;128:92–105.

111. Martin JA, Brown TD, Heiner AD, Buckwalter JA. Chondrocyte senescence, joint loading and osteoarthritis. Clin Orthop Relat Res. 2004;427:S96–103.

112. Martin JA, Buckwalter JA. Aging, articular cartilage chondrocyte senescence and osteoarthritis. Biogerontology. 2002;3(5):257–64.

113. GBD 2015 DALYs and HALE Collaborators. Global, regional, and national disability-adjusted life-years (DALYs) for 315 diseases and injuries and healthy life expectancy (HALE), 1990–2015: a systematic analysis for the Global Burden of Disease Study 2015. Lancet. 2016;388:1603–58.

114. Dieleman JL, Baral R, Birger M, et al. US spending on personal health care and public health, 1996–2013. JAMA. 2016;316:2627–46.

115. Kennon JC, Awad ME, Chutkan N, DeVine J, Fulzele S. Current insights on use of growth factors as therapy for Intervertebral Disc Degeneration. Biomol Concepts. 2018;9:43–52.

116. Sakai D, Grad S. Advancing the cellular and molecular therapy for intervertebral disc disease. Adv Drug Deliv Rev. 2015;84:159–71.

117. Dowdell J, Erwin M, Choma T, Vaccaro A, Iatridis J, Cho SK. Intervertebral disk degeneration and repair. Neurosurgery. 2017;80:S46–54.

118. Zhao C-Q, Wang L-M, Jiang L-S, Dai L-Y. The cell biology of intervertebral disc aging and degeneration. Ageing Res Rev. 2007;6:247–61.

119. Adams MA, Roughley PJ. What is intervertebral disc degeneration, and what causes it? Spine. 2006;31:2151–61.
120. James R, Kesturu G, Balian G, Chhabra AB. Tendon: biology, biomechanics, repair, growth factors, and evolving treatment options. J Hand Surg Am. 2008;33:102–12.
121. Longo UG, Ronga M, Maffulli N. Achilles tendinopathy. Sports Med Arthrosc. 2009;17:112–26.
122. Xu Y, Murrell GAC. The basic science of tendinopathy. Clin Orthop Relat Res. 2008;466:1528–38.
123. Magnusson SP, Kjaer M. The impact of loading, unloading, ageing and injury on the human tendon. J Physiol Lond. 2019;597:1283–98.
124. Cook JL, Purdam CR. Is tendon pathology a continuum? A pathology model to explain the clinical presentation of load-induced tendinopathy. Br J Sports Med. 2009;43:409–16.
125. Cook JL, Rio E, Purdam CR, Docking SI. Revisiting the continuum model of tendon pathology: what is its merit in clinical practice and research? Br J Sports Med. 2016;50:1187–91.
126. Rudavsky A, Cook J. Physiotherapy management of patellar tendinopathy (jumper's knee). J Physiother. 2014;60:122–9.
127. Puddu G, Ippolito E, Postacchini F. A classification of Achilles tendon disease. Am J Sports Med. 1976;4:145–50.
128. Rees JD, Stride M, Scott A. Tendons–time to revisit inflammation. Br J Sports Med. 2014;48:1553–7.
129. Schubert TEO, Weidler C, Lerch K, Hofstädter F, Straub RH. Achilles tendinosis is associated with sprouting of substance P positive nerve fibres. Ann Rheum Dis. 2005;64:1083–6.
130. Millar NL, Hueber AJ, Reilly JH, Xu Y, Fazzi UG, Murrell GAC, McInnes IB. Inflammation is present in early human tendinopathy. Am J Sports Med. 2010;38:2085–91.
131. Matthews TJW, Hand GC, Rees JL, Athanasou NA, Carr AJ. Pathology of the torn rotator cuff tendon. Reduction in potential for repair as tear size increases. J Bone Joint Surg Br. 2006;88:489–95.
132. Barbe MF, Barr AE, Gorzelany I, Amin M, Gaughan JP, Safadi FF. Chronic repetitive reaching and grasping results in decreased motor performance and widespread tissue responses in a rat model of MSD. J Orthop Res. 2003;21:167–76.
133. Dakin SG, Martinez FO, Yapp C, et al. Inflammation activation and resolution in human tendon disease. Sci Transl Med. 2015;7:311ra173.
134. Millar NL, Murrell GAC, McInnes IB. Inflammatory mechanisms in tendinopathy – towards translation. Nat Rev Rheumatol. 2017;13:110–22.
135. Tang C, Chen Y, Huang J, Zhao K, Chen X, Yin Z, Heng BC, Chen W, Shen W. The roles of inflammatory mediators and immunocytes in tendinopathy. J Orthop Translat. 2018;14:23–33.

Chapter 3
Viscosupplementation

Krutika Parasar Raulkar

Introduction

Osteoarthritis (OA) is a major source of disability worldwide, causing progressive pain and functional decline [1] (see Fig. 3.1). In the United States, 10–20% of people above the age of 60 suffer from clinically significant OA [2]. Patients make more than 5.5 million physician visits for OA-related treatment per year. Non-modifiable risk factors include advanced age, post-menopausal status, female gender (45% higher incidence than male gender [3]), and European ancestry [4] (see Fig. 3.2). Modifiable risk factors include obesity, injury, anatomic abnormalities, significant running history, and tobacco and alcohol use. Symptoms have insidious onset and include stiffness, pain, and swelling. Incidence of knee OA in adults is 6% [4], making knee OA twice as common as hip OA [2]. In viscosupplementation, lubricating fluid is injected with the immediate goal of adding support to arthritic joints, relieving pain, and improving mobility and the ultimate goal of slowing disease progression [1]. The most common injectate is hyaluronic acid (HA), also known as HA, hyaluronan, or hyaluronate, which is a natural substance in the joint capsule that allows cartilages to glide against each other, minimizing friction and absorbing force during weight-bearing activities. Patients with radiographic evidence of osteoarthritis (OA) who fail to benefit from conservative methods such as physical therapy and oral pain medications can be considered candidates for HA injections [1].

K. P. Raulkar (✉)
Department of Physical Medicine and Rehabilitation, New York-Presbyterian Hospital – The University Hospital of Columbia and Cornell, New York, NY, USA
e-mail: krutika_parasar@alumni.brown.edu

© Springer Nature Switzerland AG 2020
G. Cooper et al. (eds.), *Regenerative Medicine for Spine and Joint Pain*,
https://doi.org/10.1007/978-3-030-42771-9_3

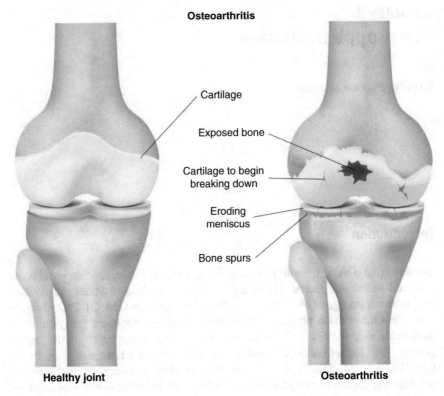

Fig. 3.1 Osteoarthritis

History

HA is a glycosaminoglycan like chondroitin that is formed inside cell plasma membranes [5]. It was originally used in the 1960s in eye surgeries, when it was harvested from human umbilical cords and rooster combs in the form of hyaluronan [6] (see Fig. 3.3). In the 1970s, the sodium hyaluronan product NIF-NaHA Healon was formed. These first-generation products were used by veterinarians to treat canine and racehorse injuries.

Over the following two decades, 2nd-generation hylans were developed. Hyalgan was produced for use in humans in Italy in the 1980s and was officially approved by the FDA for use in Canada (1992) and the United States (1997) for the treatment of knee OA [1]. It has since been approved and marked under the brand names Hyalgan (1997), Synvisc (1997), Supartz (2001), Orthovisc (2004), and Euflexxa (2004) [5] (see Fig. 3.4). Of these products, Synvisc One is available in a single formulation. Hyalgan in available as a series of two injections, and the remainder as series of three to five injections. Nonavian products include Euflexxa and Orthovisc, which are derived from bacterial fermentation. Generic formulations can also be prescribed. Treatment courses should be completed within 8 weeks.

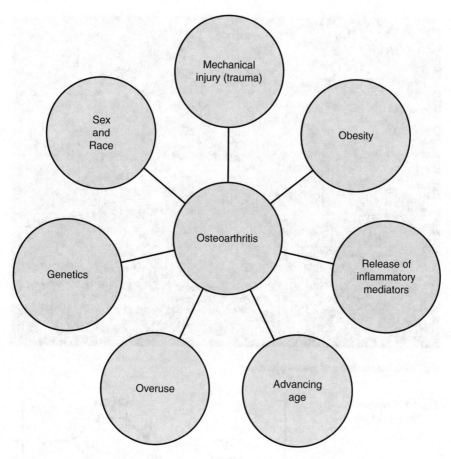

Fig. 3.2 OA risk factors

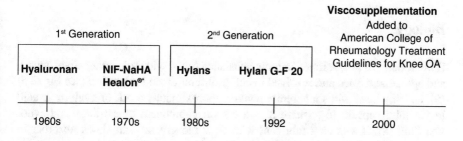

*Healon is a registered trademark of Pharmacia, Inc.

Fig. 3.3 History of viscosupplementation

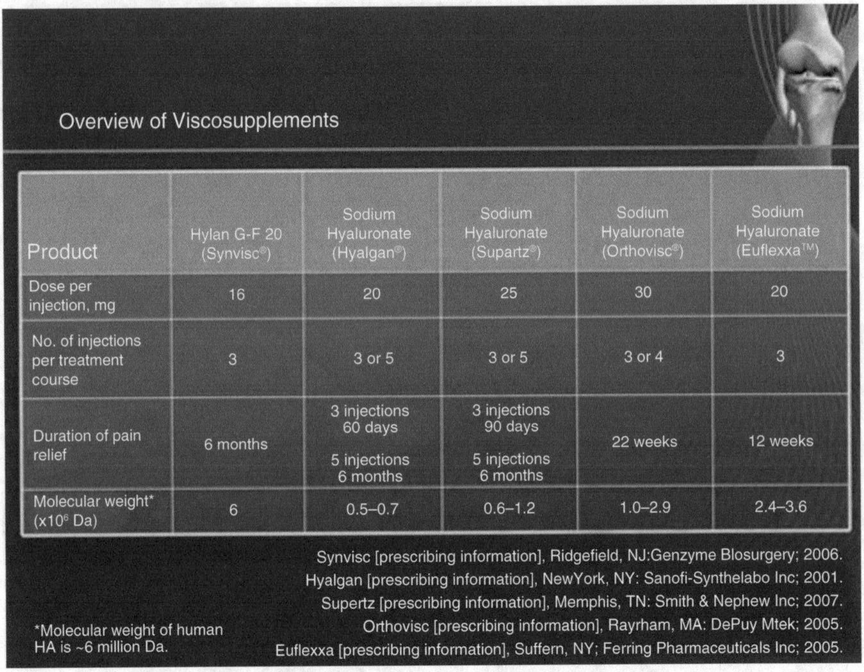

Product	Hylan G-F 20 (Synvisc®)	Sodium Hyaluronate (Hyalgan®)	Sodium Hyaluronate (Supartz®)	Sodium Hyaluronate (Orthovisc®)	Sodium Hyaluronate (Euflexxa™)
Dose per injection, mg	16	20	25	30	20
No. of injections per treatment course	3	3 or 5	3 or 5	3 or 4	3
Duration of pain relief	6 months	3 injections 60 days / 5 injections 6 months	3 injections 90 days / 5 injections 6 months	22 weeks	12 weeks
Molecular weight* (x10⁶ Da)	6	0.5–0.7	0.6–1.2	1.0–2.9	2.4–3.6

Overview of Viscosupplements

*Molecular weight of human HA is ~6 million Da.

Synvisc [prescribing information], Ridgefield, NJ:Genzyme Biosurgery; 2006.
Hyalgan [prescribing information], NewYork, NY: Sanofi-Synthelabo Inc; 2001.
Supertz [prescribing information], Memphis, TN: Smith & Nephew Inc; 2007.
Orthovisc [prescribing information], Rayrham, MA: DePuy Mtek; 2005.
Euflexxa [prescribing information], Suffern, NY; Ferring Pharmaceuticals Inc; 2005.

Fig. 3.4 Characteristics of viscosupplements

Fig. 3.5 Chemical structure of HA [4]

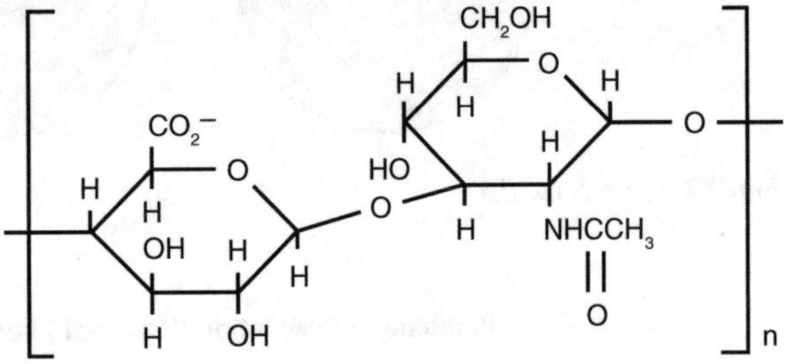

Biology

Hyaluronan is a non-sulfated anionic substance found widely in connective, neural, and epithelial tissues and involved in cell proliferation and migration (see Fig. 3.5) [5]. Healthy knee joints inherently contain approximately 4 mL of hyaluronic acid in the joint capsule [6], where it is a central component of cartilage and synovial fluid [8]. It acts as a lubricant with slow movements and shock absorber in fast motion. In OA, the molecular weight and concentration of HA decreases by 33–50%. Supplementation with HA may decrease pain-triggering molecules [7] and inflammatory matrix metalloproteinases (MMP) [8] while enhancing normal

HA production [7]. Man-made derivatives of hyaluronic acid are often used in injections and are known as hylans. Currently research suggests the effects of natural hyaluronic acid and its synthetic form to be comparable [6].

Indications

Viscosupplementation is indicated for patients with function-limiting pain refractory to NSAIDs, aspirations, and corticosteroid (CS) injections. Ideal candidates include elderly patients, younger patients with mild to moderate OA, patients with radiographic findings classified as 1–3 on the Kellgren-Lawrence Scale (see Fig. 3.6), and patients with stage 4 OA who want to delay total knee replacement (TKR) [8]. It can be considered as first-line treatment in patients with comorbidities, for example, in diabetics who cannot tolerate CS injections, patients with CAD in whom NSAIDs are not recommended, or patients on anticoagulation for whom surgery could be dangerous. Contraindications include allergy to hylan, active infection, bleeding disorder, or venous stasis [7]. Some products are made from rooster combs and should not be administered to patients with egg allergies [6].

Despite the 2008 Osteoarthritis Research Society International guidelines stating that IA HA is an acceptable treatment for both hip and knee OA [2], currently viscosupplementation is only FDA approved for the treatment of knee OA, for which injections are typically approved every 6 months. Nevertheless, it can still be considered

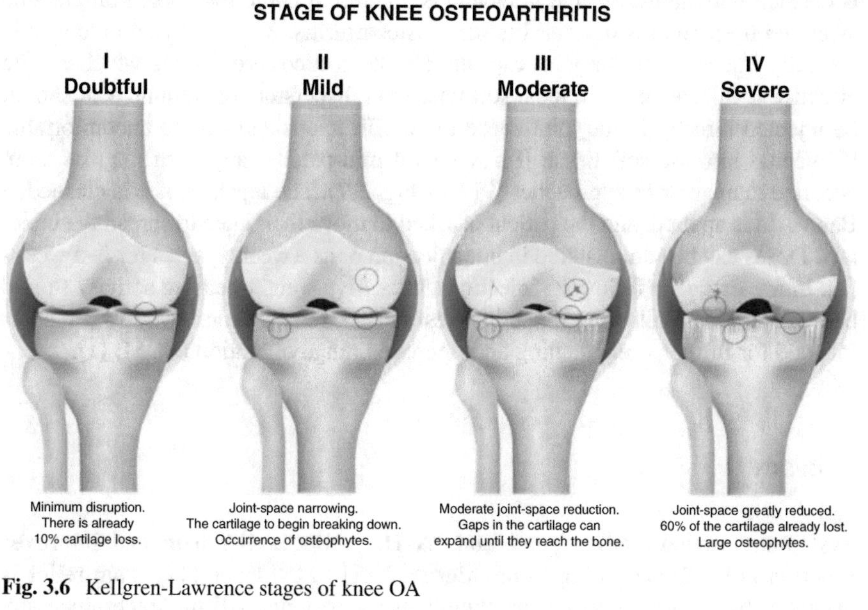

STAGE OF KNEE OSTEOARTHRITIS

| I | II | III | IV |
| Doubtful | Mild | Moderate | Severe |

| Minimum disruption. There is already 10% cartilage loss. | Joint-space narrowing. The cartilage to begin breaking down. Occurrence of osteophytes. | Moderate joint-space reduction. Gaps in the cartilage can expand until they reach the bone. | Joint-space greatly reduced. 60% of the cartilage already lost. Large osteophytes. |

Fig. 3.6 Kellgren-Lawrence stages of knee OA

as a treatment option for other joints but is usually not covered by insurance in these cases [4]. Preliminary research has shown efficacy in treating ankle OA [8]. For OA of the hip, one study found moderate improvement in pain and function at 3–6 months after HA injections without significant adverse side effects [4]. Conversely, a 2018 meta-analysis of 8 RTCs concluded that there was little difference between hyaluronic acid and placebo at 3 and 6 months, but that it was no different than methylprednisolone for pain relief or in terms of adverse events at 1 month [9]. Thus, it could potentially be an alternative to methylprednisolone for hip OA as well.

Efficacy of viscosupplementation in the treatment of acute injuries such as anterior cruciate ligament and chondral injuries has also been demonstrated, delaying the need for total knee arthroplasty (TKA) [2]. In one study of patients with stage 4 OA who were candidates for TKA, 75% were able to delay the need for TKA after 3.8 years following IA HA injections [8].

There is still little published research regarding efficacy of viscosupplementation for joints other than the knee and such use is considered off-label and usually require out-of-pocket expense from the patient [1].

Procedure

Injections can take place in an office and usually take 5 min. Patients should be positioned supine with knees flexed to 20–30° [1]. Ultrasound guidance has been shown to increase optimal placement and thus injection efficacy. The injection site is cleaned with antiseptic and lidocaine is applied to numb the knee. Fluid can be aspirated if effusion is present. For knee osteoarthritis, 2 mL of hyaluronic acid is typically injected into the joint capsule. Unlike corticosteroid shots which can be effective if injected even in local soft tissue via dispersion, hyaluronic acid should be injected directly in the joint space to be efficacious and can be uncomfortable if injected into the soft tissue [8]. A lateral mid-patellar approach may be more accurate than anterior approaches [9] (see Fig. 3.7). The injection site is cleaned, a Band-Aid is applied, and the patient is asked to move their knee to spread the injectate. Doses can be administered in one injection or as a weekly series for 3–5 weeks [1]. In the first 48 h following injections, excessive weight-bearing activity should be avoided [11]. Following this initial rest period, rehabilitation therapy is recommended for further strengthening and improved range of motion (ROM) [1].

Efficacy

Systematic reviews have found that IA HA reduces OA pain and improves function [11, 12] according to the highest level of evidence [12]. Pain relief is expected for 3 months to 1 year, though some patients will not experience any

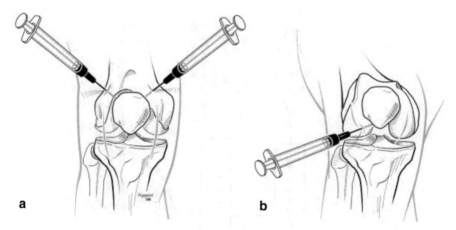

Fig. 3.7 Common injection approaches [10]. (**a**) Anterior approaches. (**b**) Lateral mid-patellar approach

relief and some will have longer-lasting effects. Maximal effect has been demonstrated between 5 and 13 weeks with benefits persisting to 26 weeks [13]. A 2006 Cochrane Database review of 76 trials cited the average pain improvement to be between 28% and 54% and with functional improvement between 9% and 32%, which is comparable to the effects of non-steroidal anti-inflammatories (NSAIDs). Benefits were found to be longer term than corticosteroid injections [14]. If first injections are without efficacy, then it is not recommended to repeat the series. Even if initially efficacious, repeat injections may be less and less effective as OA progresses [1]. Multiple studies of repeat HA injections have demonstrated the additive benefits of repeat injections in reducing pain with minimal side effects [15]. Obesity and very severe joint space narrowing are associated with decreased efficacy of viscosupplementation. Experts have suggested that patellofemoral OA is less responsive to viscosupplementation, but there is little evidence in the literature to support this.

Treatment Algorithms

If effective at 6 months, retreatment is not recommended unless patients experience recurrence of pain, they are professional sports players, they are at high risk for progression, they have severe comorbidities, or they have risk factors that prevent TKR (see Fig. 3.8) [15]. If adequate protocol and imaging guidance (ultrasound or fluoroscopy) was used but injections are not effective, retreatment is not recommended. The evidence regarding soluble biomarkers is currently not robust enough to include them in retreatment decision-making.

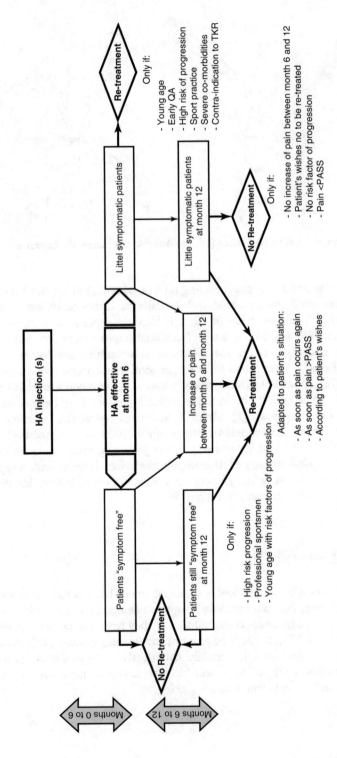

Fig. 3.8 Treatment algorithm after success with HA (PASS patient acceptable symptom state) [15]

Safety

Although viscosupplementation is considered a safe procedure, 1–3% of patients can have typical injection associated side effects of erythema, stiffness, soreness, and swelling. These are usually mild and last 1–2 days. More severe side effects include allergic reaction, bursitis, infection, or significant swelling; though uncommon, these effects may warrant more immediate medical attention. A more comprehensive list of side effects is included in Table 3.1.

Comparison to Alternative Treatments

Evidence regarding the effectiveness of HA injections has been mixed. A 2009 review found no clinically meaningful improvement following treatment for knee OA with glucosamine or chondroitin oral supplements, viscosupplementation, or arthroscopic lavage with or without debridement [2]. A 2015 meta-analysis of only double-blinded, sham-controlled trials with at least 60 patients did not find HA more clinically effective than placebo [17]. A 2015 systematic review of 137 randomized control trials found hyaluronic acid injections to be more effective in treating OA treatment than corticosteroid injections, NSAIDs, and Tylenol [18]. Corticosteroids have been shown to be more effective in the first 4 weeks whereas HA provides better relief from 4 to 26 weeks [4, 16]. Thus, there could be a synergistic benefit from administration of both medications and co-administration could reduce inflammation in part of early OA treatment [4]. Corticosteroid injections

Table 3.1 Viscosupplementation side effects [16]

Mild	Moderate (all are rare)	Severe (all are very rare)	Life-threatening (all very rate)
Local pain[a]	Acute pseudoseptic arthritis (aka "flare" reaction or chemical synovitis)	Septic arthritis	Hypotension
Transient inflammatory response[a]	Granulomatous inflammation	Reactivation of complex regional pain syndrome	Air embolism
Local tissue atrophy	Hemarthrosis	Seizures	Anaphylactic reaction
Cramps and restless legs	Vertigo	Crystal deposition arthritis	Laryngeal edema
	Adjacent structure injury (nerves, vessels)	Adjacent structure injury (nerves, vessels)	Apnea
	Urticaria, pruritus		Vasomotor collapse

[a]Common

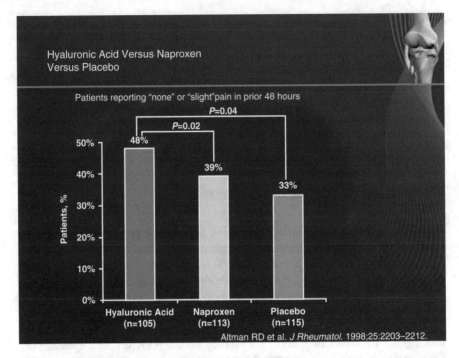

Fig. 3.9 HA provides greater pain relief than naproxen [20]

have been in common use in humans for approximately 65 years versus 35 years for HA but have more adverse side effects such as damage to cartilage, osteoporosis, hyperglycemia, immunosuppression, skin atrophy, depigmentation, Charcot arthropathy, Nicolau syndrome, and tendinopathy [7].

A 1998 comparison to naproxen and placebo showed that patients who received HA were significantly more likely to report no or slight pain in the past 48 h (see Fig. 3.9) [20]. Platelet-rich plasma has been found to be more effective than hyaluronic acid injections and with longer symptomatic relief in the treatment of knee OA [21–23]. Insurance coverage can still be a barrier for some patients to obtain IA HA injections.

Glucosamine and Chondroitin

Glucosamine and chondroitin are substrates proposed to be involved in the formation of hyaluronic acid and thus have possibly similar joint-preserving potential. Glucosamine is a precursor to glycosaminoglycan, whereas chondroitin is part of a large proteoglycan molecule that confers flexibility to cartilage and inhibits its enzymatic breakdown. They are theorized to increase the rate of new cartilage formation [2], and both are sold as dietary supplements that some short-term studies have found to be efficacious in treating OA [23]. Glucosamine derivatives are typically purified from crustacean shells and chondroitin from shark and cow cartilage [2]. In 2004, $730 million was spent on these products and while marked as a supplement in the United States and Canada, glucosamine is marketed as a drug in Europe [24]. The Glucosamine/Chondroitin Arthritis Intervention Trial (GAIT) studied 1583 patients with knee OA who received either glucosamine, chondroitin, a combination of both, celecoxib, or a placebo [2]. It found improvement of global pain and joint function in all groups without more clinically significant improvement from glucosamine and chondroitin versus placebo. However, in the subgroup of patients with moderate to severe OA, glucosamine and chondroitin did improve pain and functionality as compared to placebo. Both supplements have not been shown to have more adverse effects than placebo. It is still unknown whether the salts of glucosamine sulfate differ from glucosamine chondroitin and further investigation is needed.

Market

The market for viscosupplementation is predicted to steadily increase over the next decade [25] (see Fig. 3.10).

In 2016, the US market for viscosupplementation was valued at 3 billion, and a compound annual growth rate of 9.04% is expected until 2025 due to increasing geriatric population and rates of osteoarthritis. North American and Asia Pacific comprised the majority of the market share (Fig. 3.11). In the United States, economic impact of OA treatment was estimated to be 185.5 billion in a 2009 study, and a large portion of this was allocated to knee OA.

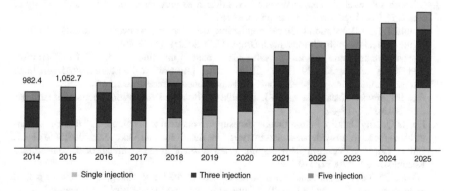

Fig. 3.10 US viscosupplementation market projections by product 2014–2025 [25]

Fig. 3.11 Viscosupplementation market share by geography [25]

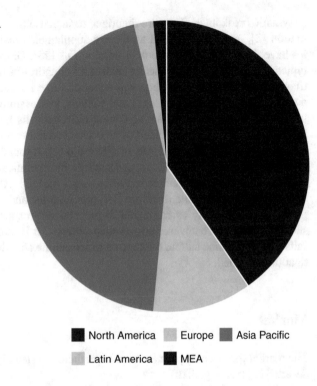

North America ■ Europe ■ Asia Pacific
■ Latin America ■ MEA

References

1. Vad VB. Viscosupplementation for knee osteoarthritis. Arthritis-Health. Accessed 28 Sept 2018 from https://www.arthritis-health.com/treatment/injections/viscosupplementation-knee-osteoarthritis.
2. Eisenberg Center at Oregon Health & Science University. Three treatments for osteoarthritis of the knee. Comparative effective review summary guides for clinicians 2009.
3. Srikanth VK, et al. A meta-analysis of sex differences prevalence, incidence and severity of osteoarthritis. Osteoarthr Cartil. 2005;13(9):769–81.
4. Iannitti T, Lodi D, Palmieri B. Intra-articular injections for the treatment of osteoarthritis: focus on the clinical use of hyaluronic acid. Drugs R&D. 2011;11(1):13–27.
5. Viscosupplementation with hyaluronic acid injections for knee arthritis. SlideShare. Accessed 29 Dec 2018 from https://www.slideshare.net/oldcadre4669/viscosupplementation-with-hyaluronic-acid-injections-for-knee-arthritis.
6. Axe JM, Snyder-Mackler L, Axe MJ. The role of viscosupplementation. Sports Med Arthrosc Rev. 2013;21(1):18–22.
7. Health Quality Ontario. Intra-articular viscosupplementation with hylan g-f 20 to treat osteoarthritis of the knee: an evidence-based analysis. Ont Health Technol Assess Ser. 2005;5(10):1–66.
8. Balazs EA, et al. Viscosupplementation: a new concept in the treatment of osteoarthritis. J Rheumatol. 1993;20(39):3–9.
9. Medscape. Viscosupplementation for osteoarthritis of the knee: strategies to improve patient outcomes 2018. Accessed 8 Dec 2018 from https://www.medscape.org/viewarticle/581361_2.
10. Wind WM, Smolinski RJ. Reliability of common new injection sites with low volume injections. J Arthroplasty. 2004;19(7):858–61.

11. OrthoInfo. Viscosupplementation treatment for knee arthritis. Accessed 14 Dec 2018 from https://orthoinfo.aaos.org/en/treatment/viscosupplemntation-treatment-for-knee-arthritis/.
12. Richette P, et al. Hyaluronan for knee osteoarthritis: an updated meta-analysis of trials with a low risk of bias. RMD Open. 2015;1(1):e000071.
13. Lubowitz JH. Editorial commentary: knee hyaluronic acid viscosupplementation reduces osteo-arthritis pain. Arthroscopy. 2015;31(10):2046. https://doi.org/10.1016/j.arthro.2015.07.005.
14. Campbell KA, Erickson BJ, Saltzman BM, Mascarenhas R, Bach BR Jr, Cole BJ, Verma NN. Is local viscosupplementation injection clinically superior to other therapies in the treatment of osteoarthritis of the knee: a systematic review of overlapping meta-analyses. Arthroscopy. 2015;31(10):2036–45. https://doi.org/10.1016/j.arthro.2015.03.030. Epub 2015 May 19.
15. Raman R, et al. Decision algorithms for the re-treatment with viscosupplementation in patients suffering from knee osteoarthritis. Osteoarthr Cartil. 2017;25(1):S357–8.
16. Leite VF, et al. Viscosupplementation for hip OA: a systematic review and meta-analysis of the efficacy on pain and disability, and the occurrence of adverse events. Arch Phys Med Rehabil. 2018;99(3):574–83.
17. Peterson C, Hodler J. Adverse events from diagnostic and therapeutic joint injections: a litera-ture review. Skelet Radiol. 2009;40(1):5–12.
18. Jevsevar D, et al. Viscosupplementation for osteoarthritis of the knee: a systematic review of the evidence. J Bone Joint Surg. 2015;97(24):2047–60.
19. Bellamy N, Campbell J, Robinson V, et al (2005).Viscosupplementation for the treatment of osteoarthritis of the knee. BMJ Evidence Based Medicine (11): 1.
20. Altman RD, et al. Intraarticular sodium hyaluronate (Hyalgan) in the treatment of patients with osteoarthritis of the knee: a randomized clinical trial. Hyalgan Study group. J Rheumatol. 1998;25:2203–12.
21. Bannuru RR, et al. Comparative effectiveness of pharmacologic interventions for knee osteo-arthritis. Ann Intern Med. 2015;162(1):46–55.
22. Kon E, et al. Platelet-rich plasma intra-articular injection versus hyaluronic acid viscosup-plementation as treatments for cartilage pathology: from early degeneration to osteoarthritis. Arthroscopy. 2011;27(11):1490–501.
23. Campbell KA, et al. Does intra-articular platelet-rich plasma injection provide clinically supe-rior outcomes compared with other therapies in the treatment of knee osteoarthritis? A system-atic review of overlapping meta-analyses. Arthroscopy. 2015;31(11):2213–21.
24. Khosla SK, Baumhauer JF. Dietary and viscosupplementation in ankle arthritis. Foot Ankle Clin. 2008;13(3):353–61.
25. Grand View Research. Viscosupplementation market by product (single injection, three injec-tion, five injection), by region (North America, Europe, Asia Pacific, Latin America, MEA) and segment forecasts, 2018–2025 2017.

Chapter 4
Stem Cells

Nadia N. Zaman and Dayna McCarthy

Introduction

Musculoskeletal pain is a common type of chronic pain often resulting from osteoarthritis and chronic tendinopathy that affects various joints in the body. Osteoarthritis is characterized by a degenerative and inflammatory process that leads to joint pain and stiffness, causing a decrease in functional mobility and joint destruction over time. Because articular hyaline cartilage is avascular with poor regenerative capabilities, chondral injuries have very little stimulus to produce inflammation and healing. According to data from the National Health Interview Survey, over 52 million Americans were reported to have been diagnosed with some form of arthritis, with over 22 million having some level of arthritis-related activity limitation; both numbers are expected to grow by 2030 [1]. Tendinopathy accounts for 30–50% of sports-related injuries and is a multifactorial condition characterized by tendon thickening and localized tendon pain that may result from trauma, or more commonly, overuse [2]. For example, nontraumatic rotator cuff tendinopathy can be a significant source of morbidity among those with shoulder pain and can lead to long-term disability if left undertreated [3]. In the past decade, the body of knowledge regarding the use of stem cells to treat musculoskeletal conditions has grown as physicians have taken an active role in the research, education, and clinical use of this regenerative technique. While there is a literature regarding the different types of stem cells and their use in various arthritic and tendinopathic processes, there is still a lack of uniformity in composition, concentration, and results post-injection.

N. N. Zaman (✉) · D. McCarthy
Sports Medicine and Interventional Spine, Department of Rehabilitation and Human Performance, Icahn School of Medicine at Mount Sinai, New York, NY, USA

© Springer Nature Switzerland AG 2020
G. Cooper et al. (eds.), *Regenerative Medicine for Spine and Joint Pain*,
https://doi.org/10.1007/978-3-030-42771-9_4

History

Prior to the availability of orthobiologics, the mainstay of nonoperative symptomatic management was intra-articular or peri-articular corticosteroid injection; however, recent research has shown only short-term benefit, with patients requiring numerous injections as the effects wear off. Repeated injections can lead to tendon and cartilage toxicity over time, with magnetic resonance imaging (MRI) showing evidence of cartilage volume loss [4]. As a result, the need for more effective treatment options for osteoarthritis and chronic tendinopathies has grown as the average man and woman continues to stay active and live longer.

While hyaluronic acid viscosupplementation has been around for some time, and regenerative therapies such as platelet-rich plasma and prolotherapy have provided alternatives to corticosteroids, stem cell therapy is another innovative technique becoming more and more available today. Stem cell therapies have been used in veterinary medicine since the early 2000s, but only more recently has the clinical efficacy been explored [5]. While the least studied of the available regenerative medicine treatments because of the often restrictive regulatory guidelines, the body of literature regarding stem cell therapy continues to grow.

Scientists Ernest A. McCulloch and James E. Till first published data regarding the clonal nature of marrow cells in the 1960s [6]. The first clinical trial of mesenchymal stem cells (MSCs) was completed in 1995 when a small number of patients were injected with cultured MSCs to test for safety [7]. Since then, hundreds of clinical trials have been registered at http://clinicaltrials.gov studying the effects of MSCs as treatment. As a result, in 2006, the International Society for Cellular Therapy recommended that cells must fulfill the following criteria to be considered MSCs: the cells must be plastic-adherent when maintained under standard culture conditions; they must express CD73, CD90, and CD105 markers and should not express CD34, CD45, CD14, HLA-DR, CD11b, or CD19; and they should be able to differentiate into osteoblasts, chondroblasts, and adipocytes in vitro [8].

MSCs are multipotent; they can be harvested from a wide variety of tissues in the body and have the ability to differentiate into many types of tissues, such as bone, cartilage, muscle, ligament, fat, and tendon as noted in Fig. 4.1 [9–11]. MSCs have been used in animal studies both in vivo and in vitro to demonstrate chondrogenesis, osteogenesis, and tendon healing in osteochondral defects, fractures, and tendinopathies, respectively [12–15]. Nonetheless, stem cells are regarded as advanced therapy medicinal products by regulatory bodies, thus requiring a time-consuming process of assessment for quality, safety, and efficacy protocols [16]. The development of processes to harvest human stem cells through minimally invasive means and prepare them using "minimal manipulation" has allowed for the use of stem cells for various musculoskeletal pathologies. Although there is no standardization of protocols, patients are required to discontinue any corticosteroids or anti-inflammatory medications for at least 7 days prior to the harvesting of cells to allow for the proper pro-inflammatory mediators in the cells to proliferate. Post procedure, patients are advised to not use any anti-inflammatory medications because these will essentially cancel out the effects of the stem cells injected.

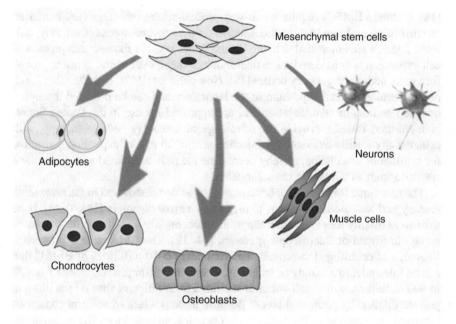

Fig. 4.1 Mesenchymal stem cells are multipotent and are believed to give rise to a number of different cell lines. (Image from Meregalli et al. [9])

This chapter will expand upon the types of stem cells currently available for soft tissue and joint pain, as well as the major indications for which they have been tested with good results.

Bone Marrow-Derived Stem Cells

Bone marrow aspirate (BMA) is a rich source of MSCs that can be isolated and concentrated to create an injectate. Once the BMA is harvested, it is prepared using centrifugation to produce bone marrow aspirate concentrate (BMAC), which is rich not only in MSCs but also other progenitor cells such as hematopoietic stem cells (HSCs), platelets, cytokines, platelet-derived growth factors, interleukin-1 receptor antagonists, and bone morphogenetic proteins 2 and 7, all of which are known to promote stem cell differentiation and proliferation [17, 18]. Although the exact mechanism of action for BMAC is not fully understood, one of the proposed theories is that progenitor cells use paracrine signaling, meaning they are able to communicate with neighboring cells to produce anti-inflammatory and immunomodulatory effects in order to stimulate growth and differentiation leading to tissue repair [19].

It is important to understand the differences between the two types of bone marrow-derived stem cells (BMSCs) that are available: cultured and non-cultured. Generally, BMSCs make up 0.001–0.01% of the total nucleated cells in BMA

[18]. Cultured BMSCs require a two-step process where cell counts are increased in vitro to several hundred- to thousand-folds over several weeks. Currently, cultured BMSCs are not available in the United States because the two-step process of cell expansion is considered more than minimal manipulation and is not approved for use by national regulatory bodies [18]. Non-cultured BMSCs, on the other hand, do not require any cell expansion in the laboratory and can be prepared through a one-step process of centrifugation and are approved for use in the United States. Non-cultured BMSCs provide the advantage of same-day bedside therapy, with cells usually readily available for injection within 30 min of aspiration and allow for autologous inoculation, thereby decreasing the risks associated with an immune response from an allogeneic transplantation.

The technique for harvesting bone marrow was first discovered in the nineteenth century and was used as a means to diagnose marrow disorders [18]. Today, bone marrow is usually harvested from the ilium under anesthesia with sterile procedure using ultrasound or fluoroscopic guidance [17, 18]. The BMA is then processed, filtered, and centrifuged to produce approximately 6–10 milliliters of BMAC that can be injected into a variety of locations. The volume aspirated can range from 30 to 400 milliliters, with small volumes aspirated from different sites on the ilium to prevent dilution by peripheral blood. Because there is a lack of uniform consensus regarding the protocol of harvesting and concentration techniques, the composition of progenitor cells in BMAC is variable; some suggest the different compositions may affect the regenerative properties that are produced. BMAC preparations from various recent studies are listed in Table 4.1.

BMAC can been used for a wide range of both bony and tendinous musculoskeletal pathologies with good results. For knee osteoarthritis, BMAC alone has been shown to be a relatively well-tolerated procedure that led to decreased pain at follow-up with no serious adverse effects reported [22, 27]. BMAC in combination with scaffold plugs in osteochondral defects of the knee showed MRI evidence of cartilage maturation with greater fill like normal hyaline cartilage than scaffolding

Table 4.1 Bone marrow aspirate concentrate preparations

Site being injected	Aspirate (mL)	Concentrate (mL)	Harvest site
Rotator cuff [16]	60–90	1–3	Posterior superior iliac crest
Rotator cuff [20]	150	12	Anterior iliac crest
Femoral head [21]	400	50	Posterior iliac crest
Knee [22]	52	6	Bilateral superior iliac crests
Femoral head [23]	60	7–10	Iliac crest
Achilles tendon [24]	30–60	6–9	Iliac crest
Patellar tendon [25]	Not reported	6–8	Anterior iliac crest
Lumbar spine [26]	100	10	Bilateral posterior iliac crests

alone [28]. BMAC injected after meniscectomy also resulted in improved pain scores in the visual analog scale, as well as increased meniscal volume quantified by MRI when compared to controls who received hyaluronic acid viscosupplementation [29]. BMAC has also been used as treatment for osteonecrosis of the femoral head with mixed results, with one particular study showing no difference in time to total hip arthroplasty; however, it has been argued in the literature that the stage of osteonecrosis was important to the ultimate results, with lower staging responding better to BMAC than higher staging [30, 31]. In the spine, posterolateral lumbar fusion has shown greater and faster bone healing with the implantation of BMAC [32].

There are limited studies in the use of BMAC as intradiscal therapy for degenerative disc disease. A randomized controlled trial reported on the safety and feasibility of using allogeneic BMAC for the treatment of low back pain secondary to degenerative disc disease, showing improved functional and pain scores [30]. Intradiscal BMAC may also lead to radiographic improvement in Pfirrmann grade and reduce the likelihood of progression to surgery in the long term [33]. Further research will elucidate whether biologic therapies for degenerative disc disease will be beneficial for patients.

The use of BMAC for rotator cuff, patellar, and Achilles tendinopathy has also been studied. Improvement in pain and disability was observed at long-term follow-up in rotator cuff tears and chronic patellar tendinopathy [16, 34]. When used in conjunction with surgical repairs, such as those done for rotator cuff and Achilles tendon pathologies, patients who received BMAC had more accelerated healing with no reported re-ruptures [29, 35]. A summary of major indications studied in the literature for BMAC are listed in Table 4.2.

Table 4.2 Major musculoskeletal indications for stem cell therapy	Bone marrow-derived stem cells	Osteonecrosis of femoral head
		Osteoarthritis of knee
		Osteochondral lesions of knee
		Osteoarthritis of shoulder
		Rotator cuff tendinopathy
		Patellar tendinopathy
		Achilles tendinopathy
	Adipose-derived stem cells	Osteoarthritis of knee
		Osteochondral lesions of talus
		Lateral epicondylosis
		Achilles tendinopathy
	Amniotic tissue-derived products	Osteoarthritis of knee
		Osteochondritis dissecans of talus
		Plantar fasciitis

Adipose-Derived Stem Cells

Subcutaneous adipose tissue is an abundant and accessible source of MSCs. Because adipose tissue is highly vascularized, it provides a large pool of undifferentiated cells with perivascular access for mobilization and relocation to injured and diseased structures [5]. Although bone marrow is currently the most studied source for MSCs, adipose tissue is considered to have a higher concentration of these cells, sometimes yielding 500–2500 times more MSCs as the same volume of bone marrow; it is also less invasive to harvest [11, 31]. Furthermore, adipose-derived stem cells (ADSCs) are considered more genetically stable and have higher proliferative and differentiation capabilities than BMSCs because it is believed that the progenitor cell concentrations are better preserved in adipose tissue as one ages [9, 11]. Injection of ADSCs stimulates recovery through paracrine signaling as well, leading to the release of cytokines and growth factors to promote healing.

There are two ways to prepare ADSCs for use. The first requires isolation, centrifugation, and culture expansion of cells to create the stromal vascular fraction (SVF), which is then resuspended for clinical use. This method allows for increasing the total number of ADSCs that can be used for treatment. However, it does not meet the requirements for "minimal manipulation" and thus is not approved for use by national regulatory bodies [35]. As a result, much of the research utilizing SVF is developed and implemented outside of the United States. The second method is a nonenzymatic mechanical method known as microfragmentation. Through this method, the adipose tissue is put through a process of mechanical filtration and agitation while protected in a liquid environment, usually saline, in order to provide the highest concentration of ADSCs without any enzymes or additives [34].

Adipose tissue is readily available and can be obtained through minimally invasive means. Approximately 50–100 milliliters of subcutaneous adipose tissue can be harvested from abdominal or buttocks fat through lipoaspiration. Once processed through filtration and centrifugation, or through enzymatic digestion, filtration, and centrifugation such as with the SVF, this can yield $1.8–9.3 \times 10^6$ stem cells in approximately 4–10 milliliters of solution [9, 29]. In vitro study of ADSCs has shown that the cells can form a biological scaffold that can provide mechanical support to the joint while helping regenerate or repair damaged cartilage [5].

ADSCs have been studied in a number of musculoskeletal pathologies. Phase I trials using injection of ADSCs for osteoarthritis have shown promising results. Individuals experienced no adverse effects from the lipoaspiration procedure or injection thereafter and showed long-term improvement in both pain and function, lasting at least 2 years [11, 32, 36]. Not only did individuals with OA experience subjective improvement; follow-up MRIs in a number of studies showed improvement in the size of the cartilage defects in the joint space [11, 31]. Intratendinous injection of ADSCs for Achilles tendinopathy showed faster improvement in pain and function than platelet-rich plasma injection, with improvement seen within 15 days [29]. In lateral epicondylosis, injection of ADSCs led to decrease in elbow pain as early as 6 weeks, with effects lasting at least 52 weeks [37]. While studies have shown good results, they were often limited due to their small sample sizes; there is still a dearth of literature regarding the use of ADSCs. A summary of major indications studied in the literature for ADSCs are listed in Table 4.2.

Amniotic Tissue-Derived Products

MSCs have also been found in abundance in cord blood, placenta, and amniotic fluid. Since these tissues are routinely discarded after birth, they do not have the same ethical concerns associated with them as the use of embryonic stem cells; thus, these are affordable and available resources for obtaining MSCs [38]. It is also important to note that because there is both a fetal and maternal component to the composition of the placenta, there has been a different terminology ascribed to the different origins of cells. Amniotic mesenchymal and epithelial cells produce and release several growth factors, cytokines, and matrix components that contribute to metabolic processes, as well as protein and collagen synthesis and collagenase activity [32, 39]. They also have an advantageous immunogenic profile because of their low levels of expression of major histocompatibility complex class I and II, thereby making them a desirable product as an allogeneic source [32]. Several preparations of amniotic tissue-derived stem cells are available in the United States, as regulated by the Food and Drug Administration (FDA) under the minimally manipulated tissue guidelines; these products can be commercially available as long as they are not marketed as stem cell products and do not contain viable cells [40].

The processing of these amniotic tissue-derived products is also varied but includes cleaning, sterilizing, screening, and testing for any pathogenic disease. The cells are then processed to preserve their efficacy through dehydration, cryopreservation, and hypothermic or fresh storage; preprocessing and postprocessing standards and guidelines are established by the American Association of Tissue Banks and the FDA. Dehydrated allograft tissue can be stored at ambient temperatures for up to 5 years; cryopreservation and hypothermic or fresh storage have a much shorter shelf life in comparison [32, 36]. The dehydrated powder can be applied directly to the site of injury or can be reconstituted into a suspension for injection [37].

Much of the current available literature on the use of amniotic tissue-derived products for musculoskeletal pathologies focuses on ankle and foot disorders. Dehydrated amniotic/chorionic membrane resuspended in saline led to improved pain and function in those suffering from chronic plantar fasciitis when injected directly at the source of pain; furthermore, the results were similar in treatment efficacy to those who received open release surgery or endoscopic plantar fasciotomy, with less follow-up office visits required [36]. When cryopreserved human amniotic membrane injection was compared to corticosteroid injection, it was found that amniotic tissue-derived products provided a safe and effective alternative treatment for chronic plantar fasciitis, but the effect may be dose-dependent with those who received a series of two injections experiencing more benefits with respect to pain and function than those who received one [41]. A small feasibility study looking at the use of amnion injections for symptomatic knee osteoarthritis found patients could tolerate the procedure and have clinical benefit up to 12 months after a single injection; however, a large-scale randomized controlled trial is not yet available [42]. A summary of major indications studied in the literature for amniotic tissue-derived products are listed in Table 4.2.

Adverse Events Associated with Stem Cell Therapy

Stem cell injections have been generally well tolerated, with little to no serious adverse effects reported in the literature. Many patients reported being completely satisfied with the procedure itself, as well as the results; when surveyed, most reported they would do it again if pain recurred or occurred at a different site [21].

The adverse effects most often reported were pain and swelling at the injection site, pain at the harvest site, discomfort on the skin overlying the injection site, or low-grade fevers, all of which usually resolved quite quickly and required little to no intervention [16, 29, 41, 42]. The use of laboratory tests, vital signs, and electrocardiograms showed no local or systemic safety concerns. As a result, it is considered safe to continue a rehabilitation protocol that includes light- to moderate-intensity exercise after a short period of relative rest, with gradual increase in activity back to baseline as the patient tolerates.

The primary theoretical concern with the use of stem cells has been whether these cells have the potential to divide spontaneously and uncontrollably into unwanted lineages of cells to produce tumors. However, studies both in vivo and in vitro, as well as in animal and human models, have shown no formation of soft tissue masses or atypical cells on fluid analysis, even on long-term follow-up [11, 20, 43]. Thus, at this time, stem cell therapies are considered to be non-tumorigenic.

Nonetheless, choosing the right patient for treatment is paramount to successful management of any disease process. While stem cell therapy can be used as treatment for musculoskeletal pathologies, it should likely be avoided in those who have bone marrow-derived cancers, such as lymphoma, are on blood thinners, or have systemic infections that put them in immunocompromised states [18].

Conclusion

While corticosteroid injections and viscosupplementation have been the longstanding choices for conservative management of many musculoskeletal pathologies, mesenchymal stem cells may provide another alternative to more costly and invasive procedures, such as surgery, when these other options fail. For example, those who have received stem cell injections for OA have often been able to avoid the need for any further procedures [22]. Moreover, stem cells may be considered the more beneficial choice as the first-line therapy for some people in order to avoid the numerous injections required with corticosteroids and viscosupplementation and the adverse effects associated over time with these treatment options.

Currently, there are no established guidelines regarding the ideal number or timing of injections, nor a standardized volume or concentration of stem cells to be injected. There is also a lack of universal consensus with respect to how stem cells are being harvested, processed, and prepared. Continued research may help elucidate some of these answers and more. Despite this, however, the literature regarding stem cell therapies grows at an exponential pace, with hundreds of clinical trials registered with governmental databases. The incredible capabilities of these multipotent cells and their accessibility through minimally invasive means make them a great addition to the clinician's arsenal of what can be done to ultimately improve the functional mobility and optimize the active lifestyles of patients.

References

1. Centers for Disease Control and Prevention. Prevalence of doctor-diagnosed arthritis and arthritis-attributable activity limitation – United States, 2010–2012. MMWR Morb Mortal Wkly Rep. 2013;62:869–73.
2. Oloff L, Elmi E, Nelson J, Crain J. Retrospective analysis of the effectiveness of platelet-rich plasma in the treatment of Achilles tendinopathy: pretreatment and posttreatment correlation of magnetic resonance imaging and clinical assessment. Foot Ankle Spec. 2015;8:490–7.
3. van der Windt DA, Koes BW, de Jong BA, Bouter LM. Shoulder disorders in general practice: incidence, patient characteristics, and management. Ann Rheum Dis. 1995;54(12):959.
4. McAlindon TE, LaValley MP, Harvey WF, et al. Effect of intraarticular triamcinolone vs saline on knee cartilage volume and pain in patients with knee osteoarthritis. JAMA. 2017;317:1967–75.
5. Bosetti M, Borrone A, Follenzi A, Messaggio F, Tremolada C, Cannas M. Human lipoaspirate as autologous injectable active scaffold for one-step repair of cartilage defects. Cell Transplant. 2016;25(6):1043–56.
6. Becker AJ, McCulloch EA, Till JE. Cytological demonstration of the clonal nature of spleen colonies derived from transplanted mouse marrow cells. Nature. 1963;197:452–4.
7. Wang S, Qu X, Zhao RC. Clinical applications of mesenchymal stem cells. J Hematol Oncol. 2012;5:19.
8. Dominici M, Le Blanc K, Mueller I, et al. Minimal criteria for defining multipotent mesenchymal stromal cells. The International Society for Cellular Therapy position statement. Cytotherapy. 2006;8(4):315–7.
9. Meregalli M, Farini A, Torrente Y. Mesenchymal stem cells as muscle reservoir. J Stem Cell Res Ther. 2011;1:105.
10. Law S, Chaudhuri S. Mesenchymal stem cell and regenerative medicine: regeneration versus immunomodulatory challenges. Am J Stem Cells. 2013;2(1):22–38.
11. Bansal H, Comella K, Leon J, Verma P, Agrawal D, Koka P, Ichim T. Intra-articular injection in the knee of adipose derived stromal cells (stromal vascular fraction) and platelet rich plasma for osteoarthritis. J Transl Med. 2017;15(1):141.
12. Han SH, Kim YH, Park MS, et al. Histological and biomechanical properties of regenerated articular cartilage using chondrogenic bone marrow stromal cells with a PLGA scaffold in vivo. J Biomed Mater Res A. 2008;87(4):850–61.
13. Chong AK, Ang AD, Goh JC, et al. Bone marrow-derived mesenchymal stem cells influence repair of tendon-healing in a rabbit Achilles tendon model. J Bone Joint Surg. 2007;89(1):74–81.

14. Berebichez-Fridman R, Gómez-García R, Granados-Montiel J, Berebichez-Fastlicht E, Olivos-Meza A, Granados J, Velasquillo C, Ibarra C. The holy grail of orthopedic surgery: mesenchymal stem cells—their current uses and potential applications. Stem Cells Int. 2017;2017:2638305.
15. Garcia D, Longo UG, Vaquero J, et al. Amniotic membrane transplant for articular cartilage repair: an experimental study in sheep. Curr Stem Cell Res Ther. 2014;10(1):77–83.
16. Poulos J. The limited application of stem cells in medicine: a review. Stem Cell Res Ther. 2018;9:1.
17. Centeno CJ, Al-Sayegh H, Bashir J, Goodyear S, Freeman MD. A prospective multi-site registry study of a specific protocol of autologous bone marrow concentrate for the treatment of shoulder rotator cuff tears and osteoarthritis. J Pain Res. 2015;8:269–76.
18. Chahla J, Mannava S, Cinque ME, Geeslin AG, Codina D, LaPrade RF. Bone marrow aspirate concentrate harvesting and processing technique. Arthrosc Tech. 2017;6(2):e441–5.
19. Sampson S, Botto-van Bemden A, Aufiero D. Autologous bone marrow concentrate: review and application of a novel intraarticular orthobiologic for cartilage disease. Phys Sports Med. 2013;41:7–18.
20. Hernigou P, Flouzat Lachaniette CH, Delambre J, et al. Biologic augmentation of rotator cuff repair with mesenchymal stem cells during arthroscopy improves healing and prevents further tears: a case-controlled study. Int Orthop. 2014;38:1811–8.
21. Hauzeur J, Maertelaer V, Baudoux E, Malaise M, Beguin Y, Gangji V. Inefficacy of autologous bone marrow concentrate in stage three osteonecrosis: a randomized controlled double-blind trial. Int Orthop. 2018;42:1429–35.
22. Shapiro S, Kazmerchak S, Heckman M, Zubair A, O'Connor M. A prospective, single-blind, placebo-controlled trial of bone marrow aspirate concentrate for knee osteoarthritis. Am J Sports Med. 2017;45(1):82–90.
23. Pilge H, Bittersohl B, Schneppendahl J, et al. Bone marrow aspirate concentrate in combination with intravenous iloprost increases bone healing in patients with avascular necrosis of the femoral head: a matched pair analysis. Orthop Rev (Pavia). 2016;8:6902.
24. Stein BE, Stroh DA, Schon LC. Outcomes of acute Achilles tendon rupture repair with bone marrow aspirate concentrate augmentation. Int Orthop. 2015;39:901–5.
25. Pascual-Garrido C, Rolón A, Makino A. Treatment of chronic patellar tendinopathy with autologous bone marrow stem cells: a 5-year-followup. Stem Cells Int. 2012;2012:953510.
26. Hart R, Komzak M, Okal F, Nahlik D, Jajtner P, Puskeiler M. Allograft alone versus allograft with bone marrow concentrate for the healing of the instrumented posterolateral lumbar fusion. Spine. 2014;14:1318–24.
27. Centeno C, Pitts J, Al-Sayegh H, Freeman M. Efficacy of autologous bone marrow concentrate for knee osteoarthritis with and without adipose graft. Biomed Res Int. 2014;2014:370621.
28. Krych AJ, Nawabi DH, Farshad-Amacker NA, et al. Bone marrow concentrate improves early cartilage phase maturation of a scaffold plug in the knee: a comparative magnetic resonance imaging analysis to platelet-rich plasma and control. Am J Sports Med. 2016;44:91–8.
29. Vangsness T, Farr J, Boyd J, Dellaero D, Mills R, Leroux-Williams M. Adult human mesenchymal stem cells delivered via intra-articular injection to the knee following partial medial meniscectomy: a randomized, double-blind, controlled study. J Bone Joint Surg. 2014;96(2):90–8.
30. Noriega DC, Ardura F, Hernández-Ramajo R, et al. Intervertebral disc repair by allogeneic mesenchymal bone marrow cells: a randomized controlled trial. Transplantation. 2017;101(8):1945–51.
31. Usuelli FG, Grassi M, Maccario C, et al. Intratendinous adipose derived stromal vascular fraction (SVF) injection provides a safe, efficacious treatment for Achilles tendinopathy: results of a randomized controlled clinical trial at a 6-month follow-up. Knee Surg Sports Traumatol Arthrosc. 2018;26:2000–10.
32. Pers Y-M, Rackwitz L, Ferreira R, Pullig O, Delfour C, Barry F, Sensebe L, Casteilla L, Fleury S, Bourih P, Noel D, Canovas F, Cyteval C, Lisignoli G, Schrauth J, Haddad D, Domergue S, Noeth U, Jorgensen C. Adipose mesenchymal stromal cell-based therapy for severe osteoarthritis of the knee: a phase I dose-escalation trial. Stem Cells Transl Med. 2016;5(7):847–56.

33. Pettine KA, Suzuki RK, Sand TT, Murphy MB. Autologous bone marrow concentrate intra-discal injection for the treatment of degenerative disc disease with three-year follow-up. Int Orthop. 2017;41(10):2097–103.
34. Bianchi F, Maioli M, Leonardi E, et al. A new nonenzymatic method and device to obtain a fat tissue derivative highly enriched in pericyte-like elements by mild mechanical forces from human lipoaspirates. Cell Transplant. 2013;22:2063–77.
35. Gimble JM, Katz AJ, Bunnell BA. Adipose-derived stem cells for regenerative medicine. Circ Res. 2007;100:1249.
36. Koh Y-G, Choi Y-J, Kwon S-K, Kim Y-S, Yeo J-E. Clinical results and second-look arthroscopic findings after treatment with adipose derived stem cells for knee osteoarthritis. Knee Surg Sports Traumatol Arthrosc. 2015;23:1308–16.
37. Lee SY, Kim W, Lim C, Chung SG. Treatment of lateral epicondylosis by using allogeneic adipose-derived mesenchymal stem cells: a pilot study. Stem Cells. 2015;33:2995–3005.
38. Friel NA, de Girolamo L, Gomoll AH, Mowry KC, Vines JB, Farr J. Amniotic fluid, cells, and membrane application. Oper Tech Sports Med. 2017;25:20–4.
39. Zelen CM, Poka A, Andrews J. Prospective, randomized, blinded, comparative study of inject-able micronized dehydrated amniotic/chorionic membrane allograft for plantar fasciitisdA feasibility study. Foot Ankle Int. 2013;34:1332–9.
40. Heckmann N, Auran RB, Mirzayan R. Application of amniotic tissue in orthopedic surgery. Am J Orthop. 2016;45:421–5.
41. Hanselman AE, Tidwell JE, Santrock RD. Cryopreserved human amniotic membrane injection for plantar fasciitis. Foot Ankle Int. 2015;36:151–8.
42. Vines JB, Aliprantis AO, Gomoll AH, Farr J. Cryopreserved amniotic suspension for the treat-ment of knee osteoarthritis. J Knee Surg. 2016;29(6):443–50.
43. Veronesi F, Giavaresi G, Tschon M, Borsari V, Nicoli Aldini N, Fini M. Clinical use of bone marrow, bone marrow concentrate, and expanded bone marrow mesenchymal stem cells in cartilage disease. Stem Cells Dev. 2013;22:181–92.

Chapter 5
Platelet-Rich Plasma

Xiaoning (Jenny) Yuan and Alfred C. Gellhorn

Introduction

In 2001, Dr. Richard Marx, an oral and maxillofacial surgeon, defined platelet-rich plasma (PRP) as a "volume of autologous plasma that has a platelet concentration above baseline" [1]. However, surgical applications of platelets and clotting factors, fibrinogen and thrombin, emerged much earlier in the 1970s and 1980 to augment healing. Yet, it was not until Dr. Marx's publication that a catalyst was in place for the development of PRP technology and commercialization.

By 2008, Hines Ward, then wide receiver for the Pittsburgh Steelers, reported to the media that he received PRP treatment for an acute grade 2 medial collateral ligament sprain, allowing him to return to play within 2 weeks, compared to the more typical 4–6-week recovery period [2]. The Steelers went on to win the Super Bowl that year. Ward's injury, treatment, and response to PRP therapy represents a key event and impetus for growing clinical interest in PRP applications in sports medicine and musculoskeletal injuries.

In this chapter, we discuss the basic science underlying PRP and clinical applications for musculoskeletal pathology. We review the diverse classification schemes and preparation methods of PRP, which relate to observed variations in clinical outcomes and efficacy of treatment, and the advantages and disadvantages of PRP therapy. We examine the regulation of PRP technology and barriers to expanding Food and Drug Administration approval for additional musculoskeletal indications. Finally, we close with future directions for PRP applications to the field of nonoperative sports medicine and spine care.

X. (J.) Yuan (✉)
Department of Rehabilitation Medicine, New York-Presbyterian Hospital, New York, NY, USA
e-mail: xiy7001@nyp.org

A. C. Gellhorn
Department of Rehabilitation Medicine, Weill Cornell Medicine, New York, NY, USA

© Springer Nature Switzerland AG 2020
G. Cooper et al. (eds.), *Regenerative Medicine for Spine and Joint Pain*,
https://doi.org/10.1007/978-3-030-42771-9_5

Basic Science of PRP and Mechanism of Action

Clinical interest in PRP lies in its regenerative properties, as well as its anti-inflammatory, anti-microbial, and analgesic actions on the tissue of interest [3]. Platelets are anucleate cytoplasmic fragments of megakaryocytes from the bone marrow, containing upward of 50–80 α-granules per platelet [4]. Physiological levels of platelets range from 150,000 to 350,000/μL. Their lifespan is approximately 10 days in circulation [5], and platelet death occurs by an intrinsic program of apoptosis [6]. Platelet activation, adhesion, and aggregation are the initial steps of the wound repair process and inflammatory cascade (Fig. 5.1). After activation, α-granules within the platelets degranulate, releasing growth factors and cytokines involved in cell proliferation and tissue remodeling, which play key roles in wound healing and repair.

The composition of PRP has been reported to contain over 300 growth factors and cytokines [8]. Growth factors present in PRP are promoters of mitogenesis and anabolism and have also been shown to suppress inflammation [9]. For example, PRP contains growth factors that have been shown to enhance chondrocyte proliferation, extracellular matrix (ECM) synthesis, and mesenchymal differentiation in laboratory studies [10, 11]. These growth factors include platelet-derived growth factors (PGDF-AA, PDGF-AB, PDGF-BB), transforming growth factors (TGF-β1,

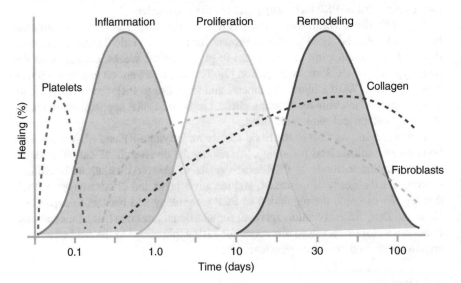

Fig. 5.1 The three overlapping phases of wound healing: inflammation, proliferation, and remodeling. Following tissue injury, platelet adhesion, aggregation, and activation occur, along with initiation of the inflammatory cascade, occurring over the first few days of healing. This is followed by the cell proliferation and tissue synthesis phase, consisting of angiogenesis, collagen deposition, granulation tissue formation, epithelization, and wound contraction. Finally, the tissue remodeling phase occurs weeks to months after injury, involving collagen and extracellular matrix maturation. Time in days presented on a logarithmic scale. (Modified from Lee et al. [7])

TGF-β2), insulin-like growth factor 1 (IGF-1), epidermal growth factor (EGF), vascular endothelial growth factor (VEGF), and fibroblast growth factor β (FGF-β) [1, 9]. PDGF in PRP has a role in early wound healing and stimulates fibroblast proliferation [12]. TGF-β1 increases collagen production by fibroblasts [13]. PRP also comprises cytokines with pro-inflammatory (interleukin 1, interleukin 6) and anti-inflammatory (interleukin 4, interleukin 10) functions. The function of major growth factors and cytokines of relevance to wound healing is summarized in Table 5.1.

Table 5.1 Composition of PRP and selected growth factors and cytokines involved in wound healing, musculoskeletal repair and regeneration

Growth factor or cytokine[a]	Role(s) in wound healing, musculoskeletal repair, and regeneration[a]	Reported concentrations in PRP	
		PRP system[b]	Concentration
Ang-2	Angiogenesis; chondrogenic and osteogenic differentiation [15–17]	PCCS	425 ± 405 pg/mL [18]
EGF	Endothelial chemotaxis and angiogenesis; MSC and epithelial cell mitogenesis; collagen synthesis; osteogenic and chondrogenic differentiation of MSCs [19, 20]	Arthrex	659.8 ± 35.9 pg/mL [4]
		Fibrinet	1.4 ± 1.2 ng/mL [21]
		GPS	470 ± 317 pg/mL [22]
		GPS III	2639.5 ± 197.7 pg/mL [23]
		PCCS	57 ± 77 pg/mL [18]
		Plateltex	1.6 ± 0.7 ng/mL [21]
		Regen	0.1 ± 0.1 ng/mL [21]
bFGF	MSC, chondrocyte, osteoblast, and capillary endothelial cells mitogenesis; chondrocyte, myoblast, and osteoblast differentiation [24, 25]	Arthrex	15.6 ± 2.4 pg/mL [23]
		Fibrinet	31 ± 27 pg/mL [21]
		GPS III	75.2 ± 21.4 pg/mL [23]
		Plateltex	3.5 ± 8 pg/mL [21]
		Regen	13 ± 10 pg/mL [21]
HGF	Angiogenesis, endothelial cell mitogenesis; anti-inflammatory effects [26]	Arthrex	645.2 ± 72.1 pg/mL [23]
		GPS III	4277.3 ± 1508.2 pg/mL [23]
IGF-1	Myoblast proliferation and differentiation; fibroblast chemotaxis and protein synthesis; osteoblast proliferation and differentiation; MSC proliferation and survival [27, 28]	AGF	132 ± 32 ng/mL [29]
		Arthrex	64.8 ± 55.4 pg/mL
		CS	100 ± 29 ng/mL [29]
		Fibrinet	27 ± 11 ng/mL [21]
		GPS	72 ± 25 pg/mL [22] 99 ± 29 ng/mL [29]
		GPS III	672.9 ± 378.4 pg/mL [23]
		MCS 3p	84 ± 23 ng/mL [30]
		PCCS	5.550 ± 2.075 ng/mL [18]
		Plateltex	88 ± 34 ng/mL [21]
		Regen	36 ± 14 ng/mL [21]
IL-1	Pro-inflammatory and catabolic effects [31]	Arthrex	IL-1β: 0.31 pg/mL [32]
		GPS III Mini	IL-1β: 3.67 pg/mL [32]

(continued)

Table 5.1 (continued)

Growth factor or cytokine[a]	Role(s) in wound healing, musculoskeletal repair, and regeneration[a]	Reported concentrations in PRP	
		PRP system[b]	Concentration
PDGF-AB	Chemotaxis of inflammatory cells; angiogenesis; fibroblast chemotaxis and proliferation; ECM synthesis; MSC and osteoblast mitogenesis [33–35]	Arthrex	16.6681 ± 5.5123 ng/mL [23] 6.4 ng/mL [32]
		Cascade	9.7 ± 3.6 ng/mL [36]
		GPS III	42.2739 ± 2.9024 ng/mL [23] 18.7 ± 12.8 ng/mL [36]
		GPS III Mini	22 ng/mL [32]
		Harvest	133 ± 29.2 ng/mL [37]
		Magellan	34.4 ± 10.7 ng/mL [36]
		MCS 3p	117 ± 63 ng/mL [30]
		PCCS	103 ± 27 ng/mL [37]
PDGF-BB		AGF	250 ± 80 pg/mL [29]
		Cascade	14.8 ± 2.5 ng/mL [36]
		CS	204 ± 53 pg/mL [29]
		Fibrinet	3.6 ± 2.4 ng/mL [21]
		GPS	17 ± 8 ng/mL [22] 191 ± 36 pg/mL [29]
		GPS III	23.1 ± 10.1 ng/mL [36]
		Magellan	33.0 ± 8.2 ng/mL [36]
		MCS 3p	10 ± 8 ng/mL [30]
		Plateltex	14.3 ± 11.3 ng/mL [21]
		Regen	2.3 ± 1.9 ng/mL [21]
MMPs	ECM remodeling and tissue degradation [38]	Arthrex	MMP-9: 40 ng/mL [32]
		GPS III Mini	MMP-9: 222 ng/mL [32]
TGF-β1	Fibroblast activation and proliferation; ECM synthesis; endothelial chemotaxis and angiogenesis; MSC proliferation; chondrogenic and osteogenic differentiation [33, 39–41]	Arthrex	66,246.2 ± 7620.4 pg/mL [23] 20 ng/mL [32]
		Cascade	0.1 ± 0.08 ng/mL [36]
		Fibrinet	8.8 ± 5.0 ng/mL [21]
		GPS	120 ± 42 ng/mL [22]
		GPS III	141.2869 ± 12.5761 ng/mL [23] 0.1 ± 0.08 ng/mL [36]
		GPS III Mini	89 ng/mL [32]
		Magellan	0.2 ± 0.1 ng/mL [36]
		MCS 3p	169 ± 84 ng/mL [30]
		Plateltex	40.4 ± 14.9 ng/mL [21]
		Regen	6.2 ± 4.0 ng/mL [21]

Table 5.1 (continued)

Growth factor or cytokine[a]	Role(s) in wound healing, musculoskeletal repair, and regeneration[a]	Reported concentrations in PRP	
		PRP system[b]	Concentration
TGF-β2	MSC proliferation; chondrogenic and osteogenic differentiation [39–41]	MCS 3p	0.4 ± 0.3 ng/mL [30]
VEGF	Angiogenesis and vasculogenesis; macrophage and granulocyte chemotaxis [42]	Arthrex	138.7 ± 11.2 pg/mL [23]
		Cascade	0.3 ± 0.3 ng/mL [36]
		Fibrinet	0.3 ± 0.3 ng/mL [21]
		GPS	955 ± 1030 pg/mL [22]
		GPS III	142.9 ± 12.5 pg/mL [23] 2.4 ± 1.1 ng/mL [36]
		Magellan	1.2 ± 0.8 ng/mL [36]
		Plateltex	0.7 ± 0.4 ng/mL [21]
		Regen	0.1 ± 0.1 ng/mL [21]

Modified from LaPrade et al. [14]

[a]*Ang-2* angiopoietin-2, *ECM* extracellular matrix, *EGF* epidermal growth factor, *bFGF* basic fibroblast growth factor, *HGF* hepatocyte growth factor, *IGF* insulin-like growth factor, *IL* interleukin, *MMP* matrix metalloproteinase, *MSC* mesenchymal stem cell, *PDGF* platelet-derived growth factor, *TGF* transforming growth factor, *VEGF* vascular endothelial growth factor

[b]AGF: Autologous Growth Factor Filter (Interpore Cross International, LLC, Irvine, CA, USA); Arteriocyte: Arteriocyte Magellan (Arteriocyte Medical Systems, Inc., Cleveland, OH, USA); Arthrex: Arthrex ACP (Autologous Conditioned Plasma) Double Syringe System (Arthrex Inc., Naples, FL, USA); CS: Electa Cell Separator (Sorin Group Italia S.r.l, Mirandola, IT); Fibrinet: Fibrinet (Cascade Medical Enterprises, LLC, Wayne, NJ, USA); GPS: Biomet Gravitational Platelet Separation (GPS) System (Biomet Inc., Warsaw, IN, USA); GPS III: Biomet GPS III (Biomet Inc.); GPS III Mini: Biomet GPS III Mini Platelet Concentrate Separation Kit (Biomet Inc.); Harvest: Harvest SmartPReP (Harvest Technologies Corporation, Plymouth, MA, USA); MCS 3p: Haemonetics Gradient Density Cell Separator (Haemonetics Corporation, München, DE); MTF: MTF Cascade PRP System (MTF Biologics, Edison, NJ, USA); PCCS: Platelet Concentrate Collection System (Implant Innovations Inc., West Palm Beach, FL, USA); Plateltex: Plateltex (Plateltex S.R.O., Bratislava, SK); Regen: RegenPRP-Kit (RegenLab SA, Mollens, CH)

PRP therapy allows for supraphysiological concentrations of these molecules to be delivered to a site of injury to optimize, accelerate, or reinitiate tissue healing, regeneration, and repair [43, 44]. Platelet activation leads to immediate secretion of growth factors, upward of 70% in the first 10 min, and over 95% of the growth factors within 1 h [1, 37]. However, an in vitro study of PRP activated by contact with collagenous tissue, explants did not demonstrate a decrease in TGF-β1 and PDGF-BB levels between 24 and 96 h (4 days) of culture [45], suggesting that platelets may continue to synthesize and secrete growth factors after initial activation. In the absence of activation, PDGF-AB release from PRP prepared by four different systems occurred steadily out to 120 h of in vitro storage at physiological temperature (37 °C) [46].

Applications of PRP leverage the function of platelets for remodeling, repair, and regeneration. Current musculoskeletal applications of PRP include treatment of tendinopathy, osteoarthritis, ligament and meniscus injury, muscle injury, and spine disorders. Although PRP has been promoted and publicized as a regenerative therapy, it is important to note that studies thus far have not demonstrated de facto tissue regeneration in clinical sports and spine applications.

Creation and Classification of PRP

The different forms and methods of preparing PRP are numerous, and its nomenclature reflects this variation. Platelet concentrate, platelet gel, platelet-rich fibrin matrix, platelet-rich in growth factors, and platelet-rich fibrin are names of products produced by various devices.

Protocols for deriving PRP involve a one- or more commonly two-step centrifugation procedure, which vary by time and speed. The first centrifugation step separates whole blood into platelet and cell fractions. The second centrifugation step, which is typically at higher speed, further refines the platelet fraction. The final volume of PRP produced from whole blood varies but is usually approximately 10% of the initial blood volume.

Preparation methods vary by platelet concentration, leukocyte concentration (leukocyte-rich versus leukocyte-poor), platelet activation, and use of anticoagulant. Platelet concentrations range from 2.5- to 8-fold compared to whole blood. Autologous conditioned plasma is a subclassification of PRP, which typically contains a lower fold increase in platelet concentration. Leukocyte concentration varies between leukocyte-rich (LR-PRP) and leukocyte-poor (LP-PRP) preparations. Tailoring PRP preparations to the treatment of specific clinical conditions is beginning to be evaluated more rigorously, with early data suggesting that LR-PRP is more effective for tendinopathy, while LP-PRP is superior for OA [47, 48].

Platelet activation serves as the first step in the inflammatory cascade. In the body, platelets are activated by agents such as thrombin, collagen, ADP, serotonin, and thromboxane A2. If desired during PRP preparation, exogenous platelet activation is typically achieved by the use of thrombin or calcium chloride. However, there remains no consensus on timing of activation, if exogenous activation is necessary at all prior to injection, or if activation should occur after injection, through interactions with collagen matrix in the native local environment. Due to the risk of life-threatening coagulopathy associated with bovine thrombin, secondary to antibodies to Factors V and XI and thrombin, recombinant human thrombin is available as an activation agent [49].

Finally, anticoagulants such as anticoagulant citrate dextrose-A (ACDA) or citrate phosphate dextrose are used to prevent blood clotting during PRP preparation.

More than 25 PRP preparation kits are currently available on the market [50]. A list summarizing representative kits, their underlying technology, and characteristics of the resulting PRP products is shown in Table 5.2. PRP systems can be categorized as plasma- or buffy coat-based. Plasma-based systems exclude leukocytes at

Table 5.2 Preparation of PRP by select devices and characteristics of their PRP products [51–55]

Technology	PRP system[a]	Centrifuge protocol Time (min)	Spins	Activation[b]	Initial blood volume (mL)	Final PRP volume (mL)	Platelet concentration from baseline	WBC content[b]	RBC content
Plasma-based	Arthrex ACP	5	1	None	16	4–7	2–3×	LP	Poor
	MTF Cascade	6	1	CaCl₂	9	4.5	1.3–1.7×	LP	Poor
Buffy coat-based	Biomet GPS III	12–15	1	AT and CaCl₂	30 or 60	3 or 6	2–8×	LR	Rich
	Harvest Smart PReP 2	12–15	2	BT or CaCl₂	20 or 60	3 or 7–10	3–7×	LR	Rich
	Arteriocyte Magellan	14–20	2	CaCl₂	30 or 60	3–10	3–7×	LR	Rich

[a]Arteriocyte Magellan: Magellan Autologous Platelet Separator System (Arteriocyte Medical Systems, Inc., Cleveland, OH, USA); Arthrex ACP: Arthrex ACP (Autologous Conditioned Plasma) Double Syringe System (Arthrex Inc., Naples, FL, USA); Biomet GPS III: Biomet GPS III (Gravitational Platelet Separation) System (Biomet Inc., Warsaw, IN, USA); Harvest Smart PReP 2: Harvest Smart PReP 2 (Harvest Technologies Corporation, Plymouth, MA, USA); MTF Cascade: Cascade PRP System (MTF Biologics, Edison, NJ, USA)

[b]AT autologous thrombin, BT bovine thrombin, CaCl₂ calcium chloride, LP leukocyte-poor, LR leukocyte-rich

the expense of some platelets, whereas buffy coat-based systems maximize platelet yield but also retain leukocytes and red blood cells (RBCs) [51].

There remains no universal classification for PRP. In 2009, Dohan Ehrenfest et al. published the first PRP classification system, based on the presence of leukocytes and fibrin architecture: leukocyte-poor or pure PRP/low-density fibrin network after activation (P-PRP), leukocyte-rich PRP/low-density fibrin network after activation (L-PRP), leukocyte-poor PRP/high-density fibrin network after activation (P-PRF), and leukocyte-rich PRP/high-density fibrin network after activation (L-PRF) [56].

In 2012, Mishra et al. added two additional classification components of platelet activation or non-activation and level of platelet enrichment [57], while Delong et al. proposed the PAW classification (P = absolute number of platelets, A = manner of platelet activation, W = presence or absence of leukocytes) [51]. The PLRA classification proposed in 2015 encompasses platelet count (P), leukocyte content (L), RBC content (R), and activation (A) [58]. The DEPA classification published by Magalon et al. encompasses four components: dose of injected platelets (D), efficiency of production (E), purity of PRP produced (P), and activation process (A) [59]. Finally, the MARSPILL classification was published in 2017, which comprises method (M; handmade or machine), activation (A; activated or not activated), red blood cells (R; rich or poor), spin (S; one or two spins), platelet number (P; folds basal), image guided (I; guided or not guided), leukocyte concentration (L; rich or poor), and light activation (L; activated or not activated) [60].

The optimal degree of fold change in platelet concentration has been debated. Early studies suggested that ideal platelet concentrations were only two- to three-fold over baseline and that higher fold changes inhibited healing. These findings are in line with in vitro studies of platelet-rich plasma, where a dose-response relationship between growth factor concentrations and cell activity existed until an asymptotic level was reached, with some growth factors exerting an inhibitory effect at sufficiently high concentrations [61]. This has been clarified by follow-up studies, which suggested that fold changes in the range of five- to sevenfold were ideal and that inhibition did not occur until up to tenfold increase over baseline [62].

Buffy coat-based PRP systems that produce higher platelet concentrations tend to produce higher leukocyte and RBC concentrations as well [51]. The controversy over leukocyte concentration has revolved around neutrophils and their association with pro-inflammatory cytokines, interleukin 1 (IL-1) and tumor necrosis factor (TNF-α), which may exacerbate inflammation in osteoarthritis or acute muscle injuries. LR-PRP has been shown to cause synoviocyte cell death in culture and increase expression of inflammatory markers [47]. Likewise, the presence of RBCs in PRP is controversial, as RBCs have been documented to cause chondrocyte death [47, 63]. However, the leukocytes in PRP also contain monocytes, which differentiate into macrophages. While the primary function of macrophages was previously thought to be only for phagocytosis, it is now recognized that different types of activated macrophages exist, which have pro-inflammatory (M1) and anti-inflammatory (M2) roles. The M2 macrophage has specific functions in wound healing, which may assist tissue repair. A PRP formulation enriched with M2 macrophages may therefore be ideal for certain tissue pathologies. Newer PRP devices are able to achieve higher platelet concentrations while minimizing both WBC and RBC content through a two-spin suspension protocol.

Differences in PRP composition are related not only to variation in preparation methods but also to variation among patients, given the autologous nature of PRP. Both age and sex are known to influence PRP composition. A study of 39 healthy patients with no history of orthopedic problems and no current NSAID, antiplatelet, or aspirin use reported significant differences in composition of LP-PRP from male versus female subjects, with sex influencing growth factor and cytokine profile more than age [64]. In this study, substantial variability in PRP composition was found within groups of male and female subjects stratified by age ("young" group aged 18–30 years, "older" group aged 45–60 years). Nevertheless, PRP from male patients consistently contained significantly higher levels of growth factors and cytokines than PRP from female patients (TGF-β1, basic fibroblast growth factor, IL-1β, interleukin 1 receptor antagonist protein, TNF-α). Variation due to age was detected only in significantly lower IGF-1 levels in PRP from "older" versus "young" patients. Extrapolation of this data from healthy subjects to patients with musculoskeletal or spine disorders is difficult, as the latter group may have various medical co-morbidities or take medications that were excluded from this study. However, donor factors such as age and gender, and processing factors such as the time of day of platelet collection [65] are variables that are recognized to influence the growth factor and cytokine composition of PRP, in addition to other variables in PRP preparation previously discussed in this section.

Clinical Applications of PRP

Over 400 clinical trials of PRP are listed on ClinicalTrials.gov for various diseases and conditions [66]. In this section, we discuss clinical applications of PRP and the current level of evidence supporting its use for musculoskeletal and spine disorders.

Tendinopathy

Tendon injuries are common in both active and more sedentary people and may occur acutely or secondary to overuse [67]. Acute injuries are classified as tendinitis during the active, acute inflammation phase and tendinosis during the chronic, non-healing phase, characterized by a lack of inflammatory cells on histology in addition to evidence of aberrant tissue repair and thickening, collagen degeneration, and neovascularization [68]. Tendinopathy is a general term for tendon disorders, and chronic tendinopathy for conditions that remain refractory to conventional treatment. Sustained or repetitive injury over time may lead to chronic pathology, disability, and loss of function. Chronic tendinopathy is postulated to be a quiescent state along the spectrum of tendon pathology, an abnormal healing response or stage of stasis, in contrast to the inflammation and inflammatory cell infiltration present in early tendinopathy [69].

In this setting, the goal of biologic agents in the treatment of chronic tendinopathy is to restore or restart the healing process within the local tissue environment, rather than decreasing inflammation in more acute or subacute injuries. In laboratory and preclinical studies, PRP enhanced ECM synthesis of tenocytes and tendon explants in vitro [45, 70, 71] and promoted patellar tendon repair in a rat model [72].

Applications of PRP for chronic tendinopathy has been investigated in multiple clinical studies. The most current evidence from a systematic review and meta-analysis of 18 randomized controlled trials (RCTs) of PRP for treatment of tendinopathy supported the use of a single injection of LR-PRP using a peppering technique intratendinously under ultrasound guidance [48]. Here we discuss specific findings of PRP for lateral epicondylar (common extensor), patellar, and Achilles tendinopathy, although the clinical use of PRP applies to rotator cuff, gluteus medius, hamstring, and other sites of tendinopathy as well.

A RCT of 100 patients with chronic lateral epicondylar tendinopathy compared PRP with corticosteroid injection, which demonstrated a significant improvement in pain and function after follow-up out to 2 years [73, 74]. Krogh et al. recruited

60 patients with chronic lateral epicondylar tendinopathy for a RCT comparing treatment by PRP, saline, or glucocorticoid injections and found no difference in pain reduction at their primary end point of 3 months [75]. A double-blind RCT of 230 patients with chronic lateral epicondylar tendinopathy, treated by dry needling with or without leukocyte-rich PRP, yielded significant improvement in elbow tenderness and pain at 24 weeks post-intervention for the PRP treatment group [76]. Most recently, a systematic review of RCTs compared clinical outcomes of PRP, autologous blood, and corticosteroid injections for lateral epicondylar tendinopathy [77]. A network meta-analysis of 10 eligible studies out of 374 identified RCTs concluded that both PRP and autologous blood injections improved pain compared to corticosteroid, but autologous blood injections had a higher risk of complications than PRP.

LR-PRP treatment for patellar tendinopathy was studied in a double-blind RCT of 23 patients and was compared to dry needling alone [78]. Both groups underwent a standardized eccentric exercise program in addition to the intervention. Subjects that received PRP demonstrated greater clinical improvement at 12 weeks post-intervention, but this early improvement did not persist, as no significant difference was found between groups after 26 weeks. In contrast, in a RCT of 46 athletes with patellar tendinopathy, where subjects were randomized to two PRP injections over 2 weeks or 3 sessions of focused extracorporeal shockwave therapy, subjects who received PRP injections demonstrated improved pain and function at later time points of 6- and 12-month follow-up [79]. The most recent evidence from a systematic review and meta-analysis of studies of nonoperative management for patellar tendinopathy (PRP, extracorporeal shockwave therapy, eccentric exercise) suggests that multiple PRP injections (≥ 2) offer more satisfactory results in terms of pain and function at follow-up ≥ 6 months [80].

However, there was no difference in pain or activity level out to 24 weeks in a double-blind RCT of 54 patients with chronic Achilles tendinopathy randomized to PRP or a saline placebo treatment, followed by an eccentric exercise program [81]. More recently, a RCT of 24 patients with chronic Achilles tendinopathy treated with PRP or saline injections did not report any improvement in pain or function at 3 months, and the study itself was limited by large dropout rate [82]. Overall, the most recent data suggest that PRP is less effective for Achilles tendinopathy than other sites. Two separate meta-analyses of PRP versus placebo (saline) injection [83] and of autologous blood-derived products [84] including PRP compared to placebo (sham injection, no injection, or PT alone) reported that PRP injections were not more effective than placebo for Achilles tendinopathy.

Table 5.3 summarizes the results of selected clinical trials of PRP for chronic tendinopathy. Although the findings are promising and generally supportive of PRP for treatment of chronic tendinopathy, inconsistencies and variation in outcomes from these studies reflect variation in PRP preparation methods, choice of control intervention, post-intervention rehabilitation protocols, and anatomic sites of pathology.

Table 5.3 Select clinical trials of PRP for lateral epicondylar, patellar, and Achilles tendinopathy (Level I evidence only)

Site of tendinopathy	Study purpose[a]	Year of publication	Sample size	Follow-up	PRP system and reported composition[b]	Injection technique	Post-procedure rehabilitation protocol[a]	Conclusions
Lateral epicondylar	LR-PRP vs. CS injections [73, 74]	2010, 2011	100 PRP: 51 CS: 49	1 [73] and 2 years [74]	Biomet Recover 3 mL LR-PRP No activation	Needling	24 h–2 weeks: Standardized stretching protocol under PT supervision	PRP significantly reduces pain and increases function out to 2-year follow-up
							2–4 weeks: Formal eccentric muscle- and tendon-strengthening	
							4 weeks: Return to activity as tolerated	
	PRP vs. CS vs. saline injections [75]	2013	60 PRP: 20 CS: 20	3 months	Biomet Recover GPS II 3–3.5 mL PRP 8× platelets	Needling Ultrasound guidance	3–4 days: Standard tennis elbow stretching and training program prescribed	No difference among PRP, CS, and saline in pain reduction at 3 months
Patellar	2 PRP injections over 2 weeks vs. 3 ESWT sessions at 48–72-h intervals [79]	2013	46 PRP: 23 ESWT: 23	12 months	MyCells 2 mL PRP $0.89–1.1 \times 10^9$ platelets/mL 3–5× platelets No activation	PRP injections with needling Ultrasound guidance	1–2 weeks: Standardized stretching and strengthening protocol	PRP injections lead to significant improvement in symptoms and pain at 12-month follow-up
							2 weeks: Water activities as tolerated	
							4 weeks: Return to previous training activity as tolerated	

(continued)

X. (J.) Yuan and A. C. Gellhorn

Table 5.3 (continued)

Site of tendinopathy	Study purpose[a]	Year of publication	Sample size	Follow-up	PRP system and reported composition[b]	Injection technique	Post-procedure rehabilitation protocol[a]	Conclusions
	LR-PRP with needling vs. dry needling [78]	2014	23 PRP: 10 Dry needling: 13	≥26 weeks	Biomet GPS III 6 mL LR-PRP	Needling Ultrasound guidance	5-phase program of eccentric exercises, supervised by PT	Ultrasound-guided LR-PRP injections with needling and standardized eccentric exercise accelerated early recovery and symptom improvement at 12 weeks, but the apparent benefit of PRP dissipated by ≥26 weeks
							Patients assessed by PT to determine appropriate starting phase	
Achilles	PRP vs. saline injections [85, 86]	2010, 2011	54 PRP: 27 Saline: 27	24 [85] and 52 [86] weeks	Biomet Recover 4 mL PRP No activation	Needling Ultrasound guidance	First 48 h: Walk short distances indoors	No difference between PRP and saline injections in pain and activity level at 24- or 52-week follow-up
							Day 3–7: Up to 30 min walks	
							1–2 weeks: Stretching exercises	
							2–14 weeks: Daily eccentric exercise program	
							4 weeks: Gradual return to sports activities	

| PRP vs. saline injections [82] | 2016 | 24 PRP: 12 Saline: 12 | 3 months | Biomet Recover GPS II 6 mL PRP 8× platelets | Needling Ultrasound guidance | First 4 days: Minimize strain Day 5: Home therapy rehabilitation protocol including strengthening, eccentric training, stretching, coordination | PRP injections did not improve pain and function at 3-month follow-up |

[a]$CaCl_2$ calcium chloride, *CS* corticosteroid, *LR-PRP* leukocyte-rich PRP, *PT* physical therapy

[b]Biomet GPS III: Biomet GPS III (Gravitational Platelet Separation) System (Biomet Inc., Warsaw, IN, USA); Biomet Recover GPS II: Recover GPS II (Gravitational Platelet Separation) System (Biomet Inc.); Biomet Recover: Recover Platelet Separation Kit (Biomet Inc.); MyCells: MyCells Autologous Platelet Preparation System (Kaylight Ltd., Ramat-Hasharon, IL)

Osteoarthritis

Osteoarthritis (OA) is a leading cause of pain and disability in adults and is multi-factorial in etiology. However, to date, there remain no disease-modifying therapies for OA that can reverse or prevent the structural changes found in later stages of disease. Laboratory studies have observed that PRP enhances chondrogenic differentiation of mesenchymal stem cells, proliferation, and ECM synthesis, leading to multiple clinical trials to assess the utility of PRP for treatment of OA, most notably of the knee and hip [87].

A systematic review of PRP injections for knee OA yielded three meta-analyses that met criteria, which compared outcomes of intra-articular PRP versus control hyaluronic acid or placebo injections [88]. Campbell et al. reported that PRP treatment led to clinically relevant improvements in symptom relief and function as early as 2 months, peaking at 6 months, and persisting up to 12 months post-intervention. They note variation in protocol, including number (1–4) of and timing (1–3 weeks) between PRP injections, PRP volume injected, one- versus two-step centrifugation, and platelet activation, as well as variation in patient profile including age, duration of pain, and severity of OA. Their findings also suggested that PRP is more effective for patients with only evidence of early radiographic evidence of OA or lower Kellgren-Lawrence grade. They were unable to determine if multiple PRP injections were helpful, although multiple injections may increase the risk of local adverse reactions. The variability across the three meta-analyses precluded conclusions regarding other protocol parameters. They did conclude that higher-quality RCTs were necessary to persuade insurance providers to provide coverage for PRP for knee OA. Most recently, a meta-analysis of RCTs reported that intra-articular PRP injection provides more pain relief and functional improvement in patients with symptomatic knee OA at 1-year follow-up compared to HA and saline [89].

While OA is traditionally described as a non-inflammatory arthritis, characterized by cartilage degeneration, it is now understood that OA affects all tissues within the joint and that inflammation plays a central role in both the onset and progression of disease. There has been much speculation that the role of PRP for clinical treatment of OA lies more in its anti-inflammatory and immunomodulatory effects for pain rather than its regenerative properties [52, 90]. In vitro studies have demonstrated that growth factors present in PRP can function in an anti-inflammatory role via the lipoxin LXA_4 [9], which acts to resolve inflammatory processes, and that PRP modulates IL-1 production by macrophages [91].

Therefore, LP-PRP has been the preferred formulation for treatment of OA, given the concern for pro-inflammatory effects of neutrophils in LR-PRP preparations. Laboratory studies have demonstrated that LP-PRP decreased catabolism and increased tissue synthesis by chondrocytes [92]. A correlation was found between increasing leukocyte concentration and elevated inflammatory cytokines (IL-1β, TNF-α, IL-6, IL-8) [93]. Synoviocytes exhibited significant cell death and pro-inflammatory response with LR-PRP treatment, further supporting recommendations of LP-PRP preparations for intra-articular applications [47].

To this end, a meta-analysis of 6 RCTs and 3 prospective studies, totaling 1055 patients, compared outcomes and adverse effects of LP- and LR-PRP against control hyaluronic acid (HA) or placebo injections for knee OA [94]. Riboh et al. detected a small improvement in functional outcome scores in favor of LP-PRP versus LR-PRP compared with HA and placebo and did not detect any significant difference in safety profile between the two PRP formulations. Both LR- and LP-PRP were associated with a higher incidence of transient reactions such as local swelling and pain compared to HA. They again noted low-quality evidence due to variation in PRP preparation methods, even among LP- and LR-PRP formulations, and variation in severity of OA between treatment groups. Moreover, the analyzed studies skewed toward younger patients with milder OA.

Few studies have been published of PRP for hip OA, and two level I studies did not demonstrate long-term benefits of PRP versus HA at 1 year [95, 96]. A meta-analysis reported that patients with hip OA treated with PRP had improvements in pain and function at 2 months, but these changes were not sustainable, as there was no difference versus HA control at 6 and 12 months [97].

Table 5.4 lists the findings of selected clinical trials of PRP for OA. Overall, for knee OA, evidence suggests that LP-PRP improves pain and provides symptom relief for upward of 1 year following intervention. Selection of candidates with earlier stages of knee OA may prove more efficacious. In contrast, studies have not demonstrated a benefit of PRP over HA in treatment of symptomatic hip OA.

Ligament and Meniscus Injuries

PRP has been studied for treatment of ligament injuries, primarily in the context of enhancing surgical outcomes of anterior cruciate ligament (ACL) reconstruction, which is outside the scope of the nonoperative applications discussed in this chapter. In vitro studies have shown that PRP enhanced ACL cell viability and collagen production [104]. Overall, there is promising evidence that PRP can improve outcomes for ACL reconstruction [105, 106]. In addition, the ongoing Bridge-Enhanced ACL Repair (BEAR) Trial led by Murray et al. is investigating biologic augmentation of surgical ACL repair by PRP [107, 108].

Scant literature exists on the nonoperative treatment of ligament injuries by PRP. Laboratory studies have demonstrated that PRP stimulated DNA and collagen synthesis in human periodontal ligament cells [109, 110], and increased gene expression and synthesis of ECM proteins in equine suspensory ligament cells [45, 111]. Preclinical animal studies have utilized PRP to augment healing of medial collateral ligament (MCL) ruptures in a rabbit model and demonstrated greater mechanical strength of MCLs treated with PRP [112].

Case reports and series have been published for partial tears of the ulnar collateral ligament of the elbow in throwing athletes, suggesting a shorter return to play (RTP) following treatment with PRP [113, 114]. A small RCT of sixteen elite athletes with high ankle sprains (anterior inferior tibiofibular ligament tears) and

Table 5.4 Select clinical trials of PRP for osteoarthritis (OA) of the knee and hip (Level I evidence only)

Site of OA	Study purpose[a]	Year of publication	Sample size	Kellgren-Lawrence grade	Follow-up	PRP system and reported composition[b]	Injection technique	Conclusions
Knee	Series of 3 weekly injections: PRP vs. HA [98, 99]	2015, 2019	192 PRP: 96 HA: 96	0–3	12 months [98], 24 months [99]	Hematology protocol with two spins 5 mL PRP $1.1 \pm 0.5\times$ WBCs $4.6 \pm 1.4\times$ platelets $CaCl_2$ activation	Intra-articular	Both PRP and HA were effective in improving symptoms and function over 24-month follow-up with no significant differences
	Series of 3 weekly injections: LP-PRP vs. saline [100]	2016	30 LP-PRP: 15 Saline: 15	2–3	1 year	Arthrex ACP 4–7.1 mL LP-PRP	Lateral parapatellar approach	LP-PRP provides pain relief and functional improvement out to 1-year follow-up
	Series of 3 weekly injections: LP-PRP vs. HA [101]	2017	99 PRP: 49 HA: 50	1–4	1 year	Arthrex ACP 4 mL LP-PRP 790 ± 0.11 WBCs/mL $1.73 \pm 0.05\times$ platelets	Intra-articular Ultrasound guidance	No difference between PRP and HA in pain, but significant improvement in function for PRP, out to 1-year follow-up
	2 PRP 1 month apart vs. 1 HA vs. 4 ozone gas injections in 1 week [102]	2017	102 patients PRP: 41 HA: 40 Ozone: 39	2–3	12 months	Ycellbio 5 mL PRP 9–13× platelets $\geq 1.5 \times 10^6/\mu L$ platelets No RBCs No activation	Intra-articular	PRP was superior to HA and ozone injections for improvement in pain and function out to 12-month follow-up

Series of 3 weekly injections: 3 PRP vs. 1 PRP and 2 saline vs. 3 HA vs. 3 saline [103]	2017	162 patients 3 PRP: 46 1 PRP: 45 3 HA: 46 Saline: 45	Early (1–3) vs. advanced (4)	6 months	Hematology protocol with 2 spins 5 mL PRP 5.2–5.3× platelets 1.1–1.2 × 10^6/ μL platelets $CaCl_2$ activation	Superolateral approach	Multiple (3) PRP injections achieve better clinical results for early OA, but no difference among injections in patients with advanced OA
Hip							
Series of 3 biweekly injections: PRP vs. HA [96]	2013	100	2–4	12 months	Hematology protocol with 2 spins 5 mL PRP 6× platelets 6–8 × 10^6/mL platelets 8300 WBCs/μL No RBCs $CaCl_2$ activation	Ultrasound guidance	Pain and function improvement detected in both groups with no significant differences between PRP and HA out to 12-month follow-up
Series of 3 weekly injections: LP-PRP vs. HA [95]	2016	43 PRP: 21 HA: 22	2–3	16 weeks	Regen 3 mL LP-PRP 1–1.5× platelets	Ultrasound guidance	PRP provided immediate improvement in pain that was not maintained at 16-week follow-up

[a] $CaCl_2$ calcium chloride, *HA* hyaluronic acid, *LP-PRP* leukocyte-poor PRP

[b] Arthrex ACP (Autologous Conditioned Plasma) Double Syringe System (Arthrex Inc., Naples, FL, USA); Regen: RegenPRP-Kit (RegenLab SA, Mollens, CH)

dynamic syndesmosis instability randomized patients to receive ultrasound-guided PRP injections with rehabilitation versus rehabilitation only [115]. Subjects from both groups followed an identical rehabilitation protocol. In this small study, the PRP group demonstrated shorter RTP, syndesmosis re-stabilization, and decreased residual pain over time. However, further studies with higher levels of evidence are necessary to support the use of PRP for ligament injuries.

PRP has also been studied as a means to augment healing of meniscal tears in the avascular zone, which intrinsically do not heal and are typically surgically resected. Over time, loss of even a portion of the meniscus through arthroscopic partial meniscectomy predisposes to development of post-traumatic OA. To this end, preclinical and clinical studies have investigated the utility of PRP for meniscal repair and regeneration and for augmentation of surgical repair outcomes. In vitro, PRP increased rabbit meniscal cell proliferation and ECM synthesis compared to platelet-poor plasma (PRP) [116]. In vivo, PRP combined with gelatin hydrogel was implanted into meniscal defects in the avascular zone using a rabbit model. Compared to hydrogel without PRP, defects treated with PRP demonstrated greater cell numbers and ECM production, suggesting PRP can enhance the healing potential of the avascular zone of the meniscus.

In a case-control study of 34 patients undergoing open meniscal repair, the group that received PRP to augment repair demonstrated slight improvement at 1 year post-operatively [117]. In a separate study of surgeons performing 35 arthroscopic meniscus repairs with or without PRP augmentation, the addition of PRP was not found to influence reoperation rate [118]. To date, there have not been studies with higher levels of evidence published on the efficacy of PRP to guide nonoperative management of meniscal tears of traumatic or degenerative etiologies, although PRP is utilized for these applications in clinical practice. Therapeutic effects observed from PRP for degenerative meniscal tears in the setting of associated OA may result indirectly from treatment of the OA rather than the meniscal pathology itself.

Muscle Injuries

There is scant literature published on the use of PRP for muscle injuries. Hammond et al. completed a laboratory study using a rat model of an acute tibialis anterior muscle strain injury, treated with PRP, PPP, or no injection [119]. They demonstrated that PRP decreased recovery time in a small animal model and postulated that this was secondary to induction of myogenesis by growth factors present in PRP. A statistically significant decrease in recovery time was also reported in a RCT of 28 patients with acute hamstring injuries who were allocated to PRP with rehabilitation (26.7 ± 7.0 days) versus rehabilitation alone (42.5 ± 20.6 days), although there was substantial variance in the results [120]. In a double-blind, placebo-controlled RCT of 80 athletes with acute hamstring injuries, subjects were allocated to PRP or placebo saline injections, but did not demonstrate benefit of PRP in return to play or reinjury rate [121]. The most current meta-analysis of PRP for acute muscle injuries concluded with limited evidence that PRP may allow earlier return to play for patients with acute grade I or II muscle strains without a significant increase in risk of reinjury out to 6 months of follow-up [122].

Follow-up laboratory studies have suggested that depletion of platelets is more favorable for myocytes. Mazzocca et al. reported that a one-spin PRP protocol yielding lower platelet concentration increased myocyte proliferation [123]. Miroshnychenko et al. studied the effects of various PRP formulations on in vitro myogenic differentiation [124], and found that LR-PRP led to myoblast proliferation, but PPP and LR-PRP subjected to a second spin to remove platelets induced myoblast differentiation. It is clear that further clinical studies with higher levels of evidence must be performed, and may require consideration of tailoring PRP formulations specifically for treatment of muscle injuries.

Spine Disorders

Low back pain is among the most common outpatient complaints. Consequently, there is particular interest in PRP for treatment of disorders associated with low back pain, such as intervertebral disc (IVD) degeneration and facet joint osteoarthritis. In vitro laboratory studies have demonstrated that PRP stimulates proliferation and matrix synthesis by cells from both the nucleus pulposus (NP) and annulus fibrosus (AF) [125, 126]. PRP has also been shown to exhibit anti-inflammatory effects on NP cells exposed to pro-inflammatory cues [127]. A preclinical study utilized a rabbit model of IVD degeneration [128], injecting PRP in gelatin hydrogel microspheres into the NP, and comparing outcomes to control saline and sham groups. At 8 weeks, the authors noted suppression of degeneration with histologic evidence of ECM synthesis in animals injected with PRP. A follow-up study demonstrated greater IVD height on MRI and decreased apoptosis in the NP after PRP injection [129]. These findings were further verified in another rabbit study of IVD degeneration, comparing intradiscal PRP versus PPP injections [130].

In this setting, a few clinical studies of intradiscal PRP injections for low back pain have been performed with early but promising results. A prospective study of 22 patients who underwent intradiscal PRP injections (single-level to as many as five levels) demonstrated early improvement in pain and function out to 6 months [131]. A prospective, double-blind RCT of 47 patients with chronic discogenic low back pain received intradiscal PRP or contrast agent [132]. The 29 patients who received intradiscal PRP injections reported significant improvement in pain and function at 8 weeks through at least 2 years of follow-up [133].

Analogous to studies of PRP for OA at other anatomic sites, two studies on intra-articular PRP injections for lumbar facet joint syndrome were published by the same group of investigators. The first is a prospective study of 19 patients who received PRP injections, which demonstrated significant improvement in pain and function within a short-term study period of 3 months [134]. This group of investigators led by Wu et al. proceeded to a prospective RCT of 46 patients with lumbar facet joint syndrome, randomized to injections of PRP versus corticosteroid with local anesthetic (LA), with up to 6 months of follow-up [135]. Subjects who received corticosteroid/LA injections experienced initial improvement in pain and function, which decreased after 6 months. In contrast, subjects treated with PRP continued to experience improvement in pain and function out to 6 months.

For radicular pain, Centeno et al. has published the results of a case series of 470 patients who received lumbar epidural injections of platelet lysate, which consists of growth factors prepared by lysing platelets and removing cell debris [136]. Within the limitations of a case series, patients reported significant improvements in pain and function through 2 years of follow-up.

Although promising so far, more rigorous studies with higher levels of evidence must be performed to further investigate the utility of PRP for spine disorders.

Advantages of PRP

The primary advantage of PRP is the ability to offer more nonoperative treatment options for patients who have failed conventional treatment, who do not want surgery, or who are poor surgical candidates and for conditions with poor surgical outcomes, such as degenerative tendinopathies or meniscal tears.

Moreover, the autologous nature of PRP is thought to eliminate or at least minimize risk of immune rejection or disease transmission. Assuming sterility in preparation, the risk of contamination is low. Potential risks of PRP administration include adverse effects arising from the use of bovine thrombin used for platelet activation, which can rarely cause coagulopathy from antibody formation. Bovine thrombin is now avoided due to these risks, although earlier studies of PRP for non-musculoskeletal applications reported its use for platelet activation during oral and maxillofacial surgery [137–140] and wound care [29, 141–145].

Although there exists immense variation in PRP protocols, the procedure can be performed during the point of care in an office setting with access to phlebotomy services and a commercial PRP system. Although the cost of commercial PRP kits is not negligible, a standard hematology protocol for PRP preparation requires a little more than a centrifuge and basic laboratory supplies. This technology has been implemented in the global arena through the creation of a PRP injection program in Tanzania at the Bugando Medical Centre [146], via a collaboration with the local blood bank, providing proof of principle that access to PRP interventions can be achieved with minimal additional cost and resources.

Disadvantages of PRP

Disadvantages of PRP lie in the variability already well described in this chapter, including the lack of standardization in PRP preparation methods and reporting of PRP composition in literature, which limits comparisons between studies, coupled with the lack of one universally accepted classification scheme. High variability exists among patients, including donor factors such as age, gender, and comorbidities, and even among underlying patient conditions. Although clinical trials study PRP for specific pathologic conditions and utilize rigorous criteria for patient selection, there remains considerable heterogeneity among patients diagnosed with the same condition in terms of chronicity of symptoms and prior treatments such as oral medications, rehabilitation, and other injections. The durability of any intervention for musculoskeletal and spine disorders depends upon the quality of post-intervention rehabilitation and patient adherence to a home exercise program. Post-PRP rehabilitation protocols are not standardized for various conditions, and variability in therapy plays a significant role in the long-term outcomes of PRP intervention.

The success of a PRP intervention hinges on clinically significant improvement in standardized but subjective patient-reported outcomes of pain and function. The burden of proof for clinical efficacy of an intervention is all the more difficult to achieve when one considers that intra-articular saline placebo injections for knee OA have been reported to have both a statistically and clinically significant effect on pain and function out to 6-month follow-up [147]. Therefore, clinical investigators are now quantifying cytokine levels in the synovial fluid before and after PRP intervention for knee OA, in order to correlate clinical outcomes with the biological mechanisms of action of PRP [148].

Contraindications to PRP therapy include cancer (tumor or metastatic disease), active infections, thrombocytopenia, and pregnancy [149]. Growth factors such as isoforms of TGF-β and hepatocyte growth factor, found in PRP, have been associated with tumor growth [150], hence the relative contraindication in patients with cancer history. However, PRP has been utilized for patients with avascular necrosis of the mandible in cancer patients with a history of bisphosphonate use [151–153] and non-musculoskeletal applications in patients undergoing surgical tumor or complications related to active chemotherapy treatment [154, 155].

Finally, PRP therapy is not covered by insurances for the applications described in this chapter, which can pose a significant financial burden for patients. Wide variability in cost is present, to upward of $2000 or more per injection [2], based on many factors including the cost of the specific kit used for preparation and other local economic influences. The cost of PRP therapy is related to its off-label use for musculoskeletal and spine disorders, which do not have FDA approval.

Regulation of PRP

The clinical applications of PRP for musculoskeletal and spine disorders discussed in this chapter are considered off-label. PRP is a biologic and falls under the regulation of the FDA Center for Biologics Evaluation and Research (CBER). Under the Code of Federal Regulations (CFR) Title 21, PRP and other blood products are exempt from the FDA Regulation of Human Cells, Tissues, and Cellular and Tissue-based Products (HCT/Ps) [156]. Instead, the 510(k) application pathway has been used for clearance of PRP preparation systems that are considered "substantially equivalent" to other existing or predicate devices already available on the market. The first PRP preparation systems were reviewed by the Office of In Vitro Diagnostics and Radiological Health, received 510(k) clearance based upon predicate centrifuge devices, and were therefore classified as centrifuges.

The 510(k) pathway for clearance of PRP devices does not strictly require clinical data for FDA approval, as they are considered lower-risk devices and "substantially equivalent" to a previously cleared device [157]. The term "clearance" designates the limitations of use of the device, only to the indications of the predicate device that it has been determined to be "substantially equivalent." This is in contrast to other regenerative therapies, which may receive "approval" through traditional FDA regulatory pathways as new drugs via new drug applications (NDA) or biologics license applications (BLA), which further require clinical data collected via investigational new drug (IND) or investigational device exemption (IDE) applications.

As early as February 2011, CBER granted 510(k) clearance to devices for mixing PRP with bone graft to improve its handling, for application to bony defects in the operative setting ("Platelet And Plasma Separator For Bone Graft Handling") [158]. Injection or implantation of PRP without mixing with bone graft materials falls outside the intended use of these PRP systems and is considered off-label use. However, a clinician may still practice off-label use of PRP for musculoskeletal and spine disorders but may not market the use of the device for these off-label applications. CBER does not require an IND or IDE application to the FDA or institutional review board (IRB) approval for off-label use [159].

In 2007, the AutoloGel™ System (Cytomedix Inc., Gaithersburg, MD) received 510(k) clearance for topical application in the management of cutaneous wounds including chronic nonhealing diabetic, pressure, or venous wounds. Mixing PRP with bone graft for defects and topical application for chronic wounds remain the sole indications of use for PRP that have received FDA approval, although these treatments are considered experimental by insurance providers including the Centers for Medicare and Medicaid Services (CMS), with limited to no coverage at this time [160].

While PRP is not subject to FDA regulation of HCT/Ps under CFR Title 21, Part 1271, further activation of PRP by exogenous agents following centrifugation alone creates a potentially tricky situation in which PRP may be considered more than "minimally manipulated" and therefore subject to further regulation. Although no changes have yet occurred that impact off-label use of PRP, clinicians should remain up-to-date with the latest FDA regulatory stance on PRP.

Future Directions

Since its inception in the early 2000s, PRP therapy has rapidly entered the mainstream for applications as diverse as musculoskeletal and spine disorders to alopecia and aesthetics. The lack of conclusive scientific evidence of clinical efficacy, FDA approval, and insurance coverage has not significantly hindered the popularity of PRP therapy or patient interest.

Regulatory approval and insurance coverage decisions depend upon demonstrating higher-level supportive evidence of both safety and clinical efficacy of PRP therapy. This in turn requires a decrease in the variability found in prior PRP studies, which can be achieved in part by adoption of one universally accepted PRP classification scheme, and standardization in preparation methods, characterization, and reporting of PRP composition across clinical trials. Delivery of PRP must also be standardized, such as number and timing of injections and concurrently performed interventions such as percutaneous tenotomy, as well as post-procedural care with pathology-specific rehabilitation protocols. FDA approval for additional indications of PRP therapy requires a BLA or premarket approval (PMA) application, which involves larger-scale clinical studies that should be designed with close consideration of these variables in mind.

Although clinicians and patients have found success with PRP for the musculoskeletal and spine disorders described in this chapter, there remains a limited understanding of the precise pathophysiology that underlie these diseases. Without this knowledge, it is difficult to determine the precise targets of PRP therapy for each disease process and what relevant characteristics in PRP impact clinical response in patients. While current evidence suggests that LR-PRP is more suitable for tendinopathy and LP-PRP for OA, future work must continue to probe and define the growth factors and cytokine cocktails that are ideal for specific pathologies and develop novel methods of PRP preparation that yield these customized formulations.

Efforts are already underway in recently published studies of PRP for OA [148], in which investigators are measuring cytokine levels in synovial fluid to better understand the local effects of PRP, further refine its mechanism of action, and identify and validate biomarkers of disease. Since PRP is believed to improve pain and function for patients with OA through anti-inflammatory effects, the goal will be to demonstrate that decreasing inflammation will in turn slow progression of OA and ultimately, that PRP is a disease-modifying therapy for early-stage OA.

Although PRP is considered a regenerative therapy, based largely upon the effects of growth factors on cells and tissues in laboratory studies, convincing evidence of tissue regeneration has yet to be demonstrated in clinical studies. Demonstration of tissue regeneration is limited in part because clinical study results typically report standardized patient-reported outcomes without biological correlates or biomarkers that can support the potential efficacy of the intervention. Incorporation of OA biomarkers developed and validated for pain and disease progression [161] allows for a more objective measurement of pain improvement due to PRP and potential disease-modifying properties.

In summary, PRP is a promising therapy that offers a nonsurgical approach to treatment of musculoskeletal and spine disorders, for patients who have failed conventional therapy or with conditions that have poor surgical outcomes. However, there remains much to elucidate in the basic science and underlying mechanism of action of PRP, in order to accelerate regulatory approval and insurance coverage and expand access to PRP treatment for patients of all socioeconomic background. In the future, PRP therapy will require a personalized approach, tailoring PRP formulations for both patient-specific and condition-specific characteristics.

References

1. Marx RE. Platelet-rich plasma (PRP): what is PRP and what is not PRP? Implant Dent. 2001;10:225–8.
2. Schwarz A. A promising treatment for athletes, in blood. New York Times. 2009.
3. McCarrel TM, Mall NA, Lee AS, Cole BJ, Butty DC, Fortier LA. Considerations for the use of platelet-rich plasma in orthopedics. Sports Med. 2014;44:1025–36.
4. Harrison P, Cramer EM. Platelet alpha-granules. Blood Rev. 1993;7:52–62.
5. Leeksma CHW, Cohen JA. Determination of the life span of human blood platelets using labelled diisopropylfluorophosphonate. J Clin Invest. 1956;35:964–9.
6. Mason KD, Carpinelli MR, Fletcher JI, et al. Programmed anuclear cell death delimits platelet life span. Cell. 2007;128:1173–86.
7. Lee KS, Wilson JJ, Rabago DP, Baer GS, Jacobson JA, Borrero CG. Musculoskeletal applications of platelet-rich plasma: fad or future? Am J Roentgenol. 2011;196:628–36.
8. Coppinger JA, Cagney G, Toomey S, Kislinger T, Belton O, McRedmond JP, Cahill DJ, Emili A, Fitzgerald DJ, Maguire PB. Characterization of the proteins released from activated platelets leads to localization of novel platelet proteins in human atherosclerotic lesions. Blood. 2004;103:2096–104.
9. El-Sharkawy H, Kantarci A, Deady J, Hasturk H, Liu H, Alshahat M, Van Dyke TE. Platelet-rich plasma: growth factors and pro- and anti-inflammatory properties. J Periodontol. 2007;78:661–9.
10. Akeda K, An HS, Okuma M, Attawia M, Miyamoto K, Thonar EJ-MA, Lenz ME, Sah RL, Masuda K. Platelet-rich plasma stimulates porcine articular chondrocyte proliferation and matrix biosynthesis. Osteoarthr Cartil. 2006;14:1272–80.
11. Vogel JP, Szalay K, Geiger F, Kramer M, Richter W, Kasten P. Platelet-rich plasma improves expansion of human mesenchymal stem cells and retains differentiation capacity and in vivo bone formation in calcium phosphate ceramics. Platelets. 2006;17:462–9.
12. Liu Y, Kalén A, Risto O, Wahlström O. Fibroblast proliferation due to exposure to a platelet concentrate in vitro is pH dependent. Wound Repair Regen. 2002;10:336–40.
13. Heldin CH, Westermark B. Mechanism of action and in vivo role of platelet-derived growth factor. Physiol Rev. 1999;79:1283–316.
14. LaPrade RF, Geeslin AG, Murray IR, Musahl V, Zlotnicki JP, Petrigliano F, Mann BJ. Biologic treatments for sports injuries II think tank – current concepts, future research, and barriers to advancement, part 1. Am J Sports Med. 2016;44:3270–83.
15. Scholz A, Plate KH, Reiss Y. Angiopoietin-2: a multifaceted cytokine that functions in both angiogenesis and inflammation. Ann N Y Acad Sci. 2015;1347:45–51.
16. Tanoue H, Morinaga J, Yoshizawa T, et al. Angiopoietin-like protein 2 promotes chondrogenic differentiation during bone growth as a cartilage matrix factor. Osteoarthr Cartil. 2018;26:108–17.
17. Yang X, Chen Z, Meng X, Sun C, Li M, Shu L, Fan D, Fan T, Huang AY, Zhang C. Angiopoietin-2 promotes osteogenic differentiation of thoracic ligamentum flavum cells via modulating the Notch signaling pathway. PLoS One. 2018;13:e0209300.
18. Fréchette J, Martineau I, Gagnon G. Platelet-rich plasmas: growth factor content and roles in wound healing. J Dent Res. 2005;84(5):434–9.
19. Tamama K, Fan VH, Griffith LG, Blair HC, Wells A. Epidermal growth factor as a candidate for ex vivo expansion of bone marrow-derived mesenchymal stem cells. Stem Cells. 2006;24:686–95.

20. Sibilia M, Wagner B, Hoebertz A, Elliott C, Marino S, Jochum W, Wagner EF. Mice humanised for the EGF receptor display hypomorphic phenotypes in skin, bone and heart. Development. 2003;130:4515–25.

21. Mazzucco L, Balbo V, Cattana E, Guaschino R, Borzini P. Not every PRP-gel is born equal. Evaluation of growth factor availability for tissues through four PRP-gel preparations: Fibrinet, RegenPRP-Kit, Plateltex and one manual procedure. Vox Sang. 2009;97:110–8.

22. Eppley BL, Woodell JE, Ph D, Higgins J. Experimental platelet quantification and growth factor analysis from platelet-rich plasma: implications for wound healing. Plast Reconstructive Surg. 2003;114(6):1502–8.

23. Mazzocca AD, McCarthy MB, Chowaniec DM, Cote MP, Romeo AA, Bradley JP, Arciero RA, Beitzel K. Platelet-rich plasma differs according to preparation method and human variability. JBJS. 2012;94:308–16.

24. Hutley L, Shurety W, Newell F, McGeary R, Pelton N, Grant J, Herington A, Cameron D, Whitehead J, Prins J. Fibroblast growth factor 1: a key regulator of human adipogenesis. Diabetes. 2004;53:3097–106.

25. Javerzat S, Auguste P, Bikfalvi A. The role of fibroblast growth factors in vascular development. Trends Mol Med. 2002;8:483–9.

26. Nomi M, Miyake H, Sugita Y, Fujisawa M, Soker S. Role of growth factors and endothelial cells in therapeutic angiogenesis and tissue engineering. Curr Stem Cell Res Ther. 2006;1:333–43.

27. Haider HK, Jiang S, Idris NM, Ashraf M. IGF-1-overexpressing mesenchymal stem cells accelerate bone marrow stem cell mobilization via paracrine activation of SDF-1alpha/CXCR4 signaling to promote myocardial repair. Circ Res. 2008;103:1300–8.

28. Longobardi L, O'Rear L, Aakula S, Johnstone B, Shimer K, Chytil A, Horton WA, Moses HL, Spagnoli A. Effect of IGF-I in the chondrogenesis of bone marrow mesenchymal stem cells in the presence or absence of TGF-beta signaling. J Bone Miner Res. 2006;21:626–36.

29. Everts PAM, Devilee RJJ, Brown Mahoney C, Eeftinck-Schattenkerk M, Box HAM, Knape JTA, van Zundert A. Platelet gel and fibrin sealant reduce allogeneic blood transfusions in total knee arthroplasty. Acta Anaesthesiol Scand. 2006;50:593–9.

30. Weibrich G, Kleis WKG, Hafner G, Hitzler WE. Growth factor levels in platelet-rich plasma and correlations with donor age, sex, and platelet count. J Craniomaxillofac Surg. 2002;30:97–102.

31. Sumanasinghe RD, Pfeiler TW, Monteiro-Riviere NA, Loboa EG. Expression of proinflammatory cytokines by human mesenchymal stem cells in response to cyclic tensile strain. J Cell Physiol. 2009;219:77–83.

32. Sundman EA, Cole BJ, Fortier LA. Growth factor and catabolic cytokine concentrations are influenced by the cellular composition of platelet-rich plasma. Am J Sports Med. 2011;39:2135–40.

33. Gothard D, Smith E, Kanczler J, Rashidi H, Qutachi O, Henstock J, Rotherham M, El Haj A, Shakesheff K, Oreffo R. Tissue engineered bone using select growth factors: a comprehensive review of animal studies and clinical translation studies in man. Eur Cell Mater. 2014;28:166–208.

34. Tokunaga A, Oya T, Ishii Y, et al. PDGF receptor beta is a potent regulator of mesenchymal stromal cell function. J Bone Miner Res. 2008;23:1519–28.

35. Ng F, Boucher S, Koh S, et al. PDGF, TGF-beta, and FGF signaling is important for differentiation and growth of mesenchymal stem cells (MSCs): transcriptional profiling can identify markers and signaling pathways important in differentiation of MSCs into adipogenic, chondrogenic, and osteogenic lineages. Blood. 2008;112:295–307.

36. Castillo TN, Pouliot MA, Kim HJ, Dragoo JL, Kim HJ, Dragoo JL. Comparison of growth factor and platelet concentration from commercial platelet-rich plasma separation systems. Am J Sports Med. 2011;39:266–71.

37. Marx RE. Platelet-rich plasma: evidence to support its use. J Oral Maxillofac Surg. 2004;62:489–96.

38. Paiva KBS, Granjeiro JM. Bone tissue remodeling and development: focus on matrix metalloproteinase functions. Arch Biochem Biophys. 2014;561:74–87.

39. Ogawa T, Akazawa T, Tabata Y. In vitro proliferation and chondrogenic differentiation of rat bone marrow stem cells cultured with gelatin hydrogel microspheres for TGF-beta1 release. J Biomater Sci Polym Ed. 2010;21:609–21.

40. Nöth U, Osyczka AM, Tuli R, Hickok NJ, Danielson KG, Tuan RS. Multilineage mesenchymal differentiation potential of human trabecular bone-derived cells. J Orthop Res. 2002;20:1060–9.

41. Joyce ME, Jingushi S, Bolander ME. Transforming growth factor-beta in the regulation of fracture repair. Orthop Clin North Am. 1990;21:199–209.

42. Grosskreutz CL, Anand-Apte B, Dupláa C, Quinn TP, Terman BI, Zetter B, D'Amore PA. Vascular endothelial growth factor-induced migration of vascular smooth muscle cells in vitro. Microvasc Res. 1999;58:128–36.

43. Anitua E, Sánchez M, Nurden AT, Zalduendo MM, De la Fuente M, Azofra J, Andía I. Platelet-released growth factors enhance the secretion of hyaluronic acid and induce hepatocyte growth factor production by synovial fibroblasts from arthritic patients. Rheumatology. 2007;46:1769–72.

44. Creaney L, Hamilton B. Growth factor delivery methods in the management of sports injuries: the state of play. Br J Sports Med. 2008;42:314–20.

45. McCarrel T, Fortier L. Temporal growth factor release from platelet-rich plasma, trehalose lyophilized platelets, and bone marrow aspirate and their effect on tendon and ligament gene expression. J Orthop Res. 2009;27:1033–42.

46. Leitner GC, Gruber R, Neumüller J, Wagner A, Kloimstein P, Höcker P, Körmöczi GF, Buchta C. Platelet content and growth factor release in platelet-rich plasma: a comparison of four different systems. Vox Sang. 2006;91:135–9.

47. Braun HJ, Kim HJ, Chu CR, Dragoo JL. The effect of platelet-rich plasma formulations and blood products on human synoviocytes. Am J Sports Med. 2014;42:1204–10.

48. Fitzpatrick J, Bulsara M, Zheng MH. The effectiveness of platelet-rich plasma in the treatment of tendinopathy. Am J Sports Med. 2017;45:226–33.

49. Zehnder JL, Leung LL. Development of antibodies to thrombin and factor V with recurrent bleeding in a patient exposed to topical bovine thrombin. Blood. 1990;76:2011–6.

50. Chahla J, Cinque ME, Piuzzi NS, Mannava S, Geeslin AG, Murray IR, Dornan GJ, Muschler GF, LaPrade RF. A call for standardization in platelet-rich plasma preparation protocols and composition reporting. JBJS. 2017;99:1769–79.

51. DeLong JM, Russell RP, Mazzocca AD. Platelet-rich plasma: the PAW classification system. Arthrosc J Arthrosc Relat Surg. 2012;28:998–1009.

52. Andia I, Maffulli N. Platelet-rich plasma for managing pain and inflammation in osteoarthritis. Nat Rev Rheumatol. 2013;9:721–30.

53. Redler LH, Thompson SA, Hsu SH, Ahmad CS, Levine WN. Platelet-rich plasma therapy: a systematic literature review and evidence for clinical use. Phys Sportsmed. 2011;39:42–51.

54. Lopez-Vidriero E, Goulding KA, Simon DA, Sanchez M, Johnson DH. The use of platelet-rich plasma in arthroscopy and sports medicine: optimizing the healing environment. Arthrosc J Arthrosc Relat Surg. 2010;26:269–78.

55. Engebretsen L, Steffen K, Alsousou J, et al. IOC consensus paper on the use of platelet-rich plasma in sports medicine. Br J Sports Med. 2010;44:1072–81.

56. Ehrenfest DM, Rasmusson L, Albrektsson T. Classification of platelet concentrates: from pure platelet-rich plasma (P-PRP) to leucocyte- and platelet-rich fibrin (L-PRF). Trends Biotechnol. 2009;27:158–67.

57. Mishra A, Harmon K, Woodall J, Vieira A. Sports medicine applications of platelet rich plasma. Curr Pharm Biotechnol. 2012;13:1185–95.

58. Mautner K, Malanga GA, Smith J, Shiple B, Ibrahim V, Sampson S, Bowen JE. A call for a standard classification system for future biologic research: the rationale for new PRP nomenclature. PM R. 2015;7:S53–9.

59. Magalon J, Chateau AL, Bertrand B, Louis ML, Silvestre A, Giraudo L, Veran J, Sabatier F. DEPA classification: a proposal for standardising PRP use and a retrospective application of available devices. BMJ Open Sport Exerc Med. 2016;2:e000060.

60. Lana JF, Purita J, Paulus C, et al. Contributions for classification of platelet rich plasma – proposal of a new classification: MARSPILL. Regen Med. 2017;12:565–74.
61. Mooren RE, Hendriks EJ, van den Beucken JJ, Merkx MA, Meijer GJ, Jansen JA, Stoelinga PJW. The effect of platelet-rich plasma in vitro on primary cells: rat osteoblast-like cells and human endothelial cells. Tissue Eng Part A. 2010;16:3159–72.
62. Giusti I, Rughetti A, D'Ascenzo S, Millimaggi D, Pavan A, Dell'Orso L, Dolo V. Identification of an optimal concentration of platelet gel for promoting angiogenesis in human endothelial cells. Transfusion. 2009;49:771–8.
63. Roosendaal G, Vianen ME, Marx JJM, Van Den Berg HM, Lafeber FPJG, Bijlsma JWJ. Blood-induced joint damage: a human in vitro study. Arthritis Rheum. 1999;42:1025–32.
64. Xiong G, Lingampalli N, Koltsov JCB, Leung LL, Bhutani N, Robinson WH, Chu CR. Men and women differ in the biochemical composition of platelet-rich plasma. Am J Sports Med. 2018;46:409–19.
65. Hartley PS. The diurnal tick-tockery of platelet biology. Platelets. 2012;23:157–60.
66. Medicine USNL of search of: platelet rich plasma – List Results 2019 ClinicalTrials.gov. https://clinicaltrials.gov/ct2/results?cond=&term=platelet+rich+plasma&cntry=&state=&city=&dist=. Accessed 27 Jan 2019.
67. Maffulli N, Wong J, Almekinders LC. Types and epidemiology of tendinopathy. Clin Sports Med. 2003;22:675–92.
68. Pingel J, Lu Y, Starborg T, Fredberg U, Langberg H, Nedergaard A, Weis M, Eyre D, Kjaer M, Kadler KE. 3-D ultrastructure and collagen composition of healthy and overloaded human tendon: evidence of tenocyte and matrix buckling. J Anat. 2014;224:548–55.
69. Millar NL, Hueber AJ, Reilly JH, Xu Y, Fazzi UG, Murrell GAC, McInnes IB. Inflammation is present in early human tendinopathy. Am J Sports Med. 2010;38:2085–91.
70. Schnabel LV, Mohammed HO, Miller BJ, McDermott WG, Jacobson MS, Santangelo KS, Fortier LA. Platelet rich plasma (PRP) enhances anabolic gene expression patterns in flexor digitorum superficialis tendons. J Orthop Res. 2007;25:230–40.
71. de Mos M, van der Windt AE, Jahr H, van Schie HT, Weinans H, Verhaar JAN, van Osch GJ. Can platelet-rich plasma enhance tendon repair? A cell culture study. Am J Sports Med. 2008;36:1171–8.
72. Aspenberg P, Virchenko O. Platelet concentrate injection improves Achilles tendon repair in rats. Acta Orthop Scand. 2004;75:93–9.
73. Peerbooms JC, Sluimer J, Bruijn DJ, Gosens T. Positive effect of an autologous platelet concentrate in lateral epicondylitis in a double-blind randomized controlled trial. Am J Sports Med. 2010;38:255–62.
74. Gosens T, Peerbooms JC, Van Laar W, Den Oudsten BL. Ongoing positive effect of platelet-rich plasma versus corticosteroid injection in lateral epicondylitis: a double-blind randomized controlled trial with 2-year follow-up. Am J Sports Med. 2011;39:1200–8.
75. Krogh TP, Fredberg U, Stengaard-Pedersen K, Christensen R, Jensen P, Ellingsen T. Treatment of lateral epicondylitis with platelet-rich plasma, glucocorticoid, or saline: a randomized, double-blind, placebo-controlled trial. Am J Sports Med. 2013;41:625–35.
76. Mishra AK, Skrepnik NV, Edwards SG, Jones GL, Sampson S, Vermillion DA, Ramsey ML, Karli DC, Rettig AC. Efficacy of platelet-rich plasma for chronic tennis elbow: a double-blind, prospective, multicenter, randomized controlled trial of 230 patients. Am J Sports Med. 2014;42:463–71.
77. Arirachakaran A, Sukthuayat A, Sisayanarane T, Laoratanavoraphong S, Kanchanatawan W, Kongtharvonskul J. Platelet-rich plasma versus autologous blood versus steroid injection in lateral epicondylitis: systematic review and network meta-analysis. J Orthop Traumatol. 2016;17:101–12.
78. Dragoo JL, Wasterlain AS, Braun HJ, Nead KT. Platelet-rich plasma as a treatment for patellar tendinopathy: a double-blind, randomized controlled trial. Am J Sports Med. 2014;42:610–8.
79. Vetrano M, Castorina A, Vulpiani MC, Baldini R, Pavan A, Ferretti A. Platelet-rich plasma versus focused shock waves in the treatment of jumper's knee in athletes. Am J Sports Med. 2013;41:795–803.

80. Andriolo L, Altamura SA, Reale D, Candrian C, Zaffagnini S, Filardo G. Nonsurgical treatments of patellar tendinopathy: multiple injections of platelet-rich plasma are a suitable option: a systematic review and meta-analysis. Am J Sports Med. 2019;47(4):1001–18.
81. de Vos RJ, Weir A, van Schie HTM, Bierma-Zeinstra SMA, Verhaar JAN, Weinans H, Tol JL. Platelet-rich plasma injection for chronic Achilles tendinopathy: a randomized controlled trial. JAMA. 2010;303:144–9.
82. Krogh TP, Ellingsen T, Christensen R, Jensen P, Fredberg U. Ultrasound-guided injection therapy of achilles tendinopathy with platelet-rich plasma or saline: a randomized, blinded, placebo-controlled trial. Am J Sports Med. 2016;44:1990–7.
83. Lin M-T, Chiang C-F, Wu C-H, Hsu H-H, Tu Y-K. Meta-analysis comparing autologous blood-derived products (including platelet-rich plasma) injection versus placebo in patients with Achilles tendinopathy. Arthroscopy. 2018;34:1966–75.
84. Zhang Y-J, Xu S-Z, Gu P-C, Du J-Y, Cai Y-Z, Zhang C, Lin X-J. Is platelet-rich plasma injection effective for chronic Achilles tendinopathy? A meta-analysis. Clin Orthop Relat Res. 2018;476:1633–41.
85. de Vos RJ, Weir A, van Schie HTM, Bierma-Zeinstra SMA, Verhaar JAN, Weinans H, Tol JL. Platelet rich plasma injection for chronic Achilles tendinopathy. JAMA. 2010;303:144–9.
86. De Jonge S, De Vos RJ, Weir A, Van Schie HTM, Bierma-Zeinstra SMA, Verhaar JAN, Weinans H, Tol JL. One-year follow-up of platelet-rich plasma treatment in chronic achilles tendinopathy: a double-blind randomized placebo-controlled trial. Am J Sports Med. 2011;39:1623–9.
87. Spreafico A, Chellini F, Frediani B, et al. Biochemical investigation of the effects of human platelet releasates on human articular chondrocytes. J Cell Biochem. 2009;108:1153–65.
88. Campbell KA, Saltzman BM, Mascarenhas R, Khair MM, Verma NN, Bach BR, Cole BJ. Does intra-articular platelet-rich plasma injection provide clinically superior outcomes compared with other therapies in the treatment of knee osteoarthritis? A systematic review of overlapping meta-analyses. Arthroscopy. 2015;31:2213–21.
89. Dai W-L, Zhou A-G, Zhang H, Zhang J. Efficacy of platelet-rich plasma in the treatment of knee osteoarthritis: a meta-analysis of randomized controlled trials. Arthrosc J Arthrosc Relat Surg. 2017;33:659–70.
90. Meheux CJ, McCulloch PC, Lintner DM, Varner KE, Harris JD. Efficacy of intra-articular platelet-rich plasma injections in knee osteoarthritis: a systematic review. Arthrosc J Arthrosc Relat Surg. 2016;32:495–505.
91. Woodall J, Tucci M, Mishra A, Benghuzzi H. Cellular effects of platelet rich plasma: a study on HL-60 macrophage-like cells. Biomed Sci Instrum. 2007;43:266–71.
92. Sundman EA, Cole BJ, Karas V, Della Valle C, Tetreault MW, Mohammed HO, Fortier LA. The anti-inflammatory and matrix restorative mechanisms of platelet-rich plasma in osteoarthritis. Am J Sports Med. 2014;42:35–41.
93. McCarrel TM, Minas T, Fortier LA. Optimization of leukocyte concentration in platelet-rich plasma for the treatment of tendinopathy. J Bone Joint Surg Am. 2012;94:e143.
94. Riboh JC, Saltzman BM, Yanke AB, Fortier L, Cole BJ. Effect of leukocyte concentration on the efficacy of platelet-rich plasma in the treatment of knee osteoarthritis. Am J Sports Med. 2016;44:792–800.
95. Di Sante L, Villani C, Santilli V, Valeo M, Bologna E, Imparato L, Paoloni M, Iagnocco A. Intra-articular hyaluronic acid vs platelet-rich plasma in the treatment of hip osteoarthritis. Med Ultrason. 2016;18:463–8.
96. Battaglia M, Guaraldi F, Vannini F, Rossi G, Timoncini A, Buda R, Giannini S. Efficacy of ultrasound-guided intra-articular injections of platelet-rich plasma versus hyaluronic acid for hip osteoarthritis. Orthopedics. 2013;36:e1501–8.
97. Ye Y, Zhou X, Mao S, Zhang J, Lin B. Platelet rich plasma versus hyaluronic acid in patients with hip osteoarthritis: a meta-analysis of randomized controlled trials. Int J Surg. 2018;53:279–87.
98. Filardo G, Di Matteo B, Di Martino A, Merli ML, Cenacchi A, Fornasari P, Marcacci M, Kon E. Platelet-rich plasma intra-articular knee injections show no superiority versus viscosupplementation: a randomized controlled trial. Am J Sports Med. 2015;43:1575–82.

99. Di Martino A, Di Matteo B, Papio T, Tentoni F, Selleri F, Cenacchi A, Kon E, Filardo G. Platelet-rich plasma versus hyaluronic acid injections for the treatment of knee osteoarthritis: results at 5 years of a double-blind, randomized controlled trial. Am J Sports Med. 2018;47(2):347–54.

100. Smith PA. Intra-articular autologous conditioned plasma injections provide safe and efficacious treatment for knee osteoarthritis: An FDA-sanctioned, randomized, double-blind, placebo-controlled clinical trial. Am J Sports Med. 2016;44:884–91.

101. Cole BJ, Karas V, Hussey K, Merkow DB, Pilz K, Fortier LA. Hyaluronic acid versus platelet-rich plasma: a prospective, double-blind randomized controlled trial comparing clinical outcomes and effects on intra-articular biology for the treatment of knee osteoarthritis. Am J Sports Med. 2017;45:339–46.

102. Duymus TM, Mutlu S, Dernek B, Komur B, Aydogmus S, Kesiktas FN. Choice of intra-articular injection in treatment of knee osteoarthritis: platelet-rich plasma, hyaluronic acid or ozone options. Knee Surgery Sport Traumatol Arthrosc. 2017;25:485–92.

103. Görmeli G, Görmeli CA, Ataoglu B, Çolak C, Aslantürk O, Ertem K. Multiple PRP injections are more effective than single injections and hyaluronic acid in knees with early osteoarthritis: a randomized, double-blind, placebo-controlled trial. Knee Surgery Sport Traumatol Arthrosc. 2017;25:958–65.

104. Fallouh L, Nakagawa K, Sasho T, Arai M, Kitahara S, Wada Y, Moriya H, Takahashi K. Effects of autologous platelet-rich plasma on cell viability and collagen synthesis in injured human anterior cruciate ligament. J Bone Joint Surg Am. 2010;92:2909–16.

105. Orrego M, Larrain C, Rosales J, Valenzuela L, Matas J, Durruty J, Sudy H, Mardones R. Effects of platelet concentrate and a bone plug on the healing of hamstring tendons in a bone tunnel. Arthroscopy. 2008;24:1373–80.

106. Radice F, Yánez R, Gutiérrez V, Rosales J, Pinedo M, Coda S. Comparison of magnetic resonance imaging findings in anterior cruciate ligament grafts with and without autologous platelet-derived growth factors. Arthroscopy. 2010;26:50–7.

107. Murray MM, Flutie BM, Kalish LA, Ecklund K, Fleming BC, Proffen BL, Micheli LJ. The bridge-enhanced anterior cruciate ligament repair (BEAR) procedure: an early feasibility cohort study. Orthop J Sport Med. 2016;4:2325967116672176.

108. Perrone GS, Proffen BL, Kiapour AM, Sieker JT, Fleming BC, Murray MM. Bench-to-bedside: bridge-enhanced anterior cruciate ligament repair. J Orthop Res. 2017;35:2606–12.

109. Okuda K, Kawase T, Momose M, Murata M, Saito Y, Suzuki H, Wolff LF, Yoshie H. Platelet-rich plasma contains high levels of platelet-derived growth factor and transforming growth factor-β and modulates the proliferation of periodontally related cells in vitro. J Periodontol. 2003;74:849–57.

110. Kawase T, Okuda K, Wolff LF, Yoshie H. Platelet-rich plasma-derived fibrin clot formation stimulates collagen synthesis in periodontal ligament and osteoblastic cells in vitro. J Periodontol. 2003;74:858–64.

111. Smith JJ, Ross MW, Smith RKW. Anabolic effects of acellular bone marrow, platelet rich plasma, and serum on equine suspensory ligament fibroblasts in vitro. Vet Comp Orthop Traumatol. 2006;19:43–7.

112. Yoshioka T, Kanamori A, Washio T, Aoto K, Uemura K, Sakane M, Ochiai N. The effects of plasma rich in growth factors (PRGF-Endoret) on healing of medial collateral ligament of the knee. Knee Surg Sports Traumatol Arthrosc. 2013;21:1763–9.

113. Podesta L, Crow SA, Volkmer D, Bert T, Yocum LA. Treatment of partial ulnar collateral ligament tears in the elbow with platelet-rich plasma. Am J Sports Med. 2013;41:1689–94.

114. Dines JS, Williams PN, ElAttrache N, Conte S, Tomczyk T, Osbahr DC, Dines DM, Bradley J, Ahmad CS. Platelet-rich plasma can be used to successfully treat elbow ulnar collateral ligament insufficiency in high-level throwers. Am J Orthop (Belle Mead NJ). 2016;45:296–300.

115. Laver L, Carmont MR, McConkey MO, Palmanovich E, Yaacobi E, Mann G, Nyska M, Kots E, Mei-Dan O. Plasma rich in growth factors (PRGF) as a treatment for high ankle sprain in elite athletes: a randomized control trial. Knee Surgery Sport Traumatol Arthrosc. 2015;23:3383–92.

116. Ishida K, Kuroda R, Miwa M, Tabata Y, Hokugo A, Kawamoto T, Sasaki K, Doita M, Kurosaka M. The regenerative effects of platelet-rich plasma on meniscal cells in vitro and its in vivo application with biodegradable gelatin hydrogel. Tissue Eng. 2007;13:1103–12.

117. Pujol N, De Chou ES, Boisrenoult P, Beaufils P. Platelet-rich plasma for open meniscal repair in young patients: any benefit? Knee Surgery Sport Traumatol Arthrosc. 2015;23:51–8.

118. Griffin JW, Hadeed MM, Werner BC, Diduch DR, Carson EW, Miller MD. Platelet-rich plasma in meniscal repair: does augmentation improve surgical outcomes? Clin Orthop Relat Res. 2015;473:1665–72.

119. Hammond JW, Hinton RY, Curl LA, Muriel JM, Lovering RM. Use of autologous platelet-rich plasma to treat muscle strain injuries. Am J Sports Med. 2009;37:1135–42.

120. A Hamid MS, Mohamed Ali MR, Yusof A, George J, LPC L. Platelet-rich plasma injections for the treatment of hamstring injuries. Am J Sports Med. 2014;42:2410–8.

121. Reurink G, Goudswaard GJ, Moen MH, Weir A, Verhaar JAN, Bierma-Zeinstra SMA, Maas M, Tol JL. Platelet-rich plasma injections in acute muscle injury. N Engl J Med. 2014;370:2546–7.

122. Sheth U, Dwyer T, Smith I, Wasserstein D, Theodoropoulos J, Takhar S, Chahal J. Does platelet-rich plasma Lead to earlier return to sport when compared with conservative treatment in acute muscle injuries? A systematic review and meta-analysis. Arthrosc – J Arthrosc Relat Surg. 2018;34:281–8.

123. Mazzocca AD, McCarthy MBR, Chowaniec DM, Dugdale EM, Hansen D, Cote MP, Bradley JP, Romeo AA, Arciero RA, Beitzel K. The positive effects of different platelet-rich plasma methods on human muscle, bone, and tendon cells. Am J Sports Med. 2012;40:1742–9.

124. Miroshnychenko O, Chang WT, Dragoo JL. The use of platelet-rich and platelet-poor plasma to enhance differentiation of skeletal myoblasts: implications for the use of autologous blood products for muscle regeneration. Am J Sports Med. 2017;45:945–53.

125. Pirvu TN, Schroeder JE, Peroglio M, Verrier S, Kaplan L, Richards RG, Alini M, Grad S. Platelet-rich plasma induces annulus fibrosus cell proliferation and matrix production. Eur Spine J. 2014;23:745–53.

126. Akeda K, An HS, Pichika R, Attawia M, Eugene JM, Lenz ME, Uchida A, Masuda K. Platelet-rich plasma (PRP) stimulates the extracellular matrix metabolism of porcine nucleus pulposus and anulus fibrosus cells cultured in alginate beads. Spine (Phila Pa 1976). 2006;31:959–66.

127. Kim H-J, Yeom JS, Koh Y-G, Yeo J-E, Kang K-T, Kang Y-M, Chang B-S, Lee C-K. Anti-inflammatory effect of platelet-rich plasma on nucleus pulposus cells with response of TNF-α and IL-1. J Orthop Res. 2014;32:551–6.

128. Nagae M, Ikeda T, Mikami Y, Hase H, Ozawa H, Matsuda K-I, Sakamoto H, Tabata Y, Kawata M, Kubo T. Intervertebral disc regeneration using platelet-rich plasma and biodegradable gelatin hydrogel microspheres. Tissue Eng. 2007;13:147–58.

129. Sawamura K, Ikeda T, Nagae M, et al. Characterization of in vivo effects of platelet-rich plasma and biodegradable gelatin hydrogel microspheres on degenerated intervertebral discs. Tissue Eng Part A. 2009;15:3719–27.

130. Obata S, Akeda K, Imanishi T, Masuda K, Bae W, Morimoto R, Asanuma Y, Kasai Y, Uchida A, Sudo A. Effect of autologous platelet-rich plasma-releasate on intervertebral disc degeneration in the rabbit anular puncture model: a preclinical study. Arthritis Res Ther. 2012;14:R241.

131. Levi D, Horn S, Tyszko S, Levin J, Hecht-Leavitt C, Walko E. Intradiscal platelet-rich plasma injection for chronic discogenic low back pain: preliminary results from a prospective trial. Pain Med. 2016;17:1010–22.

132. Tuakli-Wosornu YA, Terry A, Boachie-Adjei K, Harrison JR, Gribbin CK, LaSalle EE, Nguyen JT, Solomon JL, Lutz GE. Lumbar intradiskal platelet-rich plasma (PRP) injections: a prospective, double-blind, randomized controlled study. PM&R. 2016;8:1–10.

133. Monfett M, Harrison J, Boachie-Adjei K, Lutz G. Intradiscal platelet-rich plasma (PRP) injections for discogenic low back pain: an update. Int Orthop. 2016;40:1321–8.

134. Wu J, Du Z, Lv Y, Zhang J, Xiong W, Wang R, Liu R, Zhang G, Liu QA. New technique for the treatment of lumbar facet joint syndrome using intra-articular injection with autologous platelet rich plasma. Pain Phys. 2016;19:617–25.

135. Wu J, Zhou J, Liu C, Zhang J, Xiong W, Lv Y, Liu R, Wang R, Du Z, Zhang G, Liu Q. A prospective study comparing platelet-rich plasma and local anesthetic (LA)/corticosteroid in intra-articular injection for the treatment of lumbar facet joint syndrome. Pain Pract. 2017;17:914–24.

136. Centeno C, Markle J, Dodson E, Stemper I, Hyzy M, Williams C, Freeman M. The use of lumbar epidural injection of platelet lysate for treatment of radicular pain. J Exp Orthop. 2017;4:38.

137. Marx RE, Carlson ER, Eichstaedt RM, Schimmele SR, Strauss JE, Georgeff KR. Platelet-rich plasma: growth factor enhancement for bone grafts. Oral Surg Oral Med Oral Pathol Oral Radiol Endod. 1998;85:638–46.

138. Kassolis JD, Rosen PS, Reynolds MA. Alveolar ridge and sinus augmentation utilizing platelet-rich plasma in combination with freeze-dried bone allograft: case series. J Periodontol. 2000;71:1654–61.

139. Whitman DH, Berry RL, Green DM. Platelet gel: an autologous alternative to fibrin glue with applications in oral and maxillofacial surgery. J Oral Maxillofac Surg. 1997;55:1294–9.

140. Froum SJ, Wallace SS, Tarnow DP, Cho S-C. Effect of platelet-rich plasma on bone growth and osseointegration in human maxillary sinus grafts: three bilateral case reports. Int J Periodontics Restorative Dent. 2002;22:45–53.

141. Vang SN, Brady CP, Christensen KA, Allen KR, Anderson JE, Isler JR, Holt DW, Smith LM. Autologous platelet gel in coronary artery bypass grafting: effects on surgical wound healing. J Extra Corpor Technol. 2007;39:31–8.

142. Trowbridge CC, Stammers AH, Woods E, Yen BR, Klayman M, Gilbert C. Use of platelet gel and its effects on infection in cardiac surgery. J Extra Corpor Technol. 2005;37:381–6.

143. Khalafi RS, Bradford DW, Wilson MG. Topical application of autologous blood products during surgical closure following a coronary artery bypass graft. Eur J Cardiothorac Surg. 2008;34:360–4.

144. Driver VR, Hanft J, Fylling CP, Beriou JM, Autologel Diabetic Foot Ulcer Study Group. A prospective, randomized, controlled trial of autologous platelet-rich plasma gel for the treatment of diabetic foot ulcers. Ostomy Wound Manage. 2006;52:68–70.

145. Carter MJ, Fylling CP, Li WW, de Leon J, Driver VR, Serena TE, Wilson J. Analysis of run-in and treatment data in a wound outcomes registry: clinical impact of topical platelet-rich plasma gel on healing trajectory. Int Wound J. 2011;8:638–50.

146. Kim AE. Dr. Alfred Gellhorn and Dr. Christopher Visco present NewYork-Presbyterian's efforts in Tanzania at the United Nations | Department of Rehabilitation Medicine 2017. https://rehabmed.weill.cornell.edu/dr-alfred-gellhorn-and-dr-christopher-visco-present-newyork-presbyterians-efforts-tanzania-united. Accessed 27 Jan 2019.

147. Saltzman BM, Leroux T, Meyer MA, Basques BA, Chahal J, Bach BR, Yanke AB, Cole BJ. The therapeutic effect of intra-articular normal saline injections for knee osteoarthritis: a meta-analysis of evidence level 1 studies. Am J Sports Med. 2017;45:2647–53.

148. Cole BJ, Karas V, Hussey K, Pilz K, Fortier LA. Hyaluronic acid versus platelet-rich plasma: a prospective, double-blind randomized controlled trial comparing clinical outcomes and effects on intra-articular biology for the treatment of knee osteoarthritis. Am J Sports Med. 2017;45:339–46.

149. Bava ED, Barber FA. Platelet-rich plasma products in sports medicine. Phys Sportsmed. 2011;39:94–9.

150. Pollard JW. Tumour-stromal interactions. Transforming growth factor-beta isoforms and hepatocyte growth factor/scatter factor in mammary gland ductal morphogenesis. Breast Cancer Res. 2001;3:230–7.

151. Curi MM, Cossolin GSI, Koga DH, Araújo SR, Feher O, dos Santos MO, Zardetto C. Treatment of avascular osteonecrosis of the mandible in cancer patients with a history of bisphosphonate therapy by combining bone resection and autologous platelet-rich plasma: report of 3 cases. J Oral Maxillofac Surg. 2007;65:349–55.
152. Mozzati M, Gallesio G, Arata V, Pol R, Scoletta M. Platelet-rich therapies in the treatment of intravenous bisphosphonate-related osteonecrosis of the jaw: a report of 32 cases. Oral Oncol. 2012;48:469–74.
153. Martins MAT, Martins MD, Lascala CA, Curi MM, Migliorati CA, Tenis CA, Marques MM. Association of laser phototherapy with PRP improves healing of bisphosphonate-related osteonecrosis of the jaws in cancer patients: a preliminary study. Oral Oncol. 2012;48:79–84.
154. Aielli F, Giusti R, Rughetti A, Dell'Orso L, Ficorella C, Porzio G. Rapid resolution of refractory chemotherapy-induced oral mucositis with platelet gel-released supernatant in a pediatric cancer patient: a case report. J Pain Symptom Manag. 2014;48:e2–4.
155. Di Costanzo G, Loquercio G, Marcacci G, Iervolino V, Mori S, Petruzziello A, Barra P, Cacciapuoti C. Use of allogeneic platelet gel in the management of chemotherapy extravasation injuries: a case report. Onco Targets Ther. 2015;8:401–4.
156. U.S. Department of Health and Human Services. Regulatory considerations for human cells, tissues, and cellular and tissue-based products: minimal manipulation and homologous use 2017. https://www.fda.gov/downloads/biologicsbloodvaccines/guidancecomplianceregulatoryinformation/guidances/cellularandgenetherapy/ucm585403.pdf. Accessed 20 Jan 2019.
157. Beitzel K, Allen D, Apostolakos J, Russell R, McCarthy M, Gallo G, Cote M, Mazzocca A. US definitions, current use, and FDA stance on use of platelet-rich plasma in sports medicine. J Knee Surg. 2014;28:029–34.
158. U.S. Food and Drug Administration. 510(k) premarket notification 2019. https://www.accessdata.fda.gov/scripts/cdrh/cfdocs/cfPMN/pmn.cfm?ID=BK100058. Accessed 20 Jan 2019.
159. U.S. Food and Drug Administration. "Off-label" and investigational use of marketed drugs, biologics, and medical devices – Information Sheet 2018. https://www.fda.gov/RegulatoryInformation/Guidances/ucm126486.htm. Accessed 20 Jan 2019.
160. U.S. Centers for Medicare & Medicaid Services. Autologous platelet-rich plasma – Centers for Medicare & Medicaid Services 2015. https://www.cms.gov/Medicare/Coverage/Coverage-with-Evidence-Development/Autologous-Platelet-rich-Plasma.html. Accessed 20 Jan 2019.
161. Kraus VB, Collins JE, Hargrove D, Losina E, Nevitt M, Katz JN, Wang SX, Sandell LJ, Hoffmann SC, Hunter DJ. Predictive validity of biochemical biomarkers in knee osteoarthritis: data from the FNIH OA biomarkers consortium. Ann Rheum Dis. 2017;76:186–95.

Chapter 6
Prolotherapy

Caroline Schepker, Behnum Habibi, and Katherine V. Yao

Introduction

When practitioners use the term prolotherapy, they refer to an injection of a solution meant to rehabilitate an incompetent structure, usually by means of promoting sclerosis at the injection site [1]. It is identified as a regenerative injection therapy but differs from modern regenerative therapies such as platelet-rich plasma (PRP) and stem cell therapies because it lacks a biologic agent [2]. Hypertonic dextrose is the most commonly used prolotherapy solution and is popular in the United States and internationally. It is an inexpensive regenerative therapy option that results in great accessibility [3]. One of the earliest reports of prolotherapy for the musculoskeletal system was published in 1956 by GS Hackett, who reported that the treatment resulted in the proliferation of cells to strengthen injected tissues [4]. The most commonly used injectate is hyperosmolar dextrose (usually 10–30%) [5, 6]. This technique has been used for over 100 years [3] and many different solutions have been used to create similar effects, including phenol-glycerine-glucose (no longer used, but commonly studied previously) and sodium morrhuate (used currently, but less often than hyperosmolar glucose) [7]. Injection protocols are also varied but typically involve repeated injections on a weekly basis over several months. Anti-inflammatory medications are generally avoided after the injections to promote the expected controlled inflammatory response. Regular activity is typically resumed after resolution of possible post-injection inflammation [3].

C. Schepker · B. Habibi (✉)
New York-Presbyterian University Hospital, Columbia University Medical Center
and Weill Cornell Medical Center, New York, NY, USA
e-mail: bah9039@nyp.org

K. V. Yao
Weill Cornell Medical College, New York, NY, USA

© Springer Nature Switzerland AG 2020
G. Cooper et al. (eds.), *Regenerative Medicine for Spine and Joint Pain*,
https://doi.org/10.1007/978-3-030-42771-9_6

Mechanism of Action

The mechanism of action of prolotherapy is unclear but there have been several demonstrated effects of dextrose on cytokines in vitro. Currently discussed mechanisms include the induction of an inflammatory reaction that stimulates the wound-healing process by attracting growth factors and inducing vascular sclerosis [4, 8]. GLUT 1–4 proteins are cell surface transporters of dextrose that transport glucose into human cells and interact with cytokines to signal cell growth or repair [9]. Glucose and other sugar exposures to cells have demonstrated increased genetic expression of mesangial cell activation regulators including connective tissue growth factor (CTGF) by way of increased expression of transforming growth factor β1 (TGF- β1) and stimulating protein kinase C-dependent pathways [10]. These cytokine pathways are linked to increased production of fibroblasts [10, 11], chondrocytes [12, 13], and nerve cells in animal and human cells [14, 15].

An alternative proposed mechanism suggests that hyperosmolar dextrose opens potassium channels and thus hyperpolarizes nerve cells. This in turn decreases perceived pain by way of inhibited nociceptive fibers [8]. Another alternate mechanism suggests hyperosmolar dextrose slows osteoarthritis progression and improves cartilage regeneration, as demonstrated by multiple animal studies with small sample sizes [7, 8].

Effects of Prolotherapy on Ligaments and Tendons In Vitro and in Animal Studies

The response of tissues to prolotherapy has been studied in the rat medial collateral ligament (MCL). The results showed leukocyte and macrophage infiltration initially after prolotherapy treatment when compared to placebo, saline injections, or dry needling. This inflammatory response is hypothesized to reduce pain by limiting excessive neovascularization and neural ingrowth in the case of tendinopathy. However, the inflammatory response reported in the above MCL study varied between different prolotherapy injections [3, 16]. In the thigh muscles of guinea pigs, Harris and White demonstrated that prolotherapy induced white blood cell infiltration at 6 hours post-injection, marked edema at 24 hours post-injection, and finally the recruitment of large undifferentiated cells and fibroblasts after 24 hours [17]. Another study by Harris et al. demonstrated that within 10 months after the treatment, the thigh muscles underwent necrosis and were walled off by fibrous tissue and the necrotic tissue was then replaced entirely by thick bands of fibrous tissue [16].

The studies of the murine MCL demonstrated another interesting finding, an increase in the MCL cross-sectional area after prolotherapy. This suggests another mechanism of pain relief related to structural changes in treated tissues. However, in these studies, there were no changes in strength, stiffness, or laxity of the treated ligaments [16]. Separate work by Liu et al. on rabbit MCL did however demonstrate increased junctional strength, in addition to increased ligamentous mass, cross-sectional area, and thickness [18].

Other groups have similarly reported that the injection of sodium morrhuate into rabbit patellar and Achilles tendons increases their diameters [19]. Still others have reported increased strength in the patellar tendons of rats after prolotherapy, giving credence to the hypothesis that structural changes are responsible for the pain relief effect of prolotherapy. These results should be interpreted with caution, however, as a similar study by Harrison in murine Achilles tendons showed no difference in tendon tensile strength after injections with 18.5% dextrose compared to no intervention [19].

In conclusion, the mechanism of pain control mediated by prolotherapy at the tissue level is not well understood. It is likely multifactorial and due to both tissue displacement effects of the needle and effects of the injectate.

Osteoarthritis Clinical Studies

Osteoarthritis (OA) represents one of the most prevalent and financially burdensome health conditions worldwide; it is the fastest growing form of disability [20]. Treatment options are limited and, short of arthroplasty, typically only provide temporary relief. Prolotherapy has historically been used to address elements of laxity and instability within soft and connective tissue structures such as ligament and tendon, on the basis of increased tendon diameter, ligament hypertrophy, fibrosis, and tensile strength observed following direct injection of pro-inflammatory agents into these tissues. However, more recent research, most occurring within the twenty-first century, has sought to address whether these same prolotherapeutic injectates can address healing and/or ultimately confer anti-inflammatory effects within other tissues and regions of the musculoskeletal system—more specifically, within joints to address symptomatic osteoarthritis.

Overwhelmingly, the existing research examining this topic is limited in scope and study size and is not without methodological flaws. However, the existing body of literature suggests that intra-articular injection of prolotherapeutic injectate into symptomatic osteoarthritic joints, ranging from the small joints of the hand to large joints such as the knee, may be supported by mild to moderate evidence. The studies generally support positive effects of prolotherapy on joint pain, joint stiffness symptoms, and improvement on disability and quality of life.

Prolotherapy Effects on Small Joints

Research on prolotherapy treatment for osteoarthritis dates back to the early 2000s with small studies examining the use of 10% dextrose solution in MCP, PIP, and DIP joints of the hand [21]. Reeves and Hassanein randomized 27 patients with symptomatic hand OA for at least 6 months to either an intervention group ($n = 13$) or control group ($n = 14$). Injections were performed at 0, 2, and 4 months, with evaluation at 6 months post-initial injection. The intervention group saw a statistically significant improvement in pain with finger movement and flexion range of motion; this group also reported less pain at rest and demonstrated better grip strength; however, these latter two metrics were not statistically significant.

Prolotherapy Effects on Knee Osteoarthritis

Intrigued, this same group led by Reeves and Hassanein went on to examine the effects of dextrose injections to the knee [22]. Thirty-eight patients were selected who demonstrated at least 6 months of knee pain along with Kellgren-Lawrence radiographic evidence of knee OA. These participants were randomized into two groups: an intervention group, which underwent three injections, spaced out every 2 weeks, of a 10% dextrose/0.075% lidocaine solution, and a control group, which received an identical control solution absent the 10% dextrose. The dextrose-treated participants also underwent three further injections every 2 weeks of the 10% dextrose solution. Again, at 6 months of follow-up from the first injection, those who received the dextrose injections reported statistically significant less knee pain, swelling, buckling episodes, and greater knee flexion range of motion when compared with controls. These effects persisted at a 12-month follow-up. Secondary analysis revealed that 8 out of 13 knees treated with dextrose initially showed clinically significant ACL laxity which subsequently improved with decreased laxity at 12 months of follow-up.

Research into the use of prolotherapy in subsequent years focused primarily again on soft tissues, with a return in interest in the experimental use of prolotherapy for OA in the early 2010s. In 2012, Rabago and Patterson [23] identified 36 adults with moderate to severe knee OA and symptoms for at least 3 months; all participants received both extra-articular injections of 15% dextrose and intra-articular injections of 25% dextrose at 1, 5, and 9 weeks, with additional "as-needed" injections at weeks 13 and 17. Over 1 year of follow-up, participants reported progressively improved scores on the Western Ontario and McMaster Universities Osteoarthritis Index (WOMAC) and the validated Knee Pain Scale (KPS). Score improvement was observed as early as 4 weeks post-initial injection and demonstrated continued improvement in both measures over the 1 year of follow-up. Greater improvement was statistically significantly related to female gender, younger age (45–65 years), and BMI <25 kg/m^2. While promising, this study was severely limited methodologically by its single-arm, uncontrolled design, as well as the confounding nature associated with injecting both intra-articularly and extra-articularly. In 2013, the same group returned to the subject to perform a three-arm, blinded, randomized controlled trial [24]. Ninety adults with at least 3 months of knee OA were randomized to injection (dextrose versus saline) or a home exercise program. Again, both extra- and intra-articular injections were performed, at 1, 5, and 9 weeks. At 1 year of follow-up, all groups reported statistically significant improvements in composite WOMAC scores compared with baseline. When adjusting for sex, age, and BMI, WOMAC scores for patients receiving the dextrose injections improved significantly more, exceeding the WOMAC-based minimal clinically important difference. Individual knee pain scores also improved statistically significantly more in the prolotherapy group.

Rabago went on to attempt to further characterize the possible mechanism underlying these observed effects. In 2013, Rabago et al. examined both knee OA-specific quality of life and intra-articular cartilage volume in patients treated with intra-articular prolotherapy [25]. Knee-specific quality of life improved significantly among knee OA participants who received monthly knee prolotherapy injections over 5 months as compared with controls. Interestingly, when examining radiographic progression of knee articular cartilage degradation over time (via MRI), both groups saw interval decrease in knee articular cartilage over 1 year at about the same rate; however, the prolotherapy recipients who lost the least cartilage volume also had the greatest improvement in pain scores. Authors noted that among these participants, the change in cartilage volume and knee pain (but not stiffness or function) scores were correlated, with each 1% of cartilage volume loss being associated with 2.7% less improvement in pain score.

In 2014, Hauser et al. retrospectively evaluated the effects of both intra-articular and extra-articular knee prolotherapy injections on pain, stiffness, crepitus, and improvements in physical activity levels in 69 patients with chondromalacia patella [26]. Patients received, at one visit, 24 injections of 15% dextrose, 0.1% procaine, and 10% sarapin (total 40 cc) in the anterior knee at various locations: MCL and LCL, patellar ligament, vastus medialis and iliotibial tract, and pes anserinus, with 8 cc injected intra-articularly. Six weeks following the last injection, patients reported a statistically significant decrease in pain at rest, during ADLs, and with exercise. These patients also reported a significant decrease in stiffness and crepitus and increase in knee range of motion.

A case series performed in 2016 by Topol et al. sought to better understand if dextrose does in fact exert a chondrogenic effect to explain some of the clinical effects observed with prolotherapy injected into the joint space. Six participants with symptomatic knee OA for at least 6 months and arthroscopically confirmed medial compartment exposed subchondral bone were treated with four to six monthly 10 mL intra-articular knee injections with 12.5% dextrose. Knee articular cartilage was examined both pre-injection and at 8 months post-injection, via direct visualization (arthroscopic examination of nine standardized medial condyle zones) and biopsy of a cartilage growth area. Fifty-four total zones were examined (9 zones over 6 participants); in 19 of these, blinded arthroscopy readers reported evidence of cartilage growth post-treatment as compared with pre-treatment. Biopsy specimens showed metabolically active cartilage, with parallel fibers and cartilage typing patterns consistent with both fibrocartilage and hyaline cartilage. Additionally, compared with baseline, median WOMAC scores statistically significantly improved by 13 points [27].

Intra-articular Prolotherapy Treatment Versus Corticosteroid and Platelet-Rich Plasma Treatments

Several other groups have attempted to compare intra-articular dextrose injections with other agents, such as platelet-rich plasma (PRP) or corticosteroid. In 2014, Jahangiri et al. compared the use of hypertonic dextrose with corticosteroid for the treatment of first carpometacarpal joint OA in a randomized controlled trial [28]. Sixty patients with both symptomatic and radiographic first CMC osteoarthritis were randomized to a corticosteroid injection group ($n = 30$, received 2 monthly saline placebo injections followed by a single dose of 40 mg methylprednisolone acetate) or a prolotherapy group ($n = 30$, 20% dextrose and 2% lidocaine solution performed monthly for 3 months). At 1-month post-third injection, the corticosteroid group reported a statistically significant greater improvement in pain via Visual Analog Scale (VAS); however at 6-month follow-up, the prolotherapy group reported a statistically significant greater improvement in pain. At the 6-month follow-up, both the prolotherapy and corticosteroid groups reported improved overall hand function; however again, the prolotherapy group had a significant larger effect at this time point, overall suggesting better long-term effects of prolotherapy as compared with the expected, short-lived effects of intra-articular steroid.

In 2018, Rahimzadeh et al. compared intra-articular knee prolotherapy injections with platelet-rich plasma (PRP) injections [29]. Forty-two patients with stage 1 or 2 Kellgren-Lawrence knee OA were randomized into a PRP group (7 cc PRP solution) versus prolotherapy group (7 cc 25% dextrose solution). Participants received these injections twice, 1 month apart. All participants saw a rapid decrease in overall WOMAC score at both 1 month and 2 months following the first injection. WOMAC score then rose at the 6-month mark, but was still statistically significantly lower than baseline score. There was no statistically significant difference in these scores between the two groups, suggesting a possible comparable efficacy and underlying mechanism to both PRP and prolotherapy; however, of note was the substantially lower cost associated with performing the dextrose injections.

Intra-articular Versus Extra-articular Injections for Joint Pain

Because of the wide variation of practice and different indications of use, it has been questioned whether it is the intra-articular injection itself that results in improvements in OA symptoms or the peri-articular injection effects. Farpour performed a randomized controlled trial of 52 adults with primary knee OA (grade 2–3 Kellgren-Lawrence) for at least 3 months. Participants were randomized to either an intra-articular injection group or a peri-articular injection group. Injections were performed twice within a 2-week interval. In the peri-articular group, up to three points of tenderness surrounding the knee were identified and injected with a total of 6 cc of 25% dextrose. In the intra-articular group, 6 cc total of 25% dextrose was injected intra-articularly. Ultimately, following injections, both groups reported comparable improvements in pain and function via Visual Analog Scale, Oxford Knee Scale, and WOMAC over 4–8 weeks post-injection, without any superiority between the two methods [30].

Rezasoltani et al. did the same: in a randomized, double-blinded controlled trial, 104 patients with chronic knee OA were randomized to an intra-articular versus peri-articular injection group. In the intra-articular group, 8 cc of 10% dextrose and 2% lidocaine was injected into the knee joint. In the peri-articular group, 5 cc of 20% dextrose and 5 cc of 1% lidocaine was injected subcutaneously at 4 points in the periarticular knee. Injections were repeated at 1 and 2 weeks after the first injection. In this study, VAS was significantly lower in the peri-articular group as compared with the intra-articular group at 2-, 3-, 4-, and 5-month follow-up (but not at 1 month). Walking and stair climbing difficulty, morning stiffness, and joint locking improved in both groups and were not statistically significant between groups [31].

There has not been much investigation into efficacy of intra-articular dextrose injections past a 1-year follow-up period, and long-term outcomes are largely lacking. Only one study by Rabago et al. examined long-term outcomes in patients who had received intra-articular knee dextrose injections at 2.5 years of follow-up. Sixty-five patients who received up to 5 intra-articular injections over 17 weeks were observed to experience clinically meaningful improvements in WOMAC scores at 1 year of follow-up; these same patients reported continued improvement in WOMAC score at 2.5 years of follow-up, with an average of about 36% of improvement in WOMAC score at 2.5 years as compared with baseline. No adverse effects were observed [32].

Sacroiliac Joint and Axial Spine Prolotherapy Treatments

Very little is known about the effect of prolotherapy injections on pain within axial joints; however, several small studies exist. Kim et al. performed a prospective, randomized controlled trial comparing dextrose prolotherapy versus corticosteroid to the sacroiliac joint to address low back pain attributed primarily to SI joint dysfunction [33]. Forty-eight patients with SI joint pain (confirmed by 50% or greater improvement in response to local anesthetic block) lasting 3 months or longer were randomized to receive either intra-articular 25% dextrose or triamcinolone injections to the SI joint, performed under fluoroscopic guidance. Pain and disability scores were assessed at baseline, 2 weeks, and monthly following this injection. All scores were significantly improved from baseline in both groups at 2 weeks post-injection; however, at 15 months, the prolotherapy group had a cumulative incidence of 50% or greater improvement in symptoms of 58.7% versus 10.2% in the steroid group; this difference was found to be statistically significant. Additionally, Cusi et al. performed a prospective descriptive study of 25 patients who also received SI joint injections with dextrose and demonstrated subsequent improvements in back pain disability ratings; however, the targeted structure was not the joint space itself, but rather the dorsal interosseous ligament of the affected SI joint [34]. Finally, Hooper et al. described a retrospective case series of patients with "chronic spinal pain" treated with dextrose prolotherapy [35]. One hundred and seventy-seven patients with multi-site chronic axial back pain were treated with 20% dextrose injections to the facet capsules of the cervical, thoracic, and/or lumbar spine. Additionally, iliolumbar and dorsal sacroiliac ligaments were injected in patients with a chief complaint of lower back pain. Ninety-one percent of patients reported reductions in pain; 85% reported improvements in ADLs, and 84% reported improvements in ability to work over 2.5 years of follow-up. These patients were not compared against patients who received medical management, physical therapy, or other axial spine injections.

Given the widespread prevalence of osteoarthritis and the cost burden it imparts, dextrose injections represent an inexpensive and accessible potential tool for symptom management. However, current quality and level of evidence leaves much to be desired. There are many pitfalls associated with the research examining efficacy of prolotherapy as a viable clinical tool for osteoarthritis management. For one, there is a wide degree of heterogeneity among studies, especially with regard to sample size, blinding, controls, composition of injectate, and injection protocols. Percent of dextrose injected ranged from 10% to 25%. Injection volumes were highly variable. The number of injections performed and anatomical locations of the injections were variable. Some studies performed injections blindly, while others used ultrasound guidance for needle localization to ensure accuracy. Some injections involved additional use of anesthetic agents such as lidocaine, which have known chondrotoxic effects, potentially muddying outcomes. The vast majority of studies were performed on the knee, with overall lack of representation of other commonly affected joints in OA, such as the hip and shoulder.

Despite these limitations, existing research provides some promising insights. For example, comparable effects between dextrose and PRP injections may highlight prolotherapy as a cost-effective alternative to more expensive and time-consuming regenerative therapies. The efficacy of extra-articular injections suggests an important role of dynamic and soft tissue stabilizers as pain generators in OA. Improvements in pain observed in conjunction with increased chondral volume lend exciting evidence to the theoretical "proliferative" nature of prolotherapy, and the capacity of intra-articular injections to stimulate chondrogenesis in general. Further research is needed to corroborate these potential tissue changes, to identify ideal injectate volumes and compositions, and to identify utility and feasibility in other commonly affected joints.

Tendinopathy Clinical Studies

The most data, in terms of quantity and quality, evaluating the use of prolotherapy versus control injections exist for tendinopathies. In particular, the evidence is most robust for chronic, painful, overuse tendinopathies [36, 37]. Overuse tendinopathies secondary to repetitive motion share similar micro- and macroscopic features, suggesting shared pathologic processes. For example, tendinopathies of the common extensor tendon (lateral epicondylitis), Achilles tendon, and patellar tendon share similar histological and sonographic features, suggesting a common, noninflammatory pathophysiology [38]. Studies of prolotherapy in these cases is reviewed here.

Lateral Epicondylitis

Lateral epicondylitis (LE) is a degenerative disease caused by repetitive microtrauma that leads to angiogenesis and fibroblast proliferation [39]. There has been a hypothesis that interrupting the increased blood vessel infiltration and fibroblast proliferation may improve pain in epicondylitis. However, a study investigating purely blood vessel sclerosis did not demonstrate significant improvement. Thirty-six participants with lateral epicondylitis did not demonstrate a significant improvement after an ultrasound-guided lauromacrogol injection (lauromacrogol, or polidocanol, is not a typical prolotherapy injectate; it is a blood vessel sclerosing agent) [40].

Effects of prolotherapy have been studied for lateral epicondylitis with varied results. A double-blinded, randomized controlled study with 24 participants compared to placebo (normal saline) was conducted with three injections of hypertonic glucose, sodium morrhuate, and local anesthetic over 8 weeks. The average duration of epicondylalgia among the participants was 1.9 years. There was no significant difference in symptom improvement noted in the short term (immediately prior to the third injection), but there was a difference in the intermediate term. Of note, in this pilot study, all ten participants receiving prolotherapy reported pain at the injection site, as did all ten of the participants receiving placebo injections [41].

Another randomized controlled trial compared prolotherapy with local corticosteroid injection for LE. Seventeen participants were given two injections, 1 month apart, of either phenol-glycerine-glucose, dextrose, and sodium morrhuate or methylprednisolone. There were no clinically significant differences between groups. However, the prolotherapy group showed improvements from baseline in the Visual Analog Scale (VAS) and the Disabilities of the Arm, Shoulder, and Hand (DASH) at both 3-month and 6-month time points. The methylprednisolone group only showed improvements in the DASH at the 3-month but not 6-month time points [42].

Another randomized trial by Rabago et al. randomized patients into three groups: injections of 50% dextrose at 1, 4, and 8 weeks; 50% dextrose with 5% sodium morrhuate at 1, 4, and 8 weeks; and no intervention. The primary outcome was the Patient-Reported Tennis Elbow Evaluation score. Both experimental groups showed statistically significant improvements in the primary outcome at multiple time points in the 32-week follow-up period [43]. However, the study is limited by the lack of a control injection. Furthermore, other outcome measures in this study, including grip strength and magnetic resonance imaging severity, were mostly unchanged.

Achilles Tendinopathy

In 20 patients with Achilles tendinopathy, an ultrasound-guided lauromacrogol injection did not demonstrate a significant improvement in symptoms, though there was a suggestive trend, ($p = 0.07$) [8]. Another study of 43 participants compared prolotherapy alone, eccentric exercise alone, and a combination of the two [44]. There were no differences in the outcomes across the three groups in either the short, intermediate, or long term. However, the prolotherapy group was the quickest to achieve favorable outcomes.

In another study of 36 participants with conservative treatment refractory Achilles tendinopathy, ultrasound-guided injections of dextrose and anesthetic at 6-week intervals improved pain scores and neovascularity measured by ultrasound in 55% of the participants [45]. It is crucial to note that this study has no control group.

Rotator Cuff Tendinopathy

There have been several studies in recent literature investigating the effects of prolotherapy treatment for chronic rotator cuff tendinopathy. Rotator cuff tendinopathy is one of the most common causes of chronic shoulder pain in the absence of active inflammation. It is typically treated with exercise and physical therapy. Those that are refractory to conservative management can be difficult to treat with many techniques attempted by clinicians including corticosteroid injections, PRP injections, and prolotherapy. Results of prolotherapy treatment for rotator cuff tendinopathy have shown favorable results for pain control, particularly when compared to physiotherapy alone. But there are mixed results when compared to other injection therapies. Studies have demonstrated improvement in supraspinatus tendon structure with prolotherapy injections, but not significantly different from improvements seen with other treatments.

Comparing prolotherapy to traditional physiotherapy treatment, a few authors have found favorable outcomes for prolotherapy treatment. Lee et al. performed a retrospective case-control study of patients with nontraumatic refractory rotator cuff disease ($n = 151$) who were unresponsive to 3 months of physical therapy. The treatment group received 16.5% dextrose 10 mL solution ($n = 63$) while the control group continued with physical therapy ($n = 63$). The average number of prolotherapy injections in the treatment group were 4.8 +/− 1.3. There was significant improvement in the prolotherapy treatment group in VAS, Shoulder Pain and

Disability Index (SPADI), isometric strength of shoulder abduction, and shoulder AROM at over 1-year follow-up [46].

Seven et al. conducted a randomized controlled study ($n = 120$) of patients with chronic rotator cuff lesions for greater than 6 months. Controls treated with physical therapy 3 times a week were compared to a prolotherapy treatment group. All conducted home exercise programs. Of the 101 patients included in the study (44 in the control group, 57 in the prolotherapy group), both groups achieved significant improvements in VAS, SPADI, Western Ontario Rotator Cuff (WORC) index, and shoulder ROM ($p < 0.001$). Intergroup comparisons demonstrated significant differences in VAS, SPADI, WORC index, shoulder abduction, shoulder flexion, and shoulder internal rotation at over 1 year follow-up favoring prolotherapy treatment. Prolotherapy treatment resulted in 92.9% of patients reporting excellent or good outcomes compared to the control group with 56.8% reporting excellent or good outcomes [47].

A smaller randomized controlled prospective study by George et al. included 12 patients with focal supraspinatus tendinosis after 1 month of PT. Seven patients received 0.5–1 mL prolotherapy injection (12.5% dextrose, 0.5% lidocaine) and was compared to 5 patients who continued with standard physical therapy without interventions. He found superior and significant improvement in shoulder abduction ($p = 0.03$) and sleep score ($p = 0.027$) in the prolotherapy group. Echogenicity on ultrasound also significantly increased at the end of treatment for the prolotherapy group ($p = 0.009$). However, no significant reduction in pain score was seen in the injection group (43.5%) compared to the control group (25%) at 12 weeks ($p > 0.005$) [48].

A few authors studied prolotherapy compared to normal saline injections. Lin et al. demonstrated short-term pain relief in chronic rotator cuff tendinopathy. He conducted a double-blinded placebo-controlled trial ($n = 31$) with the treatment group receiving ultrasound-guided injection of dextrose 20% compared to a control group that received ultrasound-guided injection of normal saline 5% to the tendinopathic supraspinatus tendon. Outcome measures included VAS, SPADI, shoulder AROM, ultrasound thickness, and histogram and were measured at baseline, 2 weeks, and 6 weeks after intervention. He found that the prolotherapy group demonstrated significant improvement in VAS ($P = 0.001$), SPADI score ($P = 0.017$), shoulder AROM ($P = 0.039$), and shoulder abduction ($P = 0.043$) at 2 weeks after injection. However, the effects were not sustained at 6 weeks. No differences in ultrasound morphological changes were seen in the participants in either group [49].

Another randomized double-blinded control trial that studied the effects of prolotherapy compared to saline injections was conducted by Bertrand et al. His team studied patients with chronic moderate to severe shoulder pain due to rotator cuff tendinopathy for 7.6+/−9.6 years with ultrasound confirmation of supraspinatus tendinosis/tear ($n = 73$). Patients were stratified in to three groups, each receiving three monthly injections of dextrose into the supraspinatus enthesis, saline into the supraspinatus enthesis, and saline above the enthesis. The primary outcome was the VAS and the secondary outcome was the ultrasound shoulder pathology rating scale (USPRS). At 9-month follow-up, 59% of dextrose enthesis injection patients maintained improvement in pain, with VAS score demonstrating >2.8 improvement, compared to saline enthesis injection patients, 37% ($p = 0.088$), and superficial saline injection patients, 27% (p = 0.017). Dextrose enthesis satisfaction scores were 6.7 compared to saline, 4.7, and superficial saline, 3.9. USPRS demonstrated no difference between groups (P = 0.734). Overall, dextrose resulted in superior long-term pain improvement and satisfaction compared to blinded saline injections. All showed some improvement, but no significant differences between groups on improvement of tendinopathy were seen on ultrasound [50].

Comparing prolotherapy injections to subacromial bursa corticosteroid injections, Cole et al. performed a prospective randomized double-blinded clinical trial. His group compared prolotherapy injection into tendinopathic supraspinatus tendons (n = 17) to corticosteroid bursa injections (n = 19). There was significant reduction of pain with overhead activities at 3 months in only the prolotherapy group. By 6 months, both groups demonstrated significant reduction of pain without any difference between groups (p = 1.0). Both the prolotherapy and corticosteroid groups demonstrated significant improvement of the supraspinatus tendon on ultrasound compared to baseline at 3 months, but no significant difference between groups (p = 0.44) [51].

Finally, Lin et al. conducted a meta-analysis systematic review of randomized controlled trials comparing corticosteroid, nonsteroidal anti-inflammatory drugs (NSAIDs), hyaluronic acid, botulinum toxin, PRP, and prolotherapy in patients with RTC tendinopathy. Out of 18 studies that were included, his team found that corticosteroid was more effective only in the short term in both pain reduction and functional improvement. Prolotherapy significantly reduced pain compared with placebo in the long term (over 24 wks; SMD, 2.63; 94% CI, 1.88–3.38). PRP significantly improved shoulder function compared to placebo in the long term (24 wks; SMD, 0.44; 95% CI, 0.05–0.84) [52].

Side Effects and Adverse Events

Most adverse events associated with prolotherapy injections are related to the treatment location. In a study by Yelland et al., prolotherapy used to treat generic low back pain caused immediate pain in the low back in 88% of participants. Few patients also suffered from headaches after treatment which resolved within 1 week. Few patients suffered from leg pain with neurological features [53]. Several other studies reported similar events, most commonly, pain and stiffness at the injection site anywhere from 12 to 96 hours after the injections [54–57]. Rare adverse events in these studies include sleep disturbance due to "psychological trauma," irregular menses, lumbar puncture headache, and radicular pain. Rarer still, serious adverse events in patients receiving prolotherapy for low back pain include two cases of meningitis (both resolved with treatment) [58], adhesive arachnoiditis (requiring ventriculostomy and craniotomy ultimately resulting in post-operative death, a case report published in the Journal of the American Medical Association) [59], and encephalomyelitis (treated with ventriculojugular shunt resulting in steady improvement) [60].

References

1. Gove P. Webster's third new international dictionary, unabridged. 3rd ed. Merriam-Webster: Springfield, MA; 2002.
2. Reeves KD, Sit RWS, Rabago DP. Dextrose prolotherapy a narrative review of basic science, clinical research, and best treatment recommendations. Phys Med Rehabil Clin NA. 2016;27:783–823. https://doi.org/10.1016/j.pmr.2016.06.001.
3. Rabago D, Slattengren A, Zgierska A. Prolotherapy in primary care practice. Prim Care Clin Off Pract. 2010;37(1):65–80. https://doi.org/10.1016/J.POP.2009.09.013.
4. Hackett G. Ligament and tendon relaxation. 3rd ed. (Thomas CC, ed.). Springfield, IL; 1958.
5. Dagenais S, Ogunseitan O, Haldeman S, Wooley JR, Newcomb RL. Side effects and adverse events related to intraligamentous injection of sclerosing solutions (prolotherapy) for back and neck pain: a survey of practitioners. Arch Phys Med Rehabil. 2006;87(7):909–13. https://doi.org/10.1016/j.apmr.2006.03.017.
6. Rabago D, Best TM, Zgierska AE, Zeisig E, Ryan M, Crane D. A systematic review of four injection therapies for lateral epicondylosis: prolotherapy, polidocanol, whole blood and platelet-rich plasma. Br J Sports Med. 2009;43(7):471–81. https://doi.org/10.1136/bjsm.2008.052761.
7. Jensen KT, Rabago DP, Best TM, Patterson JJ, Vanderby R. Response of knee ligaments to prolotherapy in a rat injury model. Am J Sports Med. 2008;36(7):1347–57. https://doi.org/10.1177/0363546508314431.
8. Hoksrud A, Öhberg L, Alfredson H, Bahr R. Ultrasound-guided sclerosis of neovessels in painful chronic patellar tendinopathy. Am J Sports Med. 2006;34(11):1738–46. https://doi.org/10.1177/0363546506289168.
9. Thorens B, Mueckler M. Glucose transporters in the 21st century. Am J Physiol Endocrinol Metab. 2010;298:141–5. https://doi.org/10.1152/ajpendo.00712.2009.
10. Murphy M, Godson C, Cannon S, et al. Suppression subtractive hybridization identifies high glucose levels as a stimulus for expression of connective tissue growth factor and other genes in human mesangial cells; 1999. http://www.jbc.org/. Accessed 27 Apr 2019.
11. Pugliese G, Pricci E, Locuratolo N, et al. Increased activity of the insulin-like growth factor system in mesangial cells cultured in high glucose conditions. Relation to glucose-enhanced extracellular matrix production; 1996. https://link.springer.com/content/pdf/10.1007/s001250050510.pdf. Accessed 27 Apr 2019.
12. Mobasheri A. Glucose: an energy currency and structural precursor in articular cartilage and bone with emerging roles as an extracellular signaling molecule and metabolic regulator. Front Endocrinol (Lausanne). 2012;3(153) https://doi.org/10.3389/fendo.2012.00153.
13. Cigan AD, Nims RJ, Albro MB, et al. Insulin, ascorbate, and glucose have a much greater influence than transferrin and selenous acid on the In Vitro growth of engineered cartilage in chondrogenic media. Tissue Eng Part A. 2013;19(17–18):1941–8. https://doi.org/10.1089/ten.tea.2012.0596.
14. Russell JW, Golovoy D, Vincent AM, et al. High glucose-induced oxidative stress and mitochondrial dysfunction in neurons. FASEB J. 2002;16(13):1738–48. https://doi.org/10.1096/fj.01-1027com.
15. Stecker MM, Stevenson M. Effect of glucose concentration on peripheral nerve and its response to anoxia. Muscle Nerve. 2014;49(3):370–7. https://doi.org/10.1002/mus.23917.
16. Harris F, White A. Injection treatment of hernia. J Am Med Assoc. 1937;109(18):1456. https://doi.org/10.1001/jama.1937.02780440046017.
17. Maynard JA, Pedrini VA, Pedrini-Mille A, Romanus B, Ohlerking F. Morphological and biochemical effects of sodium morrhuate on tendons. J Orthop Res. 1985;3(2):236–48. https://doi.org/10.1002/jor.1100030214.
18. Hackett G, Henderson D. Joint stabilization; an experimental, histologic study with comments on the clinical application in ligament proliferation. – PubMed – NCBI. Am J Surg. 1955;89(5):968–73. https://www.ncbi.nlm.nih.gov/pubmed/?term=hackett%2C+henderson%2C+joint+stabilizatoin. Accessed 27 May 1955.

19. Park Y-S, Lim S-W, Lee I-H, Lee T-J, Kim J-S, Han JS. Intra-articular injection of a nutritive mixture solution protects articular cartilage from osteoarthritic progression induced by anterior cruciate ligament transection in mature rabbits: a randomized controlled trial. Arthritis Res Ther. 2007;9(1):R8. https://doi.org/10.1186/ar2114.
20. Conaghan PG, Porcheret M, Kingsbury SR, et al. Impact and therapy of osteoarthritis: the arthritis care OA nation 2012 survey. Clin Rheumatol. 2015;34(9):1581–8. https://doi.org/10.1007/s10067-014-2692-1.
21. Reeves KD, Hassanein K. Randomized, prospective, placebo-controlled double-blind study of dextrose prolotherapy for osteoarthritic thumb and finger (DIP, PIP, and trapeziometacarpal) joints: evidence of clinical efficacy. J Altern Complement Med. 2000;6(4):311–20. https://doi.org/10.1089/10755530050120673.
22. Reeves KD, Hassanein K. Randomized prospective double-blind placebo-controlled study of dextrose prolotherapy for knee osteoarthritis with or without ACL laxity. Altern Ther Health Med. 2000;6(2):68–74, 77–80. http://www.ncbi.nlm.nih.gov/pubmed/10710805. Accessed 27 May 2019.
23. Rabago D, Zgierska A, Fortney L, et al. Hypertonic dextrose injections (prolotherapy) for knee osteoarthritis: results of a single-arm uncontrolled study with 1-year follow-up. J Altern Complement Med. 2012;18(4):408–14. https://doi.org/10.1089/acm.2011.0030.
24. Rabago D, Patterson JJ, Mundt M, et al. Dextrose prolotherapy for knee osteoarthritis: a randomized controlled trial. Ann Fam Med. 2013;11(3):229–37. https://doi.org/10.1370/afm.1504.
25. Rabago D, Kijowski R, Woods M, et al. Association between disease-specific quality of life and magnetic resonance imaging outcomes in a clinical trial of prolotherapy for knee osteoarthritis. Arch Phys Med Rehabil. 2013;94(11):2075–82. https://doi.org/10.1016/j.apmr.2013.06.025.
26. Hauser RA, Sprague IS. Outcomes of prolotherapy in chondromalacia patella patients: improvements in pain level and function. Clin Med Insights Arthritis Musculoskelet Disord. 2014;7:13–20. https://doi.org/10.4137/CMAMD.S13098.
27. Topol GA, Podesta LA, Reeves KD, et al. Chondrogenic effect of intra-articular hypertonic-dextrose (prolotherapy) in severe knee osteoarthritis. PM&R. 2016;8(11):1072–82. https://doi.org/10.1016/j.pmrj.2016.03.008.
28. Jahangiri A, Moghaddam FR, Najafi S. Hypertonic dextrose versus corticosteroid local injection for the treatment of osteoarthritis in the first carpometacarpal joint: a double-blind randomized clinical trial. J Orthop Sci. 2014;19(5):737–43. https://doi.org/10.1007/s00776-014-0587-2.
29. Rahimzadeh P, Imani F, Faiz SHR, Entezary SR, Zamanabadi MN, Alebouyeh MR. The effects of injecting intra-articular platelet-rich plasma or prolotherapy on pain score and function in knee osteoarthritis. Clin Interv Aging. 2018;13:73–9. https://doi.org/10.2147/CIA.S147757.
30. Farpour HR, Fereydooni F. Comparative effectiveness of intra-articular prolotherapy versus peri-articular prolotherapy on pain reduction and improving function in patients with knee osteoarthritis: a randomized clinical trial. Electron Physician. 2017;9(11):5663–9. https://doi.org/10.19082/5663.
31. Rezasoltani Z, Taheri M, Mofrad MK, Mohajerani SA. Periarticular dextrose prolotherapy instead of intra-articular injection for pain and functional improvement in knee osteoarthritis. J Pain Res. 2017;10:1179–87. https://doi.org/10.2147/JPR.S127633.
32. Rabago D, Mundt M, Zgierska A, Grettie J. Hypertonic dextrose injection (prolotherapy) for knee osteoarthritis: long term outcomes. Complement Ther Med. 2015;23(3):388–95. https://doi.org/10.1016/j.ctim.2015.04.003.
33. Kim WM, Lee HG, Won Jeong C, Kim CM, Yoon MH. A randomized controlled trial of intra-articular prolotherapy versus steroid injection for sacroiliac joint pain. J Altern Complement Med. 2010;16(12):1285–90. https://doi.org/10.1089/acm.2010.0031.
34. Cusi M, Saunders J, Hungerford B, Wisbey-Roth T, Lucas P, Wilson S. The use of prolotherapy in the sacroiliac joint. Br J Sports Med. 2010;44(2):100–4. https://doi.org/10.1136/bjsm.2007.042044.

35. Hooper RA, Ding M. Retrospective case series on patients with chronic spinal pain treated with dextrose prolotherapy. J Altern Complement Med. 2004;10(4):670–4. https://doi.org/10.1089/acm.2004.10.670.

36. Kim SR, Stitik TP, Foye PM, Greenwald BD, Campagnolo DI. Critical review of prolotherapy for osteoarthritis, low back pain, and other musculoskeletal conditions: a psychiatric perspective. Am J Phys Med Rehabil. 2004;83(5):379–89. http://www.ncbi.nlm.nih.gov/pubmed/15100629. Accessed 27 May 2019.

37. Rabago D, Best TM, Beamsley M, Patterson J. A systematic review of prolotherapy for chronic musculoskeletal pain. Clin J Sport Med. 2005;15(5):376–80. http://www.ncbi.nlm.nih.gov/pubmed/16162983. Accessed 27 May 2019.

38. Khan KM, Cook JL, Bonar F, Harcourt P, Strom M. Histopathology of common tendinopathies. Sport Med. 1999;27(6):393–408. https://doi.org/10.2165/00007256-199927060-00004.

39. Taylor SA, Hannafin JA. Evaluation and management of elbow tendinopathy. Sport Heal Multidiscip Approach. 2012;4(5):384–93. https://doi.org/10.1177/1941738112454651.

40. Zeisig E, Fahlstrom M, Ohberg L, Alfredson H. Pain relief after intratendinous injections in patients with tennis elbow: results of a randomised study. Br J Sports Med. 2008;42(4):267–71. https://doi.org/10.1136/bjsm.2007.042762.

41. Scarpone M, Rabago DP, Zgierska A, Arbogast G, Snell E. The efficacy of prolotherapy for lateral epicondylosis: a pilot study. Clin J Sport Med. 2008;18(3):248–54. https://doi.org/10.1097/JSM.0b013e318170fc87.

42. Carayannopoulos A, Borg-Stein J, Sokolof J, Meleger A, Rosenberg D. Prolotherapy versus corticosteroid injections for the treatment of lateral epicondylosis: a randomized controlled trial. PM R. 2011;3(8):706–15. https://doi.org/10.1016/j.pmrj.2011.05.011.

43. Rabago D, Lee KS, Ryan M, et al. Hypertonic dextrose and morrhuate sodium injections (prolotherapy) for lateral epicondylosis (tennis elbow). Am J Phys Med Rehabil. 2013;92(7):587–96. https://doi.org/10.1097/PHM.0b013e31827d695f.

44. Yelland MJ, Sweeting KR, Lyftogt JA, Ng SK, Scuffham PA, Evans KA. Prolotherapy injections and eccentric loading exercises for painful Achilles tendinosis: a randomised trial. Br J Sport Med. 2011;45:421–8. https://doi.org/10.1136/bjsm.2009.057968.

45. Maxwell NJ, Ryan MB, Taunton JE, Gillies JH, Wong AD. Sonographically guided Intratendinous injection of hyperosmolar dextrose to treat chronic tendinosis of the Achilles tendon: a pilot study. Am J Roentgenol. 2007;189(4):W215–20. https://doi.org/10.2214/AJR.06.1158.

46. Lee D-H, Kwack K-S, Rah UW, Yoon S-H. Prolotherapy for refractory rotator cuff disease: retrospective case-control study of 1-year follow-up archives of physical medicine and rehabilitation. Arch Phys Med Rehabil. 2015;96:2027–32. https://doi.org/10.1016/j.apmr.2015.07.011.

47. Seven MM, Ersen O, Akpancar S, et al. Effectiveness of prolotherapy in the treatment of chronic rotator cuff lesions. Orthop Traumatol Surg Res. 2017;103(3):427–33. https://doi.org/10.1016/j.otsr.2017.01.003.

48. George J, Ch'ng Li S, Jaafar Z, Shariff M, Hamid A. Clinical study comparative effectiveness of ultrasound-guided intratendinous prolotherapy injection with conventional treatment to treat focal supraspinatus tendinosis. Scientifica (Cairo). 2018;2018:1. https://doi.org/10.1155/2018/4384159.

49. Minerva Medica E, Lin C, Huang C, Huang S-W. Effects of hypertonic dextrose injection on chronic supraspinatus tendinopathy of the shoulder: randomized placebo-controlled trial. Eur J Phys Rehabil Med. 2018. https://doi.org/10.23736/S1973-9087.18.05379-0.

50. Bertrand H, Reeves KD, Bennett CJ, Bicknell S, Cheng A-L. Dextrose prolotherapy versus control injections in painful rotator cuff tendinopathy. Arch Phys Med Rehabil. 2016;97:17–25. https://doi.org/10.1016/j.apmr.2015.08.412.

51. Cole B, Lam P, Hackett L, Murrell GAC. Ultrasound-guided injections for supraspinatus tendinopathy: corticosteroid versus glucose prolotherapy-a randomized controlled clinical trial. Shoulder Elbow. 10:170. https://doi.org/10.1177/1758573217708199.

52. Lin M-T, Chiang C-F, Wu C-H, Huang Y-T, Tu Y-K, Wang T-G. Comparative effectiveness of injection therapies in rotator cuff tendinopathy: a systematic review, pairwise and network meta-analysis of randomized controlled trials. Rev Artic Arch Phys Med Rehabil. 2019;100:336–85. https://doi.org/10.1016/j.apmr.2018.06.028.

53. Yelland MJ, Glasziou PP, Bogduk N, Schluter PJ, McKernon M. Prolotherapy injections, saline injections, and exercises for chronic low-back pain: a randomized trial. Spine (Phila Pa 1976). 2004;29(1):9–16. https://doi.org/10.1097/01.BRS.0000105529.07222.5B.

54. Peterson TH. Injection treatment for back pain. Am J Orthop. 1963;5:320–5. http://www.ncbi. nlm.nih.gov/pubmed/14082650. Accessed 27 May 2019.

55. Ongley MJ, Klein RG, Dorman TA, Eek BC, Hubert LJ. A new approach to the treatment of chronic low back pain. Lancet (London, England). 1987;2(8551):143–6. http://www.ncbi.nlm. nih.gov/pubmed/2439856. Accessed 27 May 2019.

56. Klein RG, Eek B, Delong W, Mooney V. A randomized double-blind trial of dextrose-glycerine-phenol injections for chronic, low back pain. – PubMed – NCBI. J Spinal Disord. 1993;6(1):23–33. https://www.ncbi.nlm.nih.gov/pubmed/?term=klein+rg%2C+eek+bc%2C+delong+wb. Accessed 27 May 2019.

57. Dechow E, Davies RK, Carr AJ, Thompson PW. A randomized, double-blind, placebo-controlled trial of sclerosing injections in patients with chronic low back pain. Rheumatology (Oxford). 1999;38(12):1255–9. https://doi.org/10.1093/rheumatology/38.12.1255.

58. Grayson MF. Sterile meningitis after lumbosacral ligament sclerosing injections. J Orthop Med. 1994;16(3):98–9. https://doi.org/10.1080/1355297X.1994.11719765.

59. Schneider RC, Williams JJ, Liss L. Fatality after injection of sclerosing agent to precipitate fibro-osseous proliferation. J Am Med Assoc. 1959;170(15):1768–72. http://www.ncbi.nlm. nih.gov/pubmed/13672766. Accessed 27 May 2019.

60. Hunt WE, Baird WC. Complications following injection of sclerosing agent to precipitate fibro-osseous proliferation. J Neurosurg. 1961;18(4):461–5. https://doi.org/10.3171/jns.1961.18.4.0461.

Chapter 7
Regenerative Medicine for the Spine

Anthony J. Mazzola and David A. Spinner

Introduction

The spine consists of 33 vertebrae comprising the cervical, thoracic, lumbar, sacral, and coccygeal segments. Each vertebra unit has attachments to muscles and ligaments, as well as sites of articulation with adjacent vertebrae. The typical vertebra has six joints. Due to this complex network, there are several targets where regenerative medicine can prove to be an effective treatment. This chapter will highlight the current evidence for regenerative medicine to treat common spine pathology.

Epidemiology

Back pain is among the most common patient complaints. In the adult general population, the point prevalence for low back pain is believed to be approximately 12%, the one-month prevalence 23%, the one-year prevalence 38%, and the lifetime prevalence approximately 40% [1]. In regard to neck pain, it is estimated that 20% of the adult population experiences neck pain over a one-year period and around 66% experience neck pain at one point in their lives [2]. In the United States (US), low back pain is the number one cause of years lived with disability and neck pain is ranked sixth [3]. Between 2008 and 2012, a study of the Medicare database illustrated 6,206,578 patients were diagnosed with lumbar and 3,156,215 patients were diagnosed with cervical degenerative conditions [4]. It has been estimated that 10–15% of back pain becomes chronic and, in this subset,

A. J. Mazzola · D. A. Spinner (✉)
Department of Rehabilitation and Human Performance, Icahn School of Medicine
at Mount Sinai, New York, NY, USA
e-mail: David.Spinner@mountsinai.org

© Springer Nature Switzerland AG 2020
G. Cooper et al. (eds.), *Regenerative Medicine for Spine and Joint Pain*,
https://doi.org/10.1007/978-3-030-42771-9_7

can lead to long-lasting disability. Around 80–90% of health care and social costs stemming from back pain result from this small cohort who develops chronic low back pain and disability. Just over 1% of adults in the US are permanently disabled by back pain, and another 1% are on temporary disability [5]. Those with chronic low back pain also have higher odds of unemployment [6]. With an aging population, preventative measures or treatments with the capability to reverse or halt progression are needed.

Most current treatments for back pain focus on targeting the overactive nerves responsible for the pain sensations. The most common are steroid injections and nerve ablations. In the short term many of these treatments provide significant relief; however, if the initial aggravating factors are not improved, the pain will often relapse. This leads to a population with chronic back pain. Furthermore, before the opioid crisis, many of these patients were routinely started on narcotic medications. Opioid use disorders have moved from the 11th leading cause of disability-adjusted life years in 1990 to the 7th leading cause in 2016, representing a 74.5% (95% UI, 42.8–93.9%) increase. Opioid use disorder from 1990 to 2016 went from 52nd place to 15th place on years of life lost due to premature mortality [3]. Back pain and opioid use are often linked; from one population-based survey more than 50% of opioid users reported back pain [7]. Today, the negative effects of chronic opioid use are better understood. Thus, newer treatment methods including regenerative medicine have the opportunity to provide significant relief while also proving to be safer than historical treatments. To understand the targets of regenerative medicine we will discuss the spine anatomy.

Anatomy

The spine consists of 7 cervical vertebrae, 12 thoracic vertebrae, 5 lumbar vertebrae, the sacrum (5 fused sacral vertebrae), and the coccyx (3–4 fused coccygeal vertebrae). Each vertebra unit has attachments to muscles and ligaments, as well as sites of articulation with adjacent vertebrae. The typical vertebra has two symphysis joints and four synovial joints. Each symphysis includes an intervertebral disc: one above connecting the superior vertebra and one below connecting the inferior vertebra. The synovial joints are located posteriorly and are between the articular processes. Connecting the sacrum to the lower body and distributing weight to both lower extremities is the pair of sacroiliac synovial joints. The intervertebral disc (IVD) consists of an outer annulus fibrosus and an inner nucleus pulposus. The annulus fibrosus consists of an outer ring of collagen surrounding a wider zone made of fibrocartilage and configured in a lamellar fashion. This fiber arrangement limits rotation among vertebrae. The nucleus pulposus (NP) is the center of the disc and is a gelatinous substance. It is responsible for absorbing compression forces. Between adjacent vertebra lies the intervertebral foramen through where the spinal nerve emerges from the spinal column [8].

The joints between vertebrae are supported by numerous ligaments. These ligaments reinforce the joints as they pass between vertebral bodies and interconnect structures of the vertebral arches. Along the anterior and posterior vertebral bodies lie the anterior and posterior longitudinal ligaments. The ligamenta flava connect the lamina of adjacent vertebrae. Passing along the posterior tips of the vertebra spinous processes from C7 to the sacrum is the supraspinous ligament. From C7 to the skull the ligament is known as the ligamentum nuchae as it has distinct features responsible for supporting the head. Interspinous ligaments pass between adjacent spinous processes [8].

The sacroiliac (SI) joints act to transmit forces from the lower limbs to the vertebral column. These joints are synovial joints; they lie between the L-shaped articular facets on the lateral surfaces of the sacrum and similar facets on the iliac. The joint is designed with irregular contour and interlocks to resist movement. With age the joint can become fibrous and may become completely ossified. The joint is stabilized by surrounding ligaments: the anterior sacroiliac ligament, interosseous sacroiliac ligament, and posterior sacroiliac ligament. Because this joint is weight-bearing, it is prone to degenerative changes [8].

The back musculature can be divided into the superficial group that aid in movements of the limbs, the intermediate group that may serve in respiration, and the deep group that are related to movements of the vertebral column. This deep group becomes essential for the health of the spine. Thoracolumbar fascia covers these deep muscles. The largest group of these intrinsic back muscles are the erector spinae muscles: the iliocostalis, longissimus, and spinalis. Deep to these muscles are the transversospinalis muscles which include the semispinalis, multifidus, and small rotatores muscles. The deepest group of muscles include the segmental muscles which pass between adjacent spinous processes and transverse processes. All the muscles above provide some form of stabilization or movement to the spine itself. Any derangements in these muscles, or the abdominal muscles that counteract them, can lead to abnormal function of the spine that may progress to pathology that manifests as back pain [8].

In understanding spinal pain, it is important to identify the innervated structures. These include: the vertebrae bony body (by the sinuvertebral nerve anteriorly), the zygapophyseal joint (by the medial branch of the dorsal primary ramus), the external annulus of a healthy disc (posteriorly by the sinuvertebral nerve), the anterior longitudinal ligament and anterior external annulus (by the recurrent branches of rami communicantes), posterior longitudinal ligament (by the sinuvertebral nerve), interspinous ligament (medial branch of the dorsal primary ramus), muscles (specifically the multifidus by the medial branch of the dorsal primary ramus and the paraspinal musculature by small branches of the dorsal primary ramus) and fascia (by small branches of the dorsal primary ramus), and the nerve roots themselves. The ligamentum flavum and a healthy disc's internal annulus fibrosus and nucleus pulposus are not innervated and therefore do not transmit pain signals. The posterior longitudinal ligament is often thought to be the cause of pain perception in disc herniation [9].

Overview of Back Pain Pathology and Treatment

As discussed above, the spine is composed of bones that are further supported by a network of ligaments and muscles. The spine's main role is to protect the sensitive spinal canal and support the upper body. Its secondary function is to provide mobility and movement, which is allowed by the various joint spaces along each vertebra. These include the two zygapophyseal joints (facet joints) and the intervertebral disc itself with each vertebral end plates. The spine has a natural opposing curvature pattern to soften loading forces and disperse force throughout each vertebra. Any abnormality at each of the above structures can lead to inefficient working of this spine complex that often presents as pain. As instability or increased forces target one particular location of the spine, this area often begins to generate pain.

Pain from the spine is traditionally divided into axial or radicular. Axial pain is located primarily at the spine level, where radicular pain is mostly experienced in the extremities. Radicular pain results from irritation or pinching of a spinal nerve as it exits the spinal cord. Axial back pain can be further divided into discogenic, facet mediated, or stenotic. Pain located below L5 can also be caused by the sacroiliac joint. Furthermore, fractures can occur at any boney location, most commonly at the pars interarticularis [9].

Treating back pain proves to be a challenge particularly because there is often no concrete single diagnosis and there is rarely one physical exam, laboratory, or imaging test that gives a precise answer. One study looking at MRIs of asymptomatic, pain-free individuals found that 37% of those 20 years of age showed disc degeneration and >90% of those over 60 years of age had degenerative spine changes on MRI. Similarly, 4% of the asymptomatic patients 20 years of age showed facet degeneration, while 50% of those aged 60 years old did [10]. In another MRI study, disc herniations were strongly associated with low back pain; however, annular fissures, high-intensity zone lesions, Modic changes, and spondylotic defects were all not associated with low back pain severity [11]. Thus, the pain generator often may not correlate with specific findings on imaging or other studies.

Prior to trialing a regenerative intervention, it is essential to first categorize the likely etiology of the pain. While nerve blocks and ablations target the nerves causing pain directly, regenerative medicine has the additional opportunity to target the precipitating cause of the pain. By targeting the reason why the patient has pain in the first place, it is hopeful some form of regenerative medicine will eventually be able to provide a cure, or at least halt the disease progression, rather than temporarily masking the pain.

Back pain is often multifaceted and results from a combination of pathologies. To provide a theoretical framework to highlight the effectiveness of regenerative medicine, we will group similar mechanical pain and pathology into common categories. It is important to keep in mind that the patient may suffer from multiple individual pathologies which when combined together are now the cause of presentation. Similarly, once one element of the vertebral unit is affected this often places abnormal stress on the rest further causing pathology at distinct locations. In chronic low back pain, around 42% are related to the discs, 31% related to SI joint, and 18% related to zygapophyseal joint [12].

Pain Generators of the Spine

Intervertebral Disc Pain

The intervertebral disc itself is crucial to the health of the spine. Several pathologies of the disc itself, including internal disc disruption, tears in the disc, degeneration of the disc, and loss of disc height, can predispose patients to discogenic back pain. The disc acts as a shock absorber. Degeneration often correlates with loss of disc height that can lead to excess motion and unstableness throughout the other joints of the spine. While we will focus on pain related to the disc itself, damage to the disc may lead to excess forces and damage throughout the spine. In order to illustrate the action of regenerative medicine on the disc it is important to understand the disc's histological makeup.

The disc is a central part to the complex biomechanical system of the spine, which allows for mobility and the spreading of stress. The disc is divided into four separate regions. The outer annulus is highly organized with mostly type 1 collagenous lamellae running in an alternating pattern to assist in strength. The inner annulus is larger and more fibrocartilaginous, with less collagen and lacking the lamellar structure; this collagen is mostly type II. The cells here are both fibroblasts and chondrocytes. The third layer is the transition zone made up of a thin acellular fibrous layer. The final layer, the central nucleus pulposus, is an amorphous matrix of highly hydrated proteoglycans that are embedded in now a loose network of collagen [13].

The disc itself is a sensitive environment as it is avascular at baseline. Thus, it depends on diffusion for nutrients and waste movement. This diffusion capacity is relatively poor and worsens with both age and pathology. In normal discs, nerve endings are limited to the outer one-third of the disc and are not found in the inner annulus or nucleus pulposus region [14]. In degenerated IVDs, nociceptive nerve fibers along with vasculature migrate into the central disc regions [15]. It is theorized that neurotransmitters together with changes within the extracellular matrix itself and the release of cytokines regulate this nerve ingrowth to the IVD. In addition, pain-related peptides and proinflammatory cytokines are increased.

Disc failure can be a result of overloading. Forces may lead to desiccation of the disc and annular tears. The disc itself has a limited capacity for compression and this capacity decreases with decreasing water content—as fluid is not compressible. To improve disc failure, the treatment goal is to regain disc height to reduce the axial nerve compression and to restore the tissue dynamics (fluid content) of the annulus. Secondly, the goal is to reconstitute the central nucleus with a matrix environment that can hold water and improve nutritional flow. A prosthetic disc nucleus has been designed to restore the disc height. However, it fails to fully simulate the compressibility and plasticity of the original disc. Furthermore, this implantation requires a fairly invasive procedure. Using regenerative medicine techniques, the hopes are to "regenerate" the nucleus and disc by injecting the nucleus with a complement of its original cells. In theory, these cells will reconstitute a matrix that will have the capacity to change the damaged internal environment of the disc and eventually reorganize to improve and return disc function [16].

As discussed, the IVD is composed of an interconnected unit of tissues that work together: the nucleus pulposus, annulus fibrosus supporting the nucleus pulposus, and the cartilaginous end plates that connect these tissues to the vertebral bodies providing nutrients. Thus, either of these can be targeted for potential regenerative medicine. Depending on degree of degeneration, different strategies are proposed. In early degeneration, biomolecular treatment strategies (including platelet-rich plasma (PRP), prolotherapy, and hyaluronic acid) are often considered to best support the viable cells remaining in hopes of reverting or halting progression of disease. In intermediate degeneration, cell-based therapies (articular chondrocytes, nucleus pulposus, disc chondrocytes, and stem cells) are required as the numbers of viable cells are decreased. At advanced degeneration, tissue engineering may be required as there is now structural damage and the number of viable cells is severely limited. The literature review by Moriguchi et al. suggests that protein injections are limited due to their relatively short life span. Gene therapy, which involves delivering certain genes through viral or nonviral vectors, has a promising future as it is able to induce modification of the intradiscal expression of genes for a long-term effect. Furthermore, tissue engineering advancements allow for the development of biocompatible and biomimetic scaffolding material to recover extensive loss of matrix cells and structural environment [17]. A meta-analysis by Wu et al. suggests that mesenchymal stem cell (MSC) and chondrocyte therapy for discogenic low back pain correlates with improved pain relief and function metrics. Currently, the authors conclude that there lacks an optimal cell therapy protocol. At this time, cell therapy is not considered a standard treatment; however, it has the potential to be a consideration especially in patients that have not adequately responded to nonoperative management [18].

Much of regenerative medicine studies regarding the spine focus on the intervertebral disc itself. An ex vivo experiment by Pirvu et al. on bovine annular fibrosus cells shows that platelet-rich preparations increased the matrix production and cell number after their injection into an annular fibrosus defect [19]. Another ex vivo study by Kim et al. looked at nucleus pulposus cells from human discs that were cultured in a collagen matrix. PRP administration markedly suppressed cytokine-induced pro-inflammatory degrading enzymes and mediators in the NP cell. As per the authors, it stabilized NP cell differentiation through rescued gene expression concerning matrix synthesis [20]. An additional study by Akeda et al. looked at in vitro porcine IVD cells post-PRP exposure. They concluded PRP had a mild stimulatory effect on cell proliferation. There was a significant upregulation of proteoglycans and collagen synthesis and proteoglycan accumulation compared to platelet-poor plasma [21]. These studies provide data that suggests PRP supports a regenerative-like environment at the cellular level.

One animal study by Wang et al. looked at rabbits that underwent annular needle puncture to simulate early degenerative discs. The rabbits were then injected with BMSCs and PRP, just PRP, and a control group of phosphate-buffered saline. At 8 weeks postinjection, PRP-containing bone marrow-derived mesenchymal stem cells (BMSCs) were more effective than PRP alone as evidenced by an increase in signal intensity over time, and under histological staining the extracellular matrix and cell density as well as type II collagen staining were preserved. Several other animal studies show promising results [22]. A study on platelets and BMSCs by Xu et al. demonstrated effective repair of annulus defects [23]. Another study by Hou et al. on PRP intradiscal injections post needle puncture demonstrated significant recovery of MRI signal intensity. They suggest PRP can enhance the nucleus pulposus cell's proliferation and anabolic pathway while slowing IVD degeneration in rabbits [24]. A randomized controlled trial (RCT) by Gui et al. investigated intradiscal PRP in rabbits post annulus fibrosus puncture. In the control groups, there were significant IVD height changes compared to the slight decrease in the PRP-treated group [25]. Gullung et al. looked at six rats each in a control, sham, PRP immediately post disc injury with needle, and PRP 2 weeks after disc injury. The PRP groups had fibers that were damaged with empty spaces and inflammatory cells; however overall there was maintenance of the ring structure and the nucleus appeared to keep a healthy central portion. They conclude that immediate injection has a more pronounced effect as the disc height and fluid content on MRI was significantly better in the immediate injection group compared to the sham group at 4 weeks. This study suggests that there may be a time component to treatment effects with regenerative medicine. As most patients often receive injections years after initial injury, this beneficial effect may have limited value in the clinical population [26].

While several of these above studies were RCTs and there seems to be some scientific agreement in favor of regenerative medicine, it is difficult to adopt these animal study results into clinical practice. It is important to highlight that these animals do not reflect the same stressors and pathology that is evident in patients with chronic degenerative disc disease (DDD). Often, the animals are relatively healthy and undergo a single acute stressor event to create disc pathology. Hence the environment of the disc may be more salvageable compared to that of a classic patient presenting with chronic degenerative disc disease.

Focusing on selected human trials, Miller et al. analyzed 76 consecutive patients that received intradiscal prolotherapy who suffered from internal lumbar disc derangements. These patients had undergone two epidural steroid injections (ESIs) 2 weeks apart and had initial good relief followed with later a return of symptoms. Post prolotherapy, 43.4% of patients had at least 20% reduction in pain scores and pain relief was maintained at an average of 18 months. This study provides some support in favor of intradiscal prolotherapy to treat internal disc disease [27].

Focusing on PRP, Akeda et al. led a prospective clinical study evaluating intradiscal PRP releasate in 14 patients who had positive diagnostic discography. More than 50% reduction in low back pain was seen in 71% of patients within 4 weeks of injection, and this relief was generally maintained throughout the 48-week study period. Furthermore, the authors conclude there was no change in T2 imaging and disc height which suggests no negative effects on the disc matrix [28]. In a similar prospective trial, Levi et al. injected 22 subjects intradiscally with PRP and at 2 months 41% had a successful outcome of greater than 50% decrease in visual analogue scale (VAS). At 6 months, 63% had a VAS improvement at least 20 mm [29]. An RCT by Tuakli-Wosornu et al. randomized 29 patients to intradiscal PRP and 18 to the control group receiving intradiscal contrast only. Over 8-week follow-up there were statistically significant improvements in patients who received the intradiscal PRP in pain scale, function, and patient satisfaction compared to controls. Furthermore, those who received PRP were able to maintain significant improvements in the Functional Rating Index (FRI) for at least 1-year follow-up [30].

Other studies examined PRP in patients undergoing spine surgery. Sys et al. randomized 18 patients to undergo spinal fusion with PRP-soaked autologous bone to fill the cages and 18 patients to serve as a control without the PRP soaking. The added PRP in posterior lumbar interbody fusion did not lead to a substantial improvement or deterioration when compared with autologous bone only. The PRP and autologous group trended toward improvements in VAS and Oswestry Disability Index (ODI). This study points out that there may be little improvement in using PRP during spinal fusions and it can be justified from a clinical and radiological point of view; however it may not be efficient from an economical perspective [31].

Overall PRP is generally safe and has few documented adverse effects besides from local pain temporarily post procedure. Furthermore, as patient's own blood is used this limits risks of infection and rejection. One downside to PRP is that it only provides the IVD with certain factors that may aid repair. However, if the disc cells are already severely damaged, some suggest that no amount of PRP may make a difference [32]. Thus, PRP may be more efficient when applied at an earlier stage of degeneration, in a patient that has relatively a healthy amount of functioning cells. This is where stem cells theoretically may have the advantage as they may act to replace severely degenerated cells.

Investigating stem cells, Orozco et al. reported on a case series of ten patients with chronic discogenic back pain that were treated with autologous culture-expanded bone marrow MSCs injected into the nucleus pulposus area. This study showed strong safety and feasibility. Patients exhibited improvements in both pain and disability measures. Disc height was not recovered, but water content was significantly improved on MRI [33]. Similarly, Elahd et al. studied five patients with DDD post intradiscal injection of autologous, hypoxic cultured, BMSCs. Post 4–6 years, no adverse events were reported. All patients self-reported overall improvement [34]. Pettine et al. analyzed 26 patients that were candidates for spinal fusion or total disc replacement surgery. Instead, they underwent autologous bone marrow concentrate intradiscal injection into the nucleus pulposus. After 36 months, only six patients progressed to surgery. The remaining 20 other patients reported improvements in ODI and VAS. One year MRI showed that 40% of the subjects improved one modified Pfirrmann grade and no patients worsened. Those with greater concentration of stem cells had better outcomes [35]. Furthermore, Centeno et al. studied autologous MSCs in 37 patients with DDD with secondary radicular pain. The treatments in this study included a preinjection 2 weeks before MSC injection that included a platelet lysate transforaminal epidural injection. Then, MSCs that had been cultured in platelet lysate were injected intradiscal. Two weeks later a second transforaminal epidural with platelet lysate injection was performed. At all-time points from 3 months to 24 months there was significant improvement in pain scores. FRI was statistically improved at all-time points except at 12 months. Twenty patients underwent posttreatment MRI and 85% showed reduction in disc bulge size. Due to a lack of control group, this study is limited in determining the efficacy of these interventions as it is well known that patients often improve with time regardless of treatment [36]. Although the above studies are promising, further RCTs are needed before recommendations can be made.

In an RCT by Noriega et al. 24 patients were randomized so that 12 patients received intradiscal allogeneic (from someone else) MSCs and 12 patients received sham paravertebral musculature local anesthetic treatment. This study demonstrated stem cell-treated subjects had significant improvements in algofunctional indices. However, the improvement seemed to be restricted to a group of responders representing 40% of the cohort. Degeneration graded by MRI and Pfirrmann grading improved in those treated with stem cells and worsened in the controls. This study supports the utilization of allogeneic stem cells which are more convenient than the autologous MSC treatment that must be harvested from the patient [37]. A second RCT by Bae et al. randomized a total of 100 patients to intradiscal injection treatment: 20 patients received hyaluronic acid, 30 patients received allogeneic mesenchymal precursor cells (MPCs) at 6 million dose, 30 patients received allogeneic MPCs at 18 million dose, and 20 received saline to serve as a control. The authors concluded that allogeneic MPCs showed improvements in pain and function and reduced interventions compared to the control group. However, when comparing the stem cell group to the hyaluronic acid group, the results did not reach statistical significance [38].

Secondary to the myriad of components and mixtures that can be utilized in regenerative medicine, studies comparing different mixtures or recipes of injectate present a challenge. Mochida et al. studied mixing autologous NP cells with BMSCs. Nine patients scheduled for fusion underwent harvesting of NP cells. Viable NP cells were co-cultured in direct contact with autologous BMSCs. At 1-week post fusion they underwent transplantation at adjacent levels to the fusion of the now activated NP cells. Imaging revealed improvement in one case, and functional improvement overall was minimal [39]. Studies are needed to determine the best dosage, combination, and type of injectate.

It has been shown that stem cells can also be derived from adipose cells. Kumar et al. looked at adipose tissue-derived mesenchymal stem cells combined with hyaluronic acid in ten patients who had discogenic pain with positive discography. There were no serious adverse effects at 1 year and these patients had significant improvements in VAS, ODI, and Short Form-36 (SF-36). Three of the ten patients were determined to have increased water content in their discs as determined by

MRI [40]. Similarly, Comella et al. analyzed 15 patients that underwent adipose tissue-derived stromal vascular fraction (SVF) injection directly into the nucleus pulposus. At 6 months there were no serious adverse effects, and patients improved in flexion and VAS and SF-12. ODI and Dallas pain questionnaire only showed positive trends [41].

Others have utilized stem cells from the umbilical cord. Pang et al. looked at two patients with chronic discogenic pain that were treated with human umbilical cord tissue-derived MSCs. In the two patients, pain and function improved and was maintained for a 2-year follow-up. Furthermore, the water content in the degenerative disc of one patient was found to have significant improvement. This method avoids the invasive procedures required in harvesting stem cells [42]. A separate class of stem cells include hematopoietic stem cells that have the capability to give rise to other blood cells. Huafe et al. looked at ten patients with positive discograms that received intradiscal injection of hematopoietic precursor stem cells obtained from their pelvic bone marrow. Zero patients reported improvement. This study suggests that while there may be benefit for MSCs, HSCs do not appear to have similar efficacy. The authors suggest that perhaps the HSCs are unable to survive the oxygen-poor environment of the inner disc [43]. More studies are necessary to determine which types of stem cells, if any, have the best efficacy for each diagnosis.

Fibrin is another injectate that has been trialed to help those with discogenic pain. Yin et al. reported on 15 adults with confirmed discogenic pain that underwent intradiscal injection of a fibrin sealant. Eighty-seven percent of the subjects achieved at least a 30% reduction in low back VAS compared with baseline at the 26-week primary end point. Although this was not an RCT and only evaluated 15 patients, fibrin may provide benefits in certain patients. Fibrin is composed of purified prothrombin and fibrinogen and reconstituted with aprotinin and calcium. When injected into the annular tears, it has the ability to form a matrix sealant protecting the nucleus pulposus [44].

Intradiscal methylene blue (MB) has also been trialed for patients with discogenic pain. Peng et al. looked at 72 subjects equally randomized to either the MB injection or the control group that received isotonic saline instead. In the MB group, there was a mean reduction in the numeric rating scale (NRS) of 52.4 and ODI by 35.58 and 91.6% patient satisfaction at 24 months. This was a significant improvement over the control group [45]. Once again further studies are needed to replicate these strong findings.

Others have suggested that regeneration of the disc should not be the primary goal when treating these patients with back pain. Adams et al. suggest that we should separate our focus among healing a painful disc and reversing disc degeneration, as these may be two distinct pathways. Discs are often the cause of pain as nerves in the peripheral annulus or vertebral endplate become affected by inflammation and/ or radial tears. Adams et al. conclude we should primarily focus on this peripheral region which has the cell density and metabolite transport to improve, rather than the more difficult notion of regenerating the nucleus pulposus. Regardless of the degenerative changes in the nucleus, promoting healing at the periphery can provide significant pain relief. Physical therapy, which employs mechanical loading, can act as a healing stimulus in the peripheral disc. For radial fissure, the authors recommend initial controlled mobilization toward the direction that decreases pain; then after scar formation, stretching should be directed toward the painful direction in hopes of promoting remodeling. In the case of an endplate fracture, initial therapy would include unloading followed by progressive loading and if needed intermittent traction [46].

Although the above studies (Table 7.1) are promising treatments for IVD pain, there is a general lack of comparable RCTs leading to poor overall evidence level. In examining these studies, it is crucial to acknowledge the diagnosis being treated and the precise injectate utilized. Before recommendations for treatment can be more RCTs are needed to support evidenced-based medicine.

Radiculopathy

Moving from pain resulting from the disc itself, a second generator of pain is caused by irritation or pressure on the nerve root creating a radiculopathy. This can be caused by a bulging disc, herniated disc, and/or stenosis. The classic pain felt is in the distribution of the sensory nerve root. For instance, in the lower back this shooting, electrical type of pain will be reported to be traveling down the lower extremities. Depending on which nerve root is involved, the pain often localizes to a certain extremity or dermatome. Affected cervical nerve roots often will transmit pain down the ipsilateral arm, while affected lumbar nerve roots will have symptoms from the waist down.

For acute radicular pain the routine care is commonly epidural or transforaminal steroid injection. However, although they show some short-term pain relief, they have increasingly been criticized for failure to provide lasting benefit while exposing the patient to potential risks and side effects. To better improve outcomes several clinicians have investigated the efficacy of PRP, dextrose or prolotherapy, and stem cells.

In a pilot study by Bhatia et al. ten patients with prolapsed IVD were injected with 5 ml of PRP with an interlaminar approach into the area of affected nerve root. A significant number of patients showed relief and sustained relief at 3 months. The authors conclude that PRP can be used in replace of steroids; however, a randomly controlled trial comparing the two is needed [47]. In 2017, Cameron et al. reported on PRP injections in 88 total subjects: 38 for cervical, 38 for lumbar, and 12 for both cervical and lumbar disc herniation. PRP was injected in a circumferential manner of the affected area into the lateral masses, facet joints, lateral gutters, and inter- and supraspinatus ligaments, Kambin's triangle, and spinous process. This prospective nonrandomized clinical study suggested each group of patients showed a significant improvement in pain scores [48].

Similarly, Centeno et al. analyzed a case series of 470 patients who were treated with platelet lysate and nanogram dose hydrocortisone. As per the authors, the nanogram amount of steroid used in the formation of platelet lysate is one million

Table 7.1 Regenerative medicine for intervertebral disk pain studies reviewed

Author, date [injectate]	Methodology, patients, and comparison group	Follow-up and outcome measures	Diagnosis	Injectate preparation and route	Results	Authors' conclusion	Study analysis and notes
Miller et al. [27] [prolotherapy]	Prospective consecutive patient series n = 76 Intradiscal dextrose inj. biweekly, responders received injs. up to five times biweekly	P-NRS biweekly before inj. and at 2, 6, and 18 mos. F/u (f/u) 6–41; mean of 18 mos.	Internal lumbar disc derangement who underwent two ESIs 2 wks. apart w/ initial relief followed by return of symptoms. Confirmed w/ discography	Biweekly disc space inj. 3 mL w/ final concentration of 25% dextrose and 0.125% bupivacaine. Solution 50% dextrose and 0.25% bupivacaine	43.4% (33/76) of pts. showed a sustained treatment response (≥20% reduction in pain). For responders, the avg. improvement in the PNRS was 71%	Reductions in P-NRS were maintained in pts. w/ uniformly moderate to severe disc desiccation at an avg. of 18 mos. Those pts. who experienced no appreciable improvement from the treatment were not worse in any sustained way	Level IV
Akeda et al. [28] [PRP releasate]	Prospective clinical feasibility study, primarily a safety assessment n = 14 PRP intradiscal inj. Post positive diagnostic discography	VAS and RMDQ F/u 4, 8, 16, 24, 32, 40, and 48 wks. X-ray and MRI analysis	Discogenic LBP w/o leg pain for more than 3 mos. ≥ At 1 lumbar disc w/ evidence of degenerative changes per MRI and ≥50% of normal disc height	Autologous PRP releasate, 2 mL at center of targeted disc Mean platelet count of PRP was ≈3.7 times > than whole blood. Mean WBC count of PRP was about 1/230 of whole blood. Avg. level of PDGF-BB was ≈2.1 times > autologous serum	>50% reduction of LBP was observed in 71% (10/14) of pts. within 4 wks.; generally maintained through 48 wks. Improvement in RMDQ was relatively better than that in VAS. Particularly, 79% of pts. (11/14) showed a significant reduction (>50%) in RDQ scores 4 wks. after PRP releasate inj. This was maintained for 48 wks.	Lumbar radiographs no significant change in disc height. No change in T2 imaging of AF and NP. No negative affect on the matrix of degenerated IVDs No persistent neurologic deficits	Level IV

Study	Design	Outcome measures	Population	Intervention	Results	Conclusions	Level/Comments
Levi et al. [29] [PRP]	Prospective trial n = 22 PRP inj. directly into the disc nucleus	VAS and ODI scores F/u 1, 2, and 6 mos. Successful outcome = 50% VAS improvement and a 30% ODI improvement	Discogenic pain w/o moderate to severe lumbar radiculopathy. If agreed SI and facet joint blocks were done to rule out other sources of pain	Contrast with gentamicin 16 mg injected for discitis prophylaxis Lidocaine 4%, 0.5 mL. Then, 1.5 mL of autologous WBC-rich PRP was injected intradiscal	At 2 mos. 32% and at 6 mos. 47% of pts. had a successful outcome. At 2 mos. 4 % of pts. had a >50% decrease in VAS. At 6 mos. 63% had a VAS improvement ≥20 mm	Encouraging preliminary 6-month findings, using strict categorical success criteria, for intradiscal PRP as a treatment for presumed discogenic low back pain. Randomized placebo-controlled trials are needed to further evaluate the efficacy of this treatment	Level IV Negative discography was exclusion criteria; however only presumptive discogenic pain was inclusion criteria
Tuakli-Wosornu et al. [30] [PRP]	Prospective, double-blind, randomized controlled n = 47 w/ a positive provocative discography 29 received PRP 18 received only contrast (control group)	FRI; P-NRS, SF-36; NASS Outcome Questionnaire 1, 4, and 8 wks., 6 mos., and 1 yr.	Adults w/ chronic (6 mos.), moderate-to-severe lumbar discogenic pain unresponsive to conservative treatment	1–2 ml contrast into midportion of suspected disc Only disc levels that elicited concordant pain w/ evidence of incomplete annular disruption (<2 mL) were then injected additionally w/ either 1–2 mL of PRP or contrast	Over 8 wks. of f/u, there were statistically significant improvements in participants who received intradiscal PRP w/ regard to pain (P-NRS Best Pain), function (FRI), and patient satisfaction (NASS Outcome Questionnaire) compared w/ controls	Those who received PRP maintained significant improvements in FRI scores through at least 1 year of f/u	Level II No cell counts of PRP collected. Longer f/u needed

(continued)

Table 7.1 (continued)

Author, date [injectate]	Methodology, patients, and comparison group	Follow-up and outcome measures	Diagnosis	Injectate preparation and route	Results	Authors' conclusion	Study analysis and notes
Sys et al. [31] [PRP]	Prospective randomized controlled trial $n = 36$ pts. 18 underwent spinal fusion w/ PRP-soaked autologous bone to fill the cages 18 underwent spinal fusion w/ autologous bone added w/o being soaked in PRP	VAS, ODI, SF-36. F/u at 3, 6, 12, and 24 mos. CT scans of the lumbar spine at 3, 6, and 12 mos.	Pts. scheduled for posterior lumbar interbody fusion surgery w/ single-level disc disease	PRP-soaked autograph bone used to fill the cages during spinal fusion	More pronounced improvements in VAS and the physical component summary score in pts. who received autograft w/ PRP. However, improvement was not substantial and did not reach statistical significance. CT scans showed uneventful osseous healing in all but one patient w/ no difference between groups	From a clinical and radiological point of view, the use of PRP seems to be justified in posterior lumbar interbody fusion surgery. From an economical point of view, the expense of using PRP cannot be justified until statistical significance can be reached in a larger study	Level II Showed little improvement of surgery w/ added PRP. Study limited to specific criteria and use

Orozco et al. [33] [autologous bone marrow MSC]	Case series pilot phase 1 $n = 10$ 10 pts. w/ chronic back pain treated w/ autologous expanded bone marrow MSC injected into the nucleus pulposus area	VAS, ODI, and SF-36. Clinical evolution was followed for 1 year. MRI measurements of disc height and fluid content	DDD w/ preserved external annulus fibrous and persistent LBP failing 6 mos. of conservative treatment	Inj. into IVD Autologous culture-expanded bone marrow MSCs $10 \pm 5 \times 10^6$ cells per disc from a suspension containing 10^7 cells/mL	Rapid improvement of pain and disability (85% of maximum in 3 mos.) $\approx$ 71% of optimal efficacy. Feasibility and safety were confirmed and strong indications of clinical efficacy identified. Although disc height was not recovered, water content was significantly elevated at 12 mos. No improvement in disc height, some increase in T2 signal	MSC therapy may be a valid alternative treatment for chronic back pain caused by DDD. Advantages over current gold standards include simpler and more conservative intervention w/o surgery, preservation of normal biomechanics, and same or better pain relief. This outcome compares favorably w/ spinal fusion or total disc replacement	Level IV

(continued)

Table 7.1 (continued)

Author, date [injectate]	Methodology, patients, and comparison group	Follow-up and outcome measures	Diagnosis	Injectate preparation and route	Results	Authors' conclusion	Study analysis and notes
Elabd et al. [34] [bone marrow-derived MSC]	Long-term f/u study $n = 5$ 5 pts. diagnosed w/ DDD received an intradiscal inj. of autologous, hypoxic cultured, bone marrow-derived mesenchymal stem cells as part of a previous study. These pts. were re-consented and followed for 4–6 years	Physical examination, low back MRI, and quality of life questionnaire	Lumbar degenerative disc disease associated w/ protruding discs. Pts. previously treated as per prior study	Previous inj. of 15.1–51.6 million autologous, hypoxic cultured, bone marrow-derived mesenchymal stem cells	Lower back MRI showed absence of neoplasms or abnormalities surrounding the treated region. No adverse events were reported due to the procedure or to the stem cell treatment 4–6 years post procedure. All pts. self-reported overall improvement, as well as improvement in strength, post stem cell treatment, and 4/5 pts. reported improvement in mobility	This early human clinical data suggests the safety and feasibility of the clinical use of hypoxic cultured bone marrow-derived MSCs for the treatment of LBP due to DDD and support further studies. A larger double-blind, controlled, randomized clinical study w/ significant number of pts. and implementation of validated end point measurements are next steps in order to demonstrate efficacy of this biologic	Level IV

| Pettine et al. [35] [autologous BMC] | Prospective, open-label, nonrandomized, single-arm study using the data from four FDA IDE studies as a comparative baseline $n = 26$ Pts. injected w/ intradiscal BMC in lumbar discs and followed for 3 years | ODI and VAS F/u at 3, 6, 12, 24, and 36 mos. 12-month MRI. All compared to patient demographics and BMC cellularity | DDD and candidates for spinal fusion or total disc replacement surgery | 2 ml of autologous bone marrow concentrate intradiscal inj. into nucleus pulposus Cellular analysis showed an avg. of 121 million total nucleated cells per ml. Avg. CFU-F of 2713 per ml and avg. CD34+ of 1.82 million per ml in the BMC | At 36 mos., six pts. progressed to surgery. The remaining 20 pts. reported avg. ODI and VAS improvements from 56.7 ± 3.6 to 82.1 ± 2.6 at baseline to 17.5 ± 3.2 and 21.9 ± 4.4 after 36 mos., respectively. 1-year MRI: 40% of pts. improved 1 modified Pfirrmann grade. Pts. w/ greater concentrations of CFU-F (>2000/ ml) and CD34+ cells (>2 million/ml) tended to have better clinical improvement | There were no adverse events related to marrow aspiration or inj., and this study provides evidence of safety and feasibility of intradiscal BMC therapy. No radiologic evidence of worsening. Pt. improvement and satisfaction w/ this surgical alternative supports further study of the therapy | Level III |

(continued)

Table 7.1 (continued)

Author, date [injectate]	Methodology, patients, and comparison group	Follow-up and outcome measures	Diagnosis	Injectate preparation and route	Results	Authors' conclusion	Study analysis and notes
Centeno et al. [36] [autologous MSCs]	Pilot study on safety and efficacy $n = 33$ Treated w/ culture-expanded, autologous, bone marrow–derived MSCs	P-NRS, SANE, FRI, measurement of the intervertebral disc posterior dimension, and adverse events F/u at 1, 3, 6, 12, 18, and 24 mos. and annually up to 6 yrs.	DDD and LBP w/ a posterior disc bulge diagnosed on MRI	Pre-inj. 2 wks. prior to MSC, transforaminal epidural using 3–5 cc of PL only at target Then, once MSCs had been subcultured and suspended in 10–20% PL, they were injected into disc annulus Post-inj. 2 wks. after the IVD re-inj. of MSCs, another transforaminal epidural using 3–5 cc of PL at same target	P-NRS changes relative to baseline were significant at 3, 36, 48, 60, and 72 mos. posttreatment. Avg. improvement was 2.3. The avg. SANE ratings showed a mean improvement of 60% at 3 yrs. FRI posttreatment change score avgs. exceeded the minimal clinically important difference at all-time points except 12 mos. 20 pts. treated underwent posttreatment MRI and 85% had a reduction in disc bulge size, w/ an avg. reduction size of 23% posttreatment	Pts. treated w/ autologous cultured MSCs for lower back pain w/ radicular symptoms in the setting of DDD reported minor adverse events and significant improvements in pain, function, and overall subjective improvement through 6 years of f/u. Three pts. reported pain related to procedure that resolved. No serious adverse events (i.e., death, infection, or tumor) w/the procedure	Level IV

| Noriega et al. [37] [allogeneic MSCs] | Phase I–II prospective randomized controlled clinical trial $n = 24$ 12 received intradiscal allogeneic MSCs 12 received sham paravertebral musculature local anesthetic treatment | VAS, ODI F/u 3,6,12 mos. Disc quality was followed up by magnetic resonance imaging | Lumbar LBP w/ Pfirrmann grade II–IV DDD, unresponsive to conventional treatments (physical and medical) for at least 6 mos. before recruitment | Allogeneic MSCs (25×10^6 MSC in 2 mL of saline per disc) under local anesthesia intradiscal Or sham infiltration of paravertebral musculature close to the affected disc(s) w/ 2 mL of 1% mepivacaine | MSC-treated pts. displayed a quick and significant improvement in algofunctional indices versus the controls. This improvement seemed restricted to a group of responders that included 40% of the cohort. Degeneration, quantified by Pfirrmann grading, improved in the MSC-treated pts. and worsened in the controls | Feasibility and safety were confirmed and indications of clinical efficacy were identified. Allogeneic MSC therapy may be a valid alternative for the treatment of DDD that is more logistically convenient than the autologous MSC treatment. The intervention is simple, does not require surgery, provides pain relief, and significantly improves disc quality | Level II |

(continued)

Table 7.1 (continued)

Author, date [injectate]	Methodology, patients, and comparison group	Follow-up and outcome measures	Diagnosis	Injectate preparation and route	Results	Authors' conclusion	Study analysis and notes
Bae et al. [38] [allogeneic MPCs]	Prospective, multicenter, randomized, double-blind, controlled study $n = 100$ 20 pts. injected w/ saline. 20 pts. inj. w/ HA MPC inj. groups: 30 pts. w/ 6×10^6 MPCs 30 pts. w/ 1.8×10^7 MPCs	VAS and ODI F/u at 1, 3, 6, 12, 24, and 36 mos. Success = 30% improvement in VAS, 10-point improvement in ODI. MRI and X-ray for stability	Moderate to severe chronic LBP due to moderately degenerated discs after exhausting conservative treatment options	Two control groups intradiscal inj. w/ either saline or HA MPC treatment group intradiscal injs.: 30 pts. w/ six million MPCs. 30 pts. w/ 18 million MPCs	At 12 mos., 6 million MPC group w/ 69.2% and 18 million MPC group w/ 61.5% of pts. achieving ≥50% reduction in VAS, while the saline group w/ only 31.3% and the HA group w/ 35.3% successes Three times increase in the number of MPC-treated pts. that achieved concordant pain and function treatment success at both 6 and 12 mos. relative to saline controls	Allogeneic MPCs were well tolerated, showed improvements in pain and functional improvement, and reduced interventions compared to controls. Needs randomized phase 3 studies. When compared to HA results did not reach statistical significance	Level II

| Mochida et al. [39] [NP cells and autologous MSCs] | Three-yr. result of prospective clinical phase I study, to assess the safety and efficacy of activated NP cell transplantation in the degenerate lumbar IVD $n = 9$ 1 wk. post fusion w/ NP tissue transplantation at adjacent levels to fusion | JOA back pain score 1, 2, and 4 wks., 3 and 6 mos., as well as 1, 2, and 3 yrs. X-ray and MRI | Pts. aged 20–29 yrs. who had Pfirrmann grade III disc degeneration at the level adjacent to the level scheduled for posterior lumbar intervertebral fusion. Two pts. had disc herniation and seven pts. had discopathy | Viable NP cells from the fused disc were co-cultured in direct contact w/ autologous bone marrow-derived MSCs. One million activated NP cells were transplanted into the degenerated disc adjacent to the fused level at 7 days after the first fusion surgery | No adverse effects were observed during the 3-yr. f/u period. MRI did not show any detrimental effects to the transplanted discs and revealed a mild improvement in one case. No cases reported any LBP. There was minimal functional improvement and some MRI changes | This clinical study confirmed the safety of activated NP cell transplantation, and the findings suggest the minimal efficacy of this treatment to slow the further degeneration of human intervertebral discs | Level IV |

(continued)

Table 7.1 (continued)

Author, date [injectate]	Methodology, patients, and comparison group	Follow-up and outcome measures	Diagnosis	Injectate preparation and route	Results	Authors' conclusion	Study analysis and notes
Kumar et al. [40] [AT-MSCs and HA]	Single-arm, open-label, phase I clinical trial $n = 10$ Underwent a single intradiscal inj. of combined HA derivative and AT-MSCs	VAS, ODI, SF-36 F/u 1 week and 1, 3, 6, 9, and 12 mos. Lumbar spine X-ray imaging and MRI	Chronic LBP for more than 3 mos. w/ a minimum intensity of 4/10 on VAS and disability level ≥30% on ODI. Post positive discography	Adipose tissue-derived mesenchymal stem cells at a dose of 2×10^7 cells/disc ($n = 5$) or 4×10^7 cells/disc ($n = 5$) both combine with HA	VAS, ODI, and SF-36 scores significantly improved in both groups receiving both low and high cell doses and did not differ significantly between the two groups. Among six pts. who achieved significant improvement in VAS, ODI, and SF-36, three pts. were determined to have increased water content based on an increased apparent diffusion coefficient on diffusion MRI	Combined implantation of AT-MSCs and HA derivative in chronic discogenic LBP is safe and tolerable. However, the efficacy of combined AT-MSCs and HA should be investigated in a randomized controlled trial in a larger population No procedure or stem cell-related adverse events or serious adverse events during the 1-year f/u period	Level IV

| Comella et al. [41] [SVF, fat stem cells] | Open-label study. n = 15 SVF injected directly into the nucleus pulposus | VAS, PPI, ODI, BDI, DPQ, and SF-12 F/u 2 and 6 mos. | DDD of two or three lumbar discs w/ predominant back pain after conservative treatment for at least 6 mos. | 60 ml fat aspirated, buffered in saline, and digested using collagenase and centrifuged to collect SVF pellet. Pellet then resuspended in ≈1 ccs of autologous PRP. 20–60 million cells in 1–3 cc PRP | Improvement in VAS scores from avg. of 5.6 at baseline to 3.6 at 6 mos. No severe adverse events reported. Statistically significant improvements in flexion, pain ratings, VAS, PPI, and short form questionnaires. ODI and Dallas pain questionnaire only showed positive trends | SVF proved promising; however a true evaluation of efficacy and safety would require larger phase II/III studies | Level IV |
| Pang et al. [42] [HUC-MSCs] | Clinical trial n = 2 Two pts. w/ chronic discogenic LBP were treated w/ HUC-MSC transplantation | VAS and ODI F/u at 6, 12, and 24 mos. | Pts. w/ positive discography with discogenic LBP | Human umbilical cord tissue-derived mesenchymal stem cells (HUC-MSCs) The suspension of 1 mL HUC-MSCs containing ≈1 × 10^7 cells | After transplantation, the pain and function improved immediately in the two pts. The VAS and ODI scores decreased during a 2-year f/u period. The water content in the degenerative painful disc in 1 out of 2 pts. was significantly increased at 2 years posttransplantation | The clinical outcomes indicated that HUC-MSC transplantation is a favorable alternative method for treating chronic discogenic LBP. This method avoids the invasive harvesting of stem cells. The shortcoming of this study is that it is a preliminary study w/ only two pts. | Level IV |

(continued)

Table 7.1 (continued)

Author, date [injectate]	Methodology, patients, and comparison group	Follow-up and outcome measures	Diagnosis	Injectate preparation and route	Results	Authors' conclusion	Study analysis and notes
Huafe et al. [43] [HSCs]	Prospective case report $n = 10$ Intradiscal inj. of HSCs followed by a 2-week course of hyperbaric oxygen therapy	VAS F/u at 6 and 12 mos.	Discogenic pain Attempted endoscopic discectomy w/o relief for 3 mos. w/ positive provocative discograms	Hematopoietic precursor stem cells (HSCs) obtained from pts.' pelvic bone marrow in an attempt to rejuvenate the disc. 1 cc injected into each painful disc	Of the ten pts., none reported a VAS reduction in their pain at 1-yr. post inj. After 1 year, seven of the original ten pts. underwent fusion surgery and one underwent artificial disc replacement surgery. Two continued conservative therapy	Even though MSCs have been suggested as a possible treatment for degenerative discs, this study reveals that HSCs, which are similar precursor cells, are of no benefit in living human subjects. Possibly the HSCs cannot survive in the oxygen-poor environment of the disc, even w/ hyperbaric oxygen therapy	Level IV

Yin et al. [44] [fibrin]	Prospective multicenter pilot study $n = 15$ Fibrin intradiscal inj.	VAS, RMDQ. F/u at 72 hours, and 1, 4, 13, 26, 52, and 104 wks. MRI and neurological status to evaluate for potential adverse events	Discogenic lumbar pain w/ chronic, single, or contiguous two-level lumbar discogenic pain confirmed through meticulous provocation discography	BIOSTAT BIOLOGX Fibrin Sealant w/ the Biostat Delivery Device intradiscal until sustained pressure above 100 psi, entire volume of 4 ml fibrin sealant delivered, or until pt. could not tolerate continued inj.	87% achieved ≥30% reduction in VAS score compared w/ baseline at the 26-wk. primary end point. Mean LBP VAS decreased from 72.4 at baseline to 31.7, 35.4, and 33.0; mean RMDQ score improved from 15.2 at baseline to 8.9, 6.2, and 5.6 at 26, 52, and 104 wks., respectively. Safety neurological assessments, X-ray, and MRI showed no significant changes	Intradiscal inj. of fibrin appears safe and may improve pain and function in selected pts. w/ discogenic pain. There was two instances of low back muscle spasm and one case of discitis was considered related to the procedure or product	Level IV
Peng et al. [45] [intradiscal methylene blue]	Randomized placebo-controlled trial $n = 72$ 72 subjects became eligible after discography. 36 w/ intradiscal inj. MB and 36 w/ placebo treatment	P-NRS, ODI F/u at 6, 12, and 24 mos.	Discogenic low back pain w/o radiculopathy lasting longer than 6 mos., w/ no comorbidity	1 ml of 1% MB (10 mg) inj. into the discogram-proven diseased disc, followed by inj. of 1 ml of 2% lidocaine for anesthetic. The placebo group: inj. of 1 ml of isotonic saline and 1 ml of 2% lidocaine into the painful disc	At 24 mos., the pts. in MB inj. group showed a mean reduction in P-NRS of 52.50, a mean reduction in ODI of 35.58, and satisfaction rates of 91.6%, compared w/ 6.91, 1.68, and 14.3%, respectively, in placebo treatment group, all statistically significant. No adverse effects or complications were found in the group of pts. treated w/ intradiscal MB inj.	The current clinical trial indicates that the inj. of methylene blue into the painful disc is a safe, effective, and minimally invasive method for the treatment of intractable and incapacitating discogenic low back pain	Level II

(continued)

Table 7.1 (continued)

Author, date [injectate]	Methodology, patients, and comparison group	Follow-up and outcome measures	Diagnosis	Injectate preparation and route	Results	Authors' conclusion	Study analysis and notes

Abbreviations: pt. patient, *inj.* injection, *P-NRS* Pain Numerical Rating Scale, *mos.* months, *f/u* follow-up, *ESI* epidural steroid injection, *w/* with, *wk.* week, *avg.* average, *VAS* visual analogue scale, *RMDQ* Roland-Morris Disability Questionnaire, (x-ray); *MRI* magnetic resonance imaging, *LBP* low back pain, *ODI* Oswestry Disability Index, *yr.* year, *FRI* Functional Rating Index, *SF-36* pain and physical function domains of the 36-item Short Form Health Survey, *NASS* the modified North American Spine Society, *DDD* degenerative disc disease, *FDA* Food and Drug Administration, *IDE* investigational device exemption, *SANE* modified single assessment numeric evaluation, *PL* platelet lysate, *HA* hyaluronic acid, *NP* nucleus pulposus, *JOA* Japanese Orthopaedic Association, *SVF* stromal vascular fraction obtained from a mini-lipoaspirate procedure of fat tissue, *PPI* present pain intensity, *BDI* Beck Depression Inventory, *DPQ* Dallas Pain Questionnaire, *(SF)-12* short form, *HUC-MSCs* human umbilical cord tissue–derived mesenchymal stem cells, *MB* methylene blue times less than those used in regular epidural steroid injections. At this low level, the steroid provides an anti-inflammatory effect similar to that of endogenous glucocorticoids. The patients showed significant improvements in both their numerical and functional scores. At 24 months posttreatment, patients had a 49.7% rating for their own improvement. Although this was a large study, it lacks both randomization and a control group [49].

In terms of prolotherapy and dextrose injections, Maniquis-Smigel et al. conducted an RCT that looked at 19 patients who received epidural injections of 5% dextrose and 16 who received normal saline into the caudal epidural space. Subjects who received the dextrose reported greater significant pain relief at 15 minutes and up to 48 hours, but not at 2 weeks. Although demonstrating short-term efficacy, this study suggests that dextrose may have positive results and a long-term study should investigate the effects of serial dextrose epidural injections and prolotherapy [50].

Focusing on stem cells, one RCT trial, by Bertagnoli et al., investigated the use of autologous disc-derived chondrocyte transplant in patients undergoing sequestrectomy. Only the interim analysis has been published which looked at 26 patients in each the treated and control group. The results are promising as the control group showed decreases in disc height, while the treated group did not have any cases of disc height loss. Furthermore, the discs treated with chondrocyte cells had adjacent intervertebral discs segments that appeared to retain hydration when compared to the control group. This study suggests that the autologous chondrocyte cells seem to improve disc structure and may even have beneficial effects on neighboring discs. Because the population of this study was only those undergoing discectomy, it is difficult to generalize these findings to the general patient with radicular back pain [51].

While regenerative therapy targeting herniated discs and radiculopathy seem to show promising results (Table 7.2), more long-term RCTs are needed before a general recommendation can be formulated.

Zygapophyseal Joint (Facet) Arthropathy

The current standard of care for facet-mediated pain includes directly targeting the medial branch nerve that is responsible for the innervation of this joint. This can be done with local anesthetic, steroids, and/or ablation. For each of these above procedures, often the pain returns as the medication wears off or the nerve heals. Furthermore, the root cause of the pain is not addressed. As these facet joints are synovial joints, therapies that have had success in other joints in the extremities have been further investigated. Treatments trialed include PRP, prolotherapy, and viscosupplementation.

In 2016, Wu et al. published on a new technique to treat lumbar facet pain using intra-articular injection with autologous PRP. Nineteen patients had good pain relief outcomes up to 3 months postinjection [52]. Wu later reported a prospective, randomized, controlled study of 46 subjects diagnosed with facet joint arthropathy through positive successful lidocaine blocks. Twenty three subjects underwent PRP injection

Table 7.2 Regenerative medicine for radiculopathy studies reviewed

Author, date [injectate]	Methodology, patients, and comparison group	Follow-up and outcome measures	Diagnosis	Injectate preparation and route	Results and author	Conclusions	Study analysis
Bhatia et al. [47] [PRP]	Pilot study $n = 10$ Efficacy of PRP via interlaminar epidural route in treatment of pain in pts. w/ prolapsed IVD	VAS, SLRT, and MODQ F/u at 3 wks. and 3 mos.	Lumber disc herniation / prolapse in MRI, < 65 yrs. old, w/ complaints of backache w/ or w/o radiculopathy for >4 wks. w/ a + SLRT and not responding to the conventional treatment	5 ml of autologous PRP under fluoroscopic guidance via interlaminar lumbar epidural inj. into area of affected nerve root	Pts. showed improvements in VAS and MODQ sustained during the 3-mo. study period. Apart from one pt. w/ VAS of 5, the rest showed improvement and their VAS was ≤4 at 3 mos. For most of the pts. MODQ score was <30% and SLRT improved to >70 at 3 mos. PRP was not associated with complications	Autologous PRP can be considered as a good alternative to epidural steroids and surgery in management of pts. w/ chronic prolapsed intervertebral disc. Possible alternative for steroids	Level IV
Cameron et al. [48] [PRP]	Prospective, nonrandomized, single center $n = 88$ 38 treated for cervical disc herniation. 38 for lumbar disc herniation, 12 w/ both cervical and lumbar	4 wks. to 6 wks., at 6 mos. to 12 mos., and up to 8 yrs. VAS were annually up to 8 yrs. ODI assessed in 36 pts. at least 1 yr. post procedure	Neck and/or low back pain caused by spinal disc herniation w/ or w/o radiation symptoms and failed conservative treatment for 3–6 mos. Pts. 18 to 65 yrs. old	Autologous PRP using a standardized protocol. Inj. in a circumferential manner subfascially into the lateral masses, facet joints and lateral gutters, and the inter- and supraspinatus ligaments, Kambin's triangle, and spinous processes	The duration of f/u ranged from 4 mos. to 8 yrs. (mean of 5 yrs.). 87% of pts. reported a successful outcome. Within the cervical group, the preoperative VAS showed 81% improvement. For the lumbar pts., the preoperative VAS improved by 77%. Both statically significant No complications were reported	Autologous PRP is a safe and effective treatment for neck and back pain secondary to disc herniation. Results were durable up to 8 yrs. Limitations include the multiple different time points for surveys and lack of ODI baseline scores	Level IV

							Level
Centeno et al. [49] [platelet lysate]	Case Series n = 470 Treated w/ PL epidural injs. presenting w/ symptoms of lumbar radicular pain	P-NRS; FRI; modified SANE; F/u 1, 3, 6, 12, 18, and 24 mos.; and annually thereafter	Diagnosed w/ lumbar radicular pain based on history, physical exams, and MRI findings	Either a transforaminal or interlaminar epidural 3–5 cc of PL 50% by volume, 4% lidocaine at 25% by volume, and compounded preservative-free 100–200 ng/ml hydrocortisone at 25% by volume	NPS change in score ranged from 1.6 to 2.4 Pts. treated w/ PL epidurals reported significantly lower ($p < 0.0001$) NPS and FRI change scores at all-time points compared to baseline. Avg. modified SANE ratings showed 49.7% improvement at 24 mos. posttreatment. 29 (6.3%) pts. reported mild adverse events related to treatment	PL inj. had significant improvements in pain compared to baseline, exceeded the minimal clinically important difference for FRI, and reported subjective improvement through 2-year f/u	Level IV
Maniquis-Smigel et al. [50] [prolotherapy]	Randomized double-blind (injector, participant) controlled clinical trial n = 37 19 received epidural inj. of 5% dextrose 16 received normal saline inj. into the caudal epidural space	P-NRS, F/u at 15 minutes; and 2, 4, and 48 hours and 2 wks. post-inj. 50% or more pain reduction at 4 hours	Adults w/ moderate-to-severe nonsurgical LBP w/ radiation to gluteal or leg areas for at least 6 mos.	S single 10 mL of 5% dextrose or 0.9% saline over 1 minute using a published vertical caudal inj. technique w/ pressure sensation being rate-limiting factor	Dextrose participants reported greater P-NRS change at 15 minutes ($4.4 ± 1.7$ vs $2.4 ± 2.8$ points), 2 hours ($4.6 ± 1.9$ vs $1.8 ± 2.8$ points), 4 hours ($4.6 ± 2.0$ vs $1.4 ± 2.3$ points), and 48 hours ($3.0 ± 2.3$ vs $1.0 ± 2.1$ points), but not statistically significant at 2 wks. ($2.1 ± 2.9$ vs $1.2 ± 2.4$ points) 84% (16/19) of dextrose recipients and 19% (3/16) of saline recipients reported ≥50% pain reduction at 4 hours	These findings suggest a neurogenic effect of 5% dextrose on pain at the dorsal root level; waning pain control at 2 wks. suggests the need to assess the effect of serial dextrose epidural injs. in a long-term study w/ robust outcome assessment	Level II

(continued)

Table 7.2 (continued)

Author, date [injectate]	Methodology, patients, and comparison group	Follow-up and outcome measures	Diagnosis	Injectate preparation and route	Results and author	Conclusions	Study analysis
Bertagnoli et al. [51] [autologous disc-derived chondrocyte (ADCT)	A multicenter, prospective, randomized, assessment-blinded, controlled clinical trial, EuroDISC study $n = 53$ 27 pts. within the ADCT-treated group 26 pts. control group All pts. were treated w/ a sequestrectomy	ODI, QBPD, VAS F/u 2 yrs. Disc height was assessed by MRI	Chronic back pain post lumbar disc herniation. Pts. 18–60 yrs. of age requiring surgical intervention at one level between L3 and S1	ADCT-treated group, the sequestrated disc tissue was used for disc chondrocyte isolation and their autologous propagation. 3 mos. later the disc-derived chondrocyte transplants were transplanted back into the operated discs nucleus region	During the f/u of 2 yrs., significant differences for ODI, QBPD, and VAS were found for the autologous disc-derived chondrocyte transplantation Decreases in disc height over time were only found in the control group, and of potential significance, intervertebral discs in adjacent segments appeared to retain hydration when compared to those adjacent to levels that had undergone discectomy w/o cell intervention	The interims results give strong evidence for the safety and efficiency of the disc-derived chondrocyte transplantation applied following sequestrectomy to delay or inhibit ongoing processes of disc degeneration	Level II

Abbreviations: SLRT straight leg raising test, *MODQ* Modified Oswestry Disability Questionnaire, *QBPD* Quebec Back Pain Disability, *VAS* visual analogue scale and 23 underwent standard of care lidocaine with steroid. At 1 week and 1 month the steroid group outperformed the PRP group. However, as time progressed the PRP group began to outperform the steroid group with significantly improved VAS scores from 2 months on. The steroid group peaked around 1 month and relief diminished to 6 months. The PRP group seemed to improve up to 3 months and then plateaued [53]. There seems to be promising evidence for the use of PRP to treat facet-mediated pain.

Prolotherapy has also been studied to treat facet pain. Hooper et al. reported a retrospective case review of 15 patients (three patients treated bilaterally to make 18 total facet joint sides) who were treated with intra-articular prolotherapy after confirmation of cervical facet pain post whiplash injury. This procedure significantly improved the mean neck disability index at months 2, 6, and 12. These results are promising; however this study lacks a control and furthermore may have been confounded as 13 of the patients' pain was caused by motor vehicle accidents in which they were in litigation. Furthermore, patients had concurrent physiotherapy which may have supported better outcomes [54]. Hooper et al. later reported a retrospective series on 177 patients with chronic spinal pain who each received prolotherapy to the facet capsules of the cervical, thoracic, and lumbar spine in regions that correlated with pain (in addition, the iliolumbar and dorsal sacroiliac ligaments were injected in patients with low back pain). Ninety-one percent of these patients reported reduction in pain. Lumbar and thoracic patients proved to have greater significant relief than compared to cervical [55]. These studies are in favor of prolotherapy for facet-mediated pain.

In terms of viscosupplementation, a pilot prospective study by Cleary et al. recruited 13 patients with symptomatic lumbar-facet joint pain who were treated with injection of hyaluronic acid: 18 facets of the 13 patients were injected. At 6 weeks there was no significant improvement in pain scoring. This study was limited as there was no definitive diagnostic testing for facet arthropathy [56]. A more promising study by DePalma et al. followed 15 patients with identified facet joint pain through successful trial of comparison local blocks. In this prospective uncontrolled pilot study, patients had positive results with significant improvements in VAS and ODI up to 6 months; however results were not sustained at 12 months. However, this study is flawed by its lack of control and blinding [57]. Fuchs et al. followed two groups with axial back pain: one received intra-articular sodium hyaluronate and the control received intra-articular glucocorticoids targeting the facet joints. In this observer-blinded RCT, both groups had positive results, with the hyaluronate group showing prolonged benefits in the long term at 3 and 6 months [58]. An RCT, by Annaswamy et al. investigated 30 subjects with facet pain and injected them either with hyaluronate or with steroid. While the steroid group only providing short-term functional improvement, the hyaluronate group outperformed by providing both short-term and long-term functional improvement, as well as short-term pain relief [59].

In conclusion, for PRP we identified one RCT that suggests it outperforms steroids with its longevity lasting up to 6 months. For prolotherapy, the studies seem to show improvements in pain; however an RCT is lacking. Lastly, the two viscosupplementation RCTs show hyaluronic acid to improve pain up to 6 months. The two other studies showed mixed results, with one trial confirming the positive results and the other showing no significant improvement in pain scoring. Further studies are needed that include a control group and stricter inclusion criteria confirming facet-mediated pain. Each study had a strong safety profile, suggesting these interventions (Table 7.3) can be trialed when evidence-based medicine fails to provide appropriate relief.

Sacroiliac Joint Dysfunction

Another common cause of chronic low back pain stems from the sacroiliac joints and ligaments. The SI joint acts to transmit forces from the lower limbs to the vertebral column. These synovial joints are prone to degeneration and instability. In addition, other joints of the pelvis including the sacrococcygeal joint can be a source of pain.

One case series investigated the efficacy of viscosupplementation. Srejic et al. reported on four patients treated with viscosupplementation to the SI joint. At 12–16 weeks postinjection pain was reported as 40–67% improved. The authors conclude further studies are needed to look at long-term duration and overall outcomes [60].

Others have examined the effects of prolotherapy theorized to provide stabilization of the painful instable SI joint. In a retrospective cohort study by Hoffman et al. 103 patients received prolotherapy aiming at the SI joint for a total of three injections at approximately 1 month intervals. At an average of 117 day follow-up, 23% of these patients showed a minimum clinically important improvement in ODI. Many of the responders had a median of 2 years of back pain. This suggests prolotherapy could be beneficial in a subset of patients [61]. Similarly, Mitchell et al. reported on prolotherapy in 131 patients injected around the SI joint into the deep interosseous ligament. Over 70% of patients were satisfied with the procedure. The majority of patients demonstrated at least 50% improvement in pelvic/lumbar strength. Two-thirds of patients demonstrated some pain relief with a mean of 51.6% reduction at 12 months [62]. Kim et al. investigated the current routine treatment of steroid injection and compared that to prolotherapy injection to the SI joint. Both groups (23 patients received prolotherapy and 25 patients received steroid) showed similar significant pain relief results at the 2-week follow-up. However, at 15 months the cumulative incidence of greater than 50% pain relief was 58.7% in the prolotherapy group while just 10.2% in the steroid group. This study suggests prolotherapy may have more long-term efficacy compared to steroids [63].

Examining other joints of the pelvis, Khan et al. studied patients with chronic coccygodynia and performed two injections of prolotherapy 15 days apart to the sacrococcygeal joints. Due to the good relief obtained, this prospective observational study recommends that dextrose prolotherapy should be trialed in patients with chronic, recalcitrant coccygodynia prior to undergoing coccygectomy [64].

Focusing on PRP, a case series by Ko et al. reported on four patients who had two sessions of PRP injections to the SI Joint at the three Hackett's points at the ligament-bone interface. Each of these patients showed significant reduction in pain

Table 7.3 Regenerative medicine for zygapophyseal joint (facet) arthropathy studies reviewed

Author and date [injectate]	Methodology, patients, and comparison group	Follow-up and outcome measures	Disease type	Injectate and route	Results	Author conclusions	Study analysis
Wu et al. [52] [PRP]	A prospective clinic evaluation $n = 19$ 19 pts. received lumbar facet joint inj. w/ autologous PRP	VAS at rest and flexion, RMDQ, ODI, and modified MacNab criteria F/u 1 wk., 1 mo., 2 mos., and 3 mos.	Lumbar facet joint syndrome	Intra-articular lumbar facet joint inj. w/ 0.5 ml autologous PRP tested to ensure concentration 4–5 times than in native peripheral blood	1 wk. after treatment, LBP reduced significantly compared w/ baseline pain both at rest and during flexion. The outcomes were assessed as "good" or "excellent" for 9 pts. (47%) immediately after treatment, 14 pts. (74%) at 1 wk., and 15 pts. (79%) at 1, 2, and 3 mos.	In short-term period of 3 months, PRP lumbar facet joint injections are effective and safe. Future studies would benefit from control group and longer f/u	Level IV

(continued)

Table 7.3 (continued)

Author and date [injectate]	Methodology, patients, and comparison group	Follow-up and outcome measures	Disease type	Injectate and route	Results	Author conclusions	Study analysis
Wu et al. [53] [PRP]	Prospective, randomized, controlled study $n = 46$ 23 w/ PRP 23 w/ lidocaine and steroid	VAS, RMQ, ODI, modified MacNab at 1 week, 1, 2, 3, and 6 mos.	Lumbar facet joint syndrome with continued pain 1 mo. post conservative treatment and post successful lidocaine block	Steroid group: 0.5% lidocaine and 5 mg/mL betamethasone total of 0.5 mL inj. per joint PRP group: 5–10 ml of venous blood. Centrifuged to 1–2 ml. Platelet concentration was almost 4–5 times greater than native peripheral blood 0.5 mL inj. at each joint level	Both steroid and PRP improved in VAS, RMQ, and ODI. Both groups showed improvements in VAS throughout. However, steroid group showed more significant decrease in VAS at wk. 1 and mo. 1. However, by 3 mos. after inj. and at 6 mos. pain relief, satisfaction, and functional capacity were significantly better in the PRP group	At 2 mos. the PRP group began to outperform the steroid group in terms of VAS as the steroid group peaked around 1 mo. and worsened to 6 mos. The PRP group seemed to improve to 3 mos. and then plateaued. PRP proved superior for longer duration efficacy	Level II

| Hooper et al. [54] [prolotherapy] | Retrospective case series. Consecutive pts. $n = 177$ Prolotherapy inj. done on a weekly basis for up to 3 wks. A set of three injs. was repeated in 1 mo. time if needed | Improvement in activities of daily living, level of pain, and ability to work F/u 2 mos. to 2.5 yrs. | Chronic low back pain not responding to conventional therapy and manual assessment demonstrating laxity | Pts. were treated w/ a proliferant solution containing 20% dextrose and 0.75% xylocaine. 0.5 mL of proliferant inj. into the facet capsules of the cervical, thoracic, and lumbar spine or combination. The iliolumbar and dorsal SI ligaments if LBP | 91.0% of pts. reported reduction in level of pain; 84.8% of pts. reported improvement in activities of daily living, and 84.3% reported an improvement in ability to work. Women required on avg. three more injs. than men. Cervical spine response rates were lower than thoracic or lumbar spine. No complications from treatment were noted | Dextrose prolotherapy appears to be a safe and effective method for treating chronic spinal pain that merits further investigation. Future studies need to consider differences in gender response rates | Level IV Limited by lack of definitive diagnosis of facet arthropathy by positive blocks |

(continued)

Table 7.3 (continued)

Author and date [injectate]	Methodology, patients, and comparison group	Follow-up and outcome measures	Disease type	Injectate and route	Results	Author conclusions	Study analysis
Hooper et al. [55] [prolotherapy]	Retrospective case review of prospective data n = 15 Intra-articular prolotherapy Three pts. had bilateral treatment, leaving 18 sides to analysis. Injs. repeated every 1–2 mos. if manual physiotherapy identified ongoing laxity	Mean NDI. F/u at 2, 6, and 12 mos.	Chronic whiplash-related neck pain that failed conservative and interventional procedures. Facet joint pain confirmed by diagnostic block	Intra-articular zygapophyseal joint prolotherapy by placing 0.5–1 mL of 20% dextrose solution into each zygapophyseal joint, after confirmation of intra-articular location w/ radiographic contrast. Solution was prepared by diluting D50W w/ 1% lidocaine. Treated C2–C7	Mean NDI pre-treatment was 24.7 and decreased posttreatment to 14.2 (2 mos.), 13.4 (6 mos.), and 10.9 (12 mos.). Avg. change NDI = 13.77 baseline versus 12 mos. Symptoms for 14 pts. were from motor vehicle accident, of which 13 were in litigation. Pts. attending physiotherapy over the course of treatment had better outcomes than those w/o physiotherapy. Women needed more injs. (5.4) than men (3.2)	Intra-articular prolotherapy improved pain and function. The procedure appears safe, more effective than periarticular inj., and lasted as long, or longer, than those pts. w/ previous radiofrequency neurotomy. Concurrent physiotherapy helped reduce post-inj. neck stiffness. Future trials should consider gender when deciding how many treatments to administer. Litigation was not a barrier to recovery	Level IV

Cleary et al. [56] [viscosupplementation]	Pilot study to test the potential effectiveness of HA inj. therapy in the treatment of lumbar facet joint arthritis $n = 13$ 18 facets in 13 pts. were injected w/ HA	VAS, ODI, F/u at 6 wks.	40–75 yrs. old w/ symptomatic lumbar facet joint arthritis as defined by diagnostic criteria and MRI evidence	A single inj. of HA (Suplasyn 2 mL, 10 mg) into affected facet joint was performed, w/ correct placement confirmed on fluoroscopy	At 6-wk. f/u, there was no significant improvement in pain when measured on the VAS. There was also no significant improvement in the ODI	Preliminary results from this pilot study do not demonstrate any benefit of viscosupplementation in the management of symptomatic lumbar facet arthropathy	Level IV Limited by lack of definitive diagnosis of facet arthropathy by positive blocks

(continued)

Table 7.3 (continued)

Author and date [injectate]	Methodology, patients, and comparison group	Follow-up and outcome measures	Disease type	Injectate and route	Results	Author conclusions	Study analysis
DePalma et al. [57] [viscosupplementation]	Prospective, uncontrolled, pilot study $n = 15$ 15 pts. underwent intra-articular Hylan G-F 20 injs, 10 days apart, into the painful facet joint. A third Hylan G-F 20 inj. was offered as needed	VAS, ODI, SF-36, FTF, tolerance (standing, sitting, walking), and analgesic usage F/u. 7–10 days and at 1, 3, 6, and 12 mos.	Facet joint pain diagnosed by positive local comparative blocks	1.0VmL intra-articular Hylan G-F 20 injs. performed twice 10 days apart, into the painful facet joint. A third Hylan G-F 20 inj. was offered to pts. dissatisfied w/ the results obtained w/ the first two injs.	Repeated measure mixed models indicated that VAS (avg, standing, walking), ODI, SF-36, FTF, and sitting tolerance all showed significant changes from baseline up to 6 mos. but were not sustained at 12 mos.; w/ the exception of the baseline to 12-month difference for FTF. There was no evidence of changes over time in standing ($P = 0.085$) or walking ($P = 0.084$) tolerance. Satisfaction initially increased from baseline (0%) to 7–10 days (64%) but declined over time (36% at 12 mos.)	Viscosupplementation for lumbar facet joint arthropathy w/ Hylan G-F 20 is associated w/ modest efficacy that predominately lasts up to 6 mos. As compared w/ baseline (80%), analgesic usage decreased over time showing significant decreases at 6 mos. (33%) and increased slightly at 12 mos. (45%). Limitations include a small sample size and lack of both a control and blinding. Larger RCTs are indicated to clarify its clinical safety, efficacy, and utility	Level IV

Fuchs et al. [58] [viscosupplementation]	Randomized, controlled, blind-observer clinical study *n* = 60 30 received 10 mg sodium hyaluronate (SH) 30 received 10 mg triamcinolone acetonide (TA) per facet joint	VAS, RMQ, ODI, LBOS, SF-36 F/u immediate effects, 3 and 6 mos.	Chronic nonradicular lumbar pain for at least 3 mos. Radiologic confirmation of facet osteoarthritis	The facet joints on both sides at levels S1-L5, L5-L4, and L4-L3 were treated once per wk. Each patient ultimately received six injs. of the assigned test product 10 mg/ml sodium hyaluronate or 10 mg/ml steroid (triamcinolone acetonide), max of 1 ml per facet joint	Pts. reported lasting pain relief, better function, and improved quality of life w/ both treatments. Mann-Whitney analyses of RMQ, ODQ, and LBOS very consistently showed that SH is not inferior to TA. In addition, the efficacy of SH was largely comparable w/ that of TA on the VAS and SF-36	Intra-articular SH is a very promising new option for the treatment of pts. w/ chronic nonradicular lumbar symptoms with evidence of facet osteoarthritis. No adverse effects were reported after administration of the test products. SH-treated pts. showed greater benefits in the long term at 3- and 6-month f/u	Level IV Limited by lack of confirmation testing by facet blocks

(continued)

Table 7.3 (continued)

Author and date [injectate]	Methodology, patients, and comparison group	Follow-up and outcome measures	Disease type	Injectate and route	Results	Author conclusions	Study analysis
Annaswamy et al. [59] [viscosupplementation]	Prospective double-blind randomized controlled trial $n = 25$ 13 pts. in steroid group 12 subjects in the HA group all received intra-articular facet injs.	VAS, PDQ, overall percent improvement at 6 mos. F/u at 1, 3, and 6 mos.	Symptomatic lumbar facet arthritis w/ axial chronic LBP w/o radiculopathy. Met criteria for facetogenic back pain	After randomization, bilateral L3–4, L4–5, and L5–S1 facet joints were injected. Each joint received either 1 ml of triamcinolone (10 mg/ml Kenalog) or 1 ml of Synvisc-One® (8 mg of Hylan G-F 20 per vial)	For pain, Synvisc group showed significant difference at 1 mo. (69.60 ± 19.68 to 45.15 ± 25.23). For PDQ, Kenalog group showed significant difference at 1 mo. (100.2 ± 22.93 to 77.42 ± 29.89) and Synvisc group showed significant differences at all-time points (101.93 ± 27.83 to 74.08 ± 33.90 to 74 ± 35.58 to 79 (median, 52–99.5))	Hyaluronate injs. provided statistically significant short- and long-term functional benefits and short-term pain improvement but triamcinolone injs. only provided statistically significant short-term functional benefit and no significant short- or long-term pain improvement compared to within-group baseline levels. Triamcinolone and hyaluronate injs. into facets provide similar pain and functional benefits in pts. w/ symptomatic lumbar zygapophyseal joint arthropathy causing chronic LBP	Level IV Limited by lack of facet diagnostic block and sham control. No intergroup differences were observed when comparing overall satisfaction at 6 mos.

Abbreviations: *NDI* neck disability index, *HA* hyaluronic acid, *FTF* finger to floor distance, *RMQ* Range of motion questionnaire, *ODQ* Oswestry Disability Questionnaire, *LBOS* Low Back Outcome Score and the Short Form 36 (SF-36) questionnaire, *PDQ* Pain Disability Questionnaire and improvements in quality of life [65]. A prospective randomized study by Singla et al. treated 20 patients with steroid and 20 patients with PRP to the SI joint. At 6 weeks and 3 months the PRP group had significantly better intensity of pain. The efficacy of steroid injection was reduced to only 25% at 3 months, while efficacy remained at 90% in the PRP group [66]. This study, similar to the prolotherapy study, demonstrates a longer efficacy of the regenerative medicine (PRP group) compared to steroids.

To examine the efficacy of PRP versus prolotherapy, Saunders et al. compared his prospective trial of 45 patients with PRP injection into and around the dorsal interosseous ligament to a control of a prior separate study using prolotherapy to treat presumed SI joint pain. At 3 months the PRP group had good pain and functional improvement without further improvement at 12 months. When this trial was statistically compared to a prior prolotherapy study, the PRP group had better outcomes in pain scores and function and required on average 1.6 injections compared to the three injections of the prolotherapy control group [67].

Viscosupplementation, prolotherapy, and PRP have an excellent safety profile and have shown promising results in treating SI joint pain (Table 7.4). Patient selection, injection target, and injection schedule remain significant variables lacking a gold standard. As previously noted, more well-designed comparative studies are necessary.

Back Musculature Atrophy

Pain in the back can also be related to musculature dysfunction. There are several muscles of the back that attach to the spine and act to add strength and support, often stabilizing the spine joints through various movements. When there is a misbalance, pain can result from poor mechanics and additional destructive forces. Furthermore, the general physiological response to back pain is for the muscles to disengage as they inactivate. This leads to atrophy of muscles over time, which further promotes a negative cycle.

A study by Hussein et al. analyzed 104 patients with chronic nonspecific back pain and confirmed muscle atrophy on MRI. These patients were treated with platelet leukocyte-rich plasma (PLRP) into the lumbar multifidus (LMF) muscle weekly for 6 weeks. Patients improved in pain and function as reported on questionnaires. Furthermore, 12-month MRI follow-up showed increased cross-sectional area and decreased fatty degeneration of LMF muscle. This study suggests that PLRP may better pain and function outcomes by improving LMF atrophy. One limitation includes the lack of a control group and the fact the patients were advised to remain active and walk 30 minutes per day. Thus, physical therapy targeting these muscle groups may play an important part in relieving back pain, whether in conjunction with regenerative therapy or on its own. Although this technique had promising outcomes (Table 7.5), again there is a need for RCTs [68].

Table 7.4 Regenerative medicine for sacroiliac joint dysfunction studies reviewed

Author and date [injectate]	Methodology, patients, and comparison group	Follow-up and outcome measures	Disease type	Injectate and route	Results	Author conclusions	Study analysis
Srejic et al. [60] [viscosupplementation]	Case series n = 4 Pts. received three injs. of Hylan G-F 20 in the sacroiliac joints 2 wks. apart	VAS. F/u at 12–16 wks. post inj.	SI joint syndrome by means of pt. history, physical examination, and intra-articular local anesthetic inj. Preceded by SI arthrogram	Three injs. of Hylan G-F 20 in the SI joints 2 wks. apart 1 cc (8 mg) of Hylan G-F 20 (Synvisc) into each joint	12 to 16 wks. after the injs., the pain was reported to be 40–67% better when measured on the VAS. The duration of the beneficial effect of Hylan on arthralgia and joint function was undetermined	Viscosupplementation of the SI joint induced a significant degree of analgesia in all four patients. This treatment modality could represent an option in the management of SI joint pain and dysfunction	Level IV

| Hoffman et al. [61] [prolotherapy] | Retrospective cohort study n = 103 All pts. received prolotherapy for SIJ | ODI, f/u immediately preceding each prolotherapy inj. and at 3–4 mos. | SI joint pain and instability When diagnosis uncertain, pt. underwent diagnostic inj. or positive initial prolotherapy response | Mixture of 7 ml of 1% lidocaine and 3 ml of 50% dextrose (15% dextrose solution), w/ the solution being injected aiming at the SI joint Series of three injs. at about 1 month intervals | At a median of 117 days, 24 pts. (23%) showed a minimum clinically important improvement despite an avg. of 2 years w/ LBP and a mean pre-inj. ODI of 54. Much of the improvement was seen after the first prolotherapy inj., and a 15-point improvement in ODI prior to the second inj. had a sensitivity of 92% and specificity of 80% for determining which pts. would improve | A satisfactory proportion of pts. w/ symptomatic SI joint instability as an etiology of LBP can have clinically meaningful functional gains w/ prolotherapy treatment. Those w/ abrupt onset of low back pain were unlikely to have relief | Level IV Limited by lack of pain scores and most injs. w/o imaging guidance |

(continued)

Table 7.4 (continued)

Author and date [injectate]	Methodology, patients, and comparison group	Follow-up and outcome measures	Disease type	Injectate and route	Results	Author conclusions	Study analysis
Mitchell et al. [62] [prolotherapy]	Prospective, observational study $n = 131$ Consecutive pts. undergoing prolotherapy treatment around the SIJ	Back/hip/pelvic strength, pain relief ODI, patient satisfaction and analgesic use F/u at 6 and 12 mos. post-inj.	Diagnostically confirmed SIJ instability and pain	The deep interosseous ligament injected w/ 1.5 ml Naropin 0.75% and 10 ml 50% glucose over multiple sites Injs. were repeated, on avg. three times, at 6 weekly intervals	At 12 mos., 66% of pts. reported improvements in pelvic/lumbar strength. Mean strengthening was 59.4%; 71.1% of pts. achieved ≥50% improvement. 66% also experienced at least some pain relief (mean 51.6% reduction) at 12 mos., while 80% reported they had ≥50% improved stability. Clinically meaningful mean ODI score reductions (6.58 points at 6 mos. and 8.27 points at 12 mos.) were observed	Almost half the cohort reduced their use of analgesia posttreatment and 70% of pts. were satisfied w/ the outcomes from the prolotherapy procedure. Pain relief was dependent on improved strength and correlated w/ reductions in disability score	Level IV

Kim et al. [63] [prolotherapy]	Prospective, randomized, controlled trial $n = 48$ 23 in prolotherapy group 25 in steroid group	Pain and disability scores F/u at 2 wks. and monthly for 12 mos.	SI joint pain lasting 3 mos. or longer, confirmed by ≥50% improvement in response to local anesthetic block and who failed medical treatment	Prolotherapy group, inj. 2.5 mL of 25% dextrose solution into the SIJ every other wk. up to three times. The dextrose solution 50% dextrose water w/ 0.25% levobupivacaine. Steroid inj. group 2.5 mL of triamcinolone acetonide 40 mg in 0.125% levobupivacaine	The pain and disability scores were significantly improved from baseline in both groups at the 2-week f/u, w/ no significant difference between them. The cumulative incidence of ≥50% pain relief at 15 mos. was 58.7% in the prolotherapy group and 10.2% in the steroid group. There was a statistically significant difference between the groups	Intra-articular prolotherapy provided significant relief of sacroiliac joint pain, and its effects lasted longer than those of steroid injs. Further studies are needed to confirm the safety of the procedure and to validate an appropriate inj. protocol	Level IV

(continued)

Table 7.4 (continued)

Author and date [injectate]	Methodology, patients, and comparison group	Follow-up and outcome measures	Disease type	Injectate and route	Results	Author conclusions	Study analysis
Khan et al. [64] [prolotherapy]	Prospective observational study n = 37 Pts. received two injs. of prolotherapy 15 days apart. A third inj. given 4 wks. later to eight pts. w/ pain scores >4	VAS F/u 15 days and 4 wks.	Chronic coccygodynia not responding to conservative treatment for more than 6 mos. 27 of the pts. had received local steroid injs. elsewhere	8 ml of 25% dextrose and 2 ml of 2% lignocaine into the coccyx Inj. over the most tender spot of the coccyx, using an image intensifier to locate the sacrococcygeal joint	The mean VAS before prolotherapy was 8.5. It was 3.4 after the first inj. and 2.5 after the second inj. Minimal or no improvement was noted in seven pts.; the remaining 30 pts. had good pain relief	Dextrose prolotherapy is an effective treatment option in pts. w/ chronic, recalcitrant coccygodynia and should be used before undergoing coccygectomy. Randomized studies are needed to compare prolotherapy w/ local steroid injs. or coccygectomies	Level IV Limited by lack of functional outcome studies

					Level IV
Ko et al. [65] [PRP]	Case series $n = 4$ Pts. inj. w/ PRP to SI joint for two sessions	SFM, P-NRS, ODI, f/u at 12 mos. and 48 mos.	SI joint instability diagnosed by combination of pt. history, provocative tests, or suggestive imaging	Inj. to SI joint at Hackett's points A, B (medial to PSIS), and C (inferior to the PSIS). 0.5 ml of PRP w/ each needle contact of the ligament-bone interface. Two sessions total. PRP platelet concentration was 5–6 times baseline blood	At f/u 12-mo. posttreatment, pooled data from all pts. reported a marked improvement in joint stability, a statistically significant reduction in pain, and improvement in quality of life. The clinical benefits of PRP were still significant at 4-year posttreatment	PRP therapy exhibits clinical usefulness in both pain reduction and for functional improvement in pts. with chronic SI joint pain

(continued)

Table 7.4 (continued)

Author and date [injectate]	Methodology, patients, and comparison group	Follow-up and outcome measures	Disease type	Injectate and route	Results	Author conclusions	Study analysis
Singla et al. [66] [PRP]	Prospective randomized open blinded end point (PROBE) study $n = 40$ 20 in group S received steroid inj. 20 in group P received PRP inj.	VAS, modified ODI, SF-12, and complications F/u at 2 wks., 4 wks., 6 wks., and 3 mos.	SI joint area LBP. Unilateral SIJ seen on either x-ray, MRI, or nuclear scan w/ three or more positive provocative tests	Group S received 1.5 mL of methylprednisolone (40 mg/mL) and 1.5 mL of 2% lidocaine w/ 0.5 mL of saline Group P received 3 mL of leukocyte-free PRP w/ 0.5 mL of calcium chloride into ultrasound-guided SIJ inj.	Intensity of pain was significantly lower in group PRP at 6 wks. as compared to group steroids. The efficacy of steroid inj. was reduced to only 25% at 3 mos. in group steroids, while it was 90% in group platelets. There were no serious adverse events	The intra-articular PRP inj. is an effective treatment modality in LBP involving SIJ. PRP group exhibited greater pain and functional improvements which lasted longer compared to steroid group	Level II Limited by lack of pt. blinding

| Saunders et al. [67] [PRP vs prolotherapy] | Prospective open label n = 45 45 pts. received PRP inj. The results were then compared to a matched control group who had received hypertonic glucose injs. following tertiary referral from specialized sports medicine physicians | VAS, RMDQ, and QBPD. As well as clinical tests of SIJ incompetence F/u at 3 and 12 mos. | Pain in the lumbosacral region w/ 3 of 4 positive validated clinical signs. Confirmed by the fused single photon emission computed tomography and low-dose x-ray computed tomography | Inj. into and around the dorsal interosseous ligament rather than the synovial portion of the sacroiliac joint On avg. 1.6 injs. per pt. The system used concentrate platelets 1.6 times baseline | At 3 mos. the PRP group had good pain and functional improvement w/o further improvement at 12 mos. The outcome measures of change in pain scores; improvement in function between the groups was superior for the PRP group. All PRP pts. experienced significant improvement in pain score and function. The number of injs. required was less for the PRP group (mean of 1.6) than the controls (mean 3.0) | PRP is a viable alternative to prolotherapy into the dorsal interosseous ligament in patients who have failed physiotherapy for SIJ incompetence | Level III Limited by lack of documented amount of PRP or prolotherapy injected and matched control group comparison |

Abbreviations: Inj. injection, *SFM* short-form McGill Pain Questionnaire

Table 7.5 Regenerative medicine for back musculature atrophy studies reviewed

Author and date	Methodology, patients, and comparison group	Follow-up and outcome measures	Diagnosis type	Injectate and route	Results and author conclusion	Conclusion	Study analysis
Huessein et al. [68] [PLRP]	Prospective trial $n = 104$ pts. w weekly PLRP injs. into lumbar multifidus muscle (LMF) for six wks. and followed up for 24 mos.	NRS, ODI, patient satisfaction index, and modified MacNab criteria F/u at 1 day, 6 mos., 12 mos., and 24 mos. Lumbar MRI at 12 mos.	Chronic non-specified LBP, atrophy of multifidus muscle seen in MRI scan and at least one level of degenerative disc disease	Needle targeted the deep fibers of the LMF muscle at the degenerated lumbar motion segment. Needle was withdrawn 1–2 mm from lamina and 2.5 mL of PLRP injected per side Weekly PLRP inj. for 6 wks. into the LMF muscle Platelet count ranged from 0.8 to 1.2 million/mL or 4–6 times baseline blood values	NRS significantly improved gradually from a mean of 8.8 ± 8 pre-inj. to 3.45 ± 2.9 by 12 mos. and ODI significantly improved gradually from a mean of 36.7 ± 3.9 to 14.6 ± 12.8 by 12 mos. After reaching maximum improvement between 12 and 18 mos., all outcome measures remained stable till the end of the 24 mos. 87.8% (65/74) of the satisfied pts. showed increased cross-sectional area and decreased fatty degeneration of LMF muscle on MRI at 12-mo. f/u	PLRP injs. into atrophied LMF muscle represents a safe, effective method for relieving chronic LBP and disability w/ long-term patient satisfaction and success rate of 71.2%. We recommend the use of the lumbar PLRP injs. of LMF muscle to refine the inclusion criteria of lumbar fusion to avoid failed back syndrome	Level IV Limited by lack of control group and all pts. encouraged to walk 30 minutes a day and remain active

Abbreviations: LMF lumbar multifidus muscle, *LBP* lower back pain

Back Ligament Dysfunction

Similar to the muscles of the back, the ligaments act to support the spine and its joints. Ligaments can be visualized as guy wires providing strength, reinforcement, and stability. Due to this important role, ligaments can be another target for regenerative therapy. Historically, prolotherapy has been used in theory to strengthen ligaments.

Dechow et al. reported a randomized, double-blind, placebo-controlled trial of 74 mechanical back pain patients, with 36 undergoing three once weekly dextrose injections and 38 in the control group receiving normal saline. Sites injected included the tip of the spinous process of L4 and L5 and associated supraspinous and interspinous ligaments, apophyseal joint capsules at L4–5 and L5–S1, attachment of the iliolumbar ligaments at the transverse processes of L5, attachment of the iliolumbar and dorsolumbar fascia to the iliac crest, and attachments of the long and short fibers of the posterior sacroiliac ligaments and the sacral and iliac attachments of the interosseous sacroiliac ligaments. The authors' findings showed no statistically significant differences between the control and the prolotherapy group. The authors acknowledge that their inclusion criteria did not evaluate for instability and hence the treatment sample group may not have been the ideal patient cohort that could potentially benefit from prolotherapy [69]. A retrospective case study published by Hauser et al. analyzed 140 patients that received prolotherapy to sites that included the sacroiliac, iliolumbar, sacrotuberous, lumbosacral, supraspinous and interspinous, sacrococcygeal, and sacrospinous ligaments, as well as the gluteal and pyriformis muscle attachments on the iliac crest. On an average of 12-month follow-up, 89% of these patients demonstrated more than 50% pain relief with prolotherapy. Again, this study lacks both a control and blinding [70].

Klein et al. randomized 39 chronic low back pain patients to a xylocaine/proliferant group and 40 to a xylocaine/saline (control group) that received injections into the posterior sacroiliac and interosseous ligaments, iliolumbar ligaments, and dorsolumbar fascia. Although both groups improved, the proliferant (prolotherapy) group showed a statistically significant improvement in number of patients that achieved a 50% or greater diminution in pain or disability scores at 6-month follow-up [71]. Similarly, an RCT by Yelland et al. treated 110 patients with either prolotherapy or normal saline injections into tender lumbo-pelvic ligaments and was then randomized to either flexion/extension exercises or normal activity over 6 months. Although each ligament injection group showed improvement and sustained reductions in pain and disability, no significant attributable difference was seen among the prolotherapy group. This suggests that any needling of these ligaments may provide relief; a different control group that did not receive injectate could better identify these findings [72].

These studies (Table 7.6) show promise that prolotherapy can help in cases of ligament dysfunction. Furthermore, they highlight the importance of identifying

Table 7.6 Regenerative medicine for back ligament dysfunction studies reviewed

Author, date [injectate]	Methodology, patients, and comparison group	Follow-up and outcome measures	Diagnosis	Injectate preparation and route	Results and author	Conclusions	Study analysis
Dechow et al. [69] [prolotherapy]	Randomized, double-blind, placebo-controlled trial n = 74 36 underwent three once weekly injs. of dextrose-glycerine-phenol w/ lignocaine 38 in the control group received three once weekly injs. of saline plus lignocaine	McGill Pain, the modified Somatic Pain Questionnaire, the Zung Depression Inventory, the ODI, and modified Schober to measure spinal flexion F/u at 1, 3, and 6 mos.	Mechanical back pain of more than 6 mos. duration	Treatment group: 5 ml of dextrose 25%, glycerine 25%, and phenol 2.4% made up to 100 ml w/ sterile water combined w/ 5 ml of 1% lignocaine Control group: 5 ml of the normal saline solution combined w/ 5 ml of 1% lignocaine Inj. sites: included the tip of the spinous process of L4 and L5 and associated supraspinous and interspinous ligaments, apophyseal joint capsules at L4–5 and L5–S1, attachment of the iliolumbar ligaments at the transverse processes of L5, attachment of the iliolumbar and dorsolumbar fascia to the iliac crest, and attachments of long and short fibers of the posterior sacroiliac ligaments and the sacral and iliac attachments of interosseous SI ligaments	There were no statistically significant differences in patient characteristics between the placebo and treatment groups at baseline or for any measure at f/u	Three weekly sclerosant injs. alone may not be effective treatment in many pts. w/ undifferentiated chronic back pain. Patient selection and combination w/ other treatment modalities may be factors in determining treatment success	Level II Limited by undifferentiated LBP without clear diagnosis. No clinical measures of instability were tested

					Level IV
Hauser et al. [70] [prolotherapy]	Retrospective case studies $n = 145$ Each treated quarterly w/ Hackett-Hemwall dextrose prolotherapy An avg. of four lower back treatments, given every three mos., per pt.	Pain level, physical and psychological symptoms, and activities of daily living F/u at an avg. of 12 mos., at end of treatment	Unresolved chronic low back pain for an avg. of 4 years	Each site was injected w/ 0.5–1 cc of solution of 15% dextrose, 0.2% lidocaine solution w/ a total of 60 to 90 cc of solution per lower back treatment Inj. sites included the sacroiliac, iliolumbar, sacrotuberous, lumbosacral, supraspinous and interspinous, sacrococcygeal, and sacrospinous ligaments, as well as the gluteal and pyriformis muscle attachments on the iliac crest	In the 145 pts., pain levels decreased from 5.6 to 2.7 after prolotherapy; 89% experienced more than 50% pain relief w/ prolotherapy; more than 80% showed improvements in walking and exercise ability, anxiety, depression, and overall disability; 75% were able to completely stop taking pain medications	The decrease in pain reached statistical significance including the subset of (55) pts. who were told there were no other options for their pain and those (26) who were told surgery was their only treatment option. Prolotherapy should be considered in those with unresolved LBP

(continued)

Table 7.6 (continued)

Author, date [injectate]	Methodology, patients, and comparison group	Follow-up and outcome measures	Diagnosis	Injectate preparation and route	Results and author	Conclusions	Study analysis
Klein et al. [71] [prolotherapy]	Randomized, double-blinded clinical trial $n = 79$ 39 in Xylocaine/ proliferant group 40 in control Xylocaine/saline solution group	VAS, disability, and pain grid scores and w/ objective computerized triaxial tests of lumbar function F/u at 6 mos.	Chronic LBP that had failed to respond to previous conservative care	Proliferant solution consisted of dextrose 25%, glycerine 25%, and phenol 2.4%. 15 ml w/ 15 ml of 0.5% lidocaine. Max of 30 ml at each inj. section Control group 30 ml of solution, 15 ml of 0.5% solution, 15 ml of sterile lidocaine w/ 15 ml of sterile normal saline Inj. sites: included posterior sacroiliac and interosseous ligaments, iliolumbar ligaments, and dorsolumbar fascia	30 of the 39 pts. randomly assigned to the proliferant group achieved a $\geq 50\%$ diminution in pain or disability scores at 6 mos. compared to 21 of 40 in the group receiving lidocaine. Improvements in VAS, disability, and pain grid scores were greater in the proliferant group and reached statistical significance. The MRI and CT scans showed significant abnormalities in both groups, but these did not correlate w/ subjective complaints and were not predictive of response to treatment	Objective testing of range of motion, isometric strength, and velocity of movement showed significant improvements in both groups posttreatment but did not favor either group. LBP may in part be related to injury of the fibrous posterior supporting structures of the lumbar motion segments and posterior SI ligaments. Proliferant inj. known to induce collagen proliferation appears to be a useful treatment in appropriately selects pts.	Level II

Yelland et al. [72] [prolotherapy]	RCT w/ two-by-two factorial design, triple blinded for inj. status, and single blinded for exercise status $n = 110$ 28 had repeated prolotherapy and exercise 27 had saline and exercise 26 had prolotherapy and normal activity 29 had saline and normal activity Injs. into tender lumbo-pelvic ligaments and randomized to perform either flexion/extension exercises or normal activity over 6 mos.	VAS and RMDQ. F/u at 2.5, 4, 6, 12, and 24 mos.	Chronic nonspecific low back pain	The primary guide for inj. sites was tenderness in ligaments and broad tendinous attachments (entheses) of the lumbosacral spine and pelvic girdle, w/ consideration of the patterns of local and referred pain. Injs. were performed through an anesthetized wheal of skin over each tender site Approximately 3 ml solution was infiltrated at each site (mean 7.3) and a maximum of ten sites treated at each visit If no improvement was noted by the fifth session, the deeper interosseous sacroiliac ligaments on the affected side or sides were also treated Injs. occurred every 2 wks. until six treatments. At 4 and 6 mos. were repeated if partial response. Injs. repeated from 6 to 12 mos. as needed. Mean of 7.1 treatments total Prolotherapy composition: 20% glucose/0.2% lignocaine	Ligament injs., w/ exercises and w/ normal activity, resulted in significant and sustained reductions in pain and disability throughout the trial, but no attributable effect was found for prolotherapy injs. or for saline injs. or for exercises over normal activity At 12 mos., the proportions achieving >50% reduction in pain from baseline by inj. group were glucose-lignocaine (0.46) versus saline (0.36). By activity group these proportions were exercise (0.41) versus normal activity (0.39). Corresponding proportions for >50% reduction in disability were glucose-lignocaine (0.42) versus saline (0.36) and exercise (0.36) versus normal activity (0.38)	There were no between group differences in any of the above measures In chronic nonspecific low back pain, significant and sustained reductions in pain and disability occur w/ ligament injs., irrespective of the solution injected or the concurrent use of exercises	Level II Limited by lack of significant differences found among groups and lack of control group

Abbreviations: RCT randomized controlled trial

the disease pathology one is attempting to treat. For instance, a treatment might fail in an individual patient and have success in another based on the pathology of the patient and the target of the injectate. More RCTs would hopefully define both the optimal patient selection criteria and the ideal injectate target.

Overall Levels of Evidence

When reviewing the available literature, it is important to objectively determine the evidence level that can be drawn from the authors' conclusions. It is crucial to define this evidence level prior to adopting the study outcomes into clinical practice. In order to systematically grade the evidence, Manchikanti et al. have developed an interventional specific pain management instrument used in assessing the methodological quality of trials. Randomized controlled trials are often considered the gold standard and superior evidence compared to studies without randomization and/or without controls. Case reports and observational clinical experiences or reports of expert committees are determined to be the lowest level of evidence. This qualified modified approach (Table 7.7) to grading allows us to define the level of evidence for a specific treatment [73]. However, it remains important to remember the specific patient population treated, the exact injectate utilized, and the overall magnitude of results achieved by each study. By utilizing this qualified modified approach to grading, we are better able to categorize the evidence.

Table 7.7 The qualified modified instrument developed by Manchikanti et al. in assessing the methodological quality of trials and grading the overall scientific evidence in interventional specific pain management [73]

Level I	Strong	Two or more relevant high-quality RCTs for effectiveness or four or more relevant high-quality observational studies or large case series for assessment of preventive measures, adverse, consequences, and effectiveness of other measures
Level II	Moderate	At least one relevant high-quality RCT or multiple relevant moderate- or low-quality RCTs or at least two high-quality relevant observational studies or large case series for assessment of preventive measures, adverse consequences, and effectiveness of other measures
Level III	Fair	At least one relevant high-quality nonrandomized trial or observational study with multiple moderate- or low-quality observation studies or at least one high-quality relevant observation study or large case series for assessment of preventative measures, adverse consequences, and effectiveness of other measures
Level IV	Limited	Multiple moderate- or low-quality relevant observational studies or moderate-quality observation studies or large case series for assessment of preventative measures, adverse consequences, and effectiveness of other measures
Level V	Consensus based	Opinion or consensus of a large group of clinicians for effectiveness as well as to assess preventive measures, adverse consequences, effectiveness of other measures, or single case reports

Limitations of Current Studies and Future Implications

There are several common pitfalls when analyzing regenerative medicine trials. In terms of injectate (whether stem cells, PRP, viscosupplementation, or prolotherapy), there is often not a defined common mixture or recipe. With each injectate the exact effective dose is vital, and each clinician should strive to achieve what is considered the gold standard formula. Further studies should strictly define and list the active dose of the injectate utilized. Although in certain cases the injectate cannot be standardized, for instance, where the injectate is partially derived from the patient (PRP, stem cells), a dose-response relationship should be developed. Furthermore, a combination of regenerative medicine substances should be trialed for greatest benefit. With many pain trials, a control group is essential as often seen some pain may heal with time independent of treatment. In addition, the construct of a control or sham is significant as any injectate or needling may provide some hidden benefit on its own.

The selection criteria in spine pain studies are essential to ensure that the patient has the pathology the clinician is attempting to treat. Poor selection can lead to poor results, as some patients may not have the specific disease that the intervention was designed to treat. Furthermore, injection technique is crucial to ensure the injectate reaches the precise target. Attention must be placed on the scales used to measure a positive result. Regarding pain, function, and quality of life scales it is important that a statistically significant difference makes for a clinical impact on the patient. Lastly, most studies focus on the lumbar spine likely secondary to a lower perceived risk. Although these results have the possibility to be generalized, more data and controlled studies are needed for the thoracic and cervical spine to demonstrate efficacy as well as define a risk profile.

Overall regenerative medicine for the spine appears relatively safe with few side effects or adverse reactions reported from the injectate alone. Prolotherapy, viscosupplementation, and PRP can be used with few risks. Compared to current routine treatments of local anesthetics and steroids, these regenerative treatments may have a superior safety profile with most adverse events coming from the injection technique itself. For stem cells, the safety data is also strong, but longer time frame studies are needed. Most clinical studies have not followed patients for enough time to evaluate long-term safety prognosis. One case report describes a 66-year-old male that, in hopes of curing his deficits from an ischemic stroke, traveled to three separate countries for infusions of mesenchymal, embryonic, and fetal neural stem cells into his spine. He was later found to have a spinal tumor that resulted from the intrathecally introduced exogenous stem cells [74]. Although the pluripotent stem cells this patient received are of a different cell type than those used primarily in regenerative medicine for joint and spine pain, this exceptionally rare and unfortunate case serves as a cautionary tale for possible unforeseen risks.

Regulation Concerns

Currently much of the field of regenerative medicine is regulated in the United States under section 361 by the Federal Drug Administration (FDA). Section 361 of the Public Health Service Act gives the FDA authority to make and enforce regulations if the substance meets certain specifications, is minimally manipulated, is intended for homologous use, is for autologous use, and does not involve combination of the cells or tissues with another article except for water, crystalloids, or a sterilizing, preserving, or storage. Products that do not meet these criteria fall under Section 351 and these products are to be regulated as biologicals. This includes any virus, serum, antitoxin, vaccine, blood component or derivative, allergenic product, or analogous product that is used in the medical care of patients. 351 products are either more than minimally manipulated or used in a nonhomologous manner (different from original function). To summarize, 351 products are defined as a biologic drug and require complete FDA review, including premarket approval and clearance before the biologic drug can be legally marketed. Thus, the average time to market for substances labeled under Section 351 is around 10 years costing millions of dollars similar to the requirements of more traditional chemical drug products. Substances labeled as 351 products fall under the higher regulation and therefore may currently be unattainable for routine clinical use. To the contrary, most of the regenerative medicine substances discussed fall under Section 361 making them easily accessible. One of the substances in a gray area is adipose stem cells. After harvesting the adipose stem cells, preparation requires enzymatic dissociation of the tissue. This would suggest more than minimal manipulation and classify these adipose stem cells as a biologic drug under Section 351 [75]. With advancements in regenerative medicine, it is crucial to understand and follow the evolving regulations set forth.

Future Directions

New technology and advances should allow for better efficacy of regenerative medicine. Currently 3D printing utilizing bio-ink materials creates the ability to provide an optimal artificial extracellular environment to cells which allows for ideal adhesion, proliferation, and differentiation. Cells can now be encapsulated with this 3D printed structure with high viability. Important cell building blocks can be incorporated into this matrix [76]. Furthermore, studies have analyzed the use of exosomes which are extracellular vesicles that carry microRNA, proteins, and other molecules that work to mediate biologic function through gene regulation and intercellular communication. MSC exosomes have in theory the ability to mediate functional recovery by upregulating and promoting repair utilizing the patient's own intact cells [77].

Conclusion

Traditional pain management treatments target individual pain generators with the main goal of eliminating or masking pain through interrupting the transmission of painful signals. In this approach it is essential to isolate the activated nerves. Similarly, due to this complex network of possible pain generators, there are several targets where regenerative medicine can prove to be an effective treatment. With regenerative medicine, the goal is to create a favorable environment in which the body can jumpstart the healing cascade, promote repair, and hence revitalize itself. Consequently, it may be important to view the entire spine in a holistic approach. Individually deactivating painful nerves may control pain signals, but will not improve the original cause of the pain. Idealistically, through regenerative medicine, the etiology of the pain can be corrected, and pain relief will naturally follow and sustain.

Furthermore, we must use caution with the term regenerative medicine, as the term "regenerative" may not apply to all treatments and may not accurately portray the actual science on a cellular level. While pain and function may improve, this does not necessarily prove that anything has indeed been physically "regenerated." The pain signal may resolve, but the fundamental pathology itself may remain.

As many of these interventions remain at the investigational level, more quality long-term, randomized, controlled human trials are required if these promising treatments are to become evidence-based medicine and the standard of care in everyday clinical practice. While there is a substantial amount of data on lumbar spine utilization, there is a paucity of studies analyzing intervention at the thoracic and cervical level. As regenerative medicine is a relatively new field with constantly developing technology and biologics, clinicians must continue to judiciously evaluate the evidence. With new evolving therapies, it is vital to remember the first priority remains to do no harm. Overall, due to an increase in promising evidence (Table 7.8) and a relatively good safety profile, regenerative medicine remains an important tool in the physician's armamentarium to trial on a case-by-case basis: especially (even more so) when routine medical care fails to provide acceptable results. However, at this point regenerative medicine for spinal pain remains a hopefully optimistic treatment to be perfected in the future.

Table 7.8 A summary of the overall level of evidence for the listed regenerative medicine treatments and each specific pain syndrome targeted

Evidence level for regenerative medicine based on reviewed studies				
	Prolotherapy	PRP	Hyaluronic acid	Stem cells
IVD-mediated pain	Level IV	Level II	Level V	Level III
Radicular pain	Level IV Level II (at 2 weeks)	Level IV	x	Level II (in discectomy patients)
Facet joint pain	Level IV	Level II	Level II	x
SI joint pain	Level II	Level II	Level IV	x
Musculature mediated	x	Level IV	x	x
Ligament mediated	Level II	x	x	x

References

1. Manchikanti L, Singh V, Falco FJE, Benyamin RM, Hirsch JA. Epidemiology of low back pain in adults. Neuromodulation. 2014;17:3–10. https://doi.org/10.1111/ner.12018.
2. Rubin DI. Epidemiology and risk factors for spine pain. Neurol Clin. 2007;25(2):353–71.
3. US Burden of Disease Collaborators, Mokdad AH, Ballestros K, et al. The state of US health, 1990-2016: burden of diseases, injuries, and risk factors among US states. JAMA. 2018;319(14):1444–72.
4. Buser Z, Ortega B, D'Oro A, et al. Spine degenerative conditions and their treatments: national trends in the United States of America. Global Spine J. 2018;8(1):57–67. https://doi.org/10.1177/2192568217696688.
5. Nachemson AL, Waddell G, Norlund AI. Epidemiology of neck and low back pain. In: Nachemson AL, Johnsson B, editors. Neck and back pain: the scientific evidence of causes, diagnosis, and treatment. Philadelphia: Lippincott Williams & Wilkins; 2000.
6. Shmagel A, Foley R, Ibrahim H. Epidemiology of chronic low back pain in US adults: data from the 2009-2010 National Health and Nutrition Examination Survey. Arthritis Care Res (Hoboken). 2016;68(11):1688–94.
7. Hudson TJ, Edlund MJ, Steffick DE, Tripathi SP, Sullivan MD. Epidemiology of regular prescribed opioid use: results from a national, population-based survey. J Pain Symptom Manag. 2008;36(3):280–8.
8. Drake RL, Vogl W, Mitchell AWM, Gray H. Gray's anatomy for students. 3rd ed. Philadelphia: Churchill Livingstone Elsevier; 2015.
9. Barr K, et al. Low back pain. Chapter 33. In: Braddom's physical medicine & rehabilitation. 5th ed. Philadelphia: Elsevier; 2016.
10. Brinjikji W, Luetmer PH, Comstock B, et al. Systematic literature review of imaging features of spinal degeneration in asymptomatic populations. AJNR Am J Neuroradiol. 2014;36(4):811–6.
11. Takatalo J, Karppinen J, Niinimäki J, Taimela S, Mutanen P, Sequeiros RB, et al. Association of modic changes, Schmorl's nodes, spondylolytic defects, high-intensity zone lesions, disc herniations, and radial tears with low back symptom severity among young Finnish adults. Spine (03622436). 2012;37(14):1231–9.
12. DePalma MJ, Ketchum JM, Saullo T. What is the source of chronic low back pain and does age play a role? Pain Med. 2011;12:224–33.
13. Walker MH, Anderson DG. Molecular basis of intervertebral disc degeneration. Spine J. 2004;4(6):166.
14. Buckwalter JA, Mow VC, Boden SD, Eyre DR, Weidenbaum M. Intervertebral disc structure, composition, and mechanical function. In: Buckwalter JA, Einhorn TA, Simon SR, editors. Orthopaedic basic science—biology and biomechanics for the musculoskeletal system. 2nd ed. Rosemont: American Academy of Orthopaedic Surgeons; 2000. p. 548–55.
15. García-Cosamalón J, Del Valle ME, Calavia MG, et al. Intervertebral disc, sensory nerves and neurotrophins: who is who in discogenic pain? J Anat. 2010;217(1):1–15.
16. Ganey TM, Meisel HJ. A potential role for cell-based therapeutics in the treatment of intervertebral disc herniation. Eur Spine J. 2002;11 Suppl 2(Suppl 2):S206–14.
17. Moriguchi Y, Alimi M, Khair T, et al. Biological treatment approaches for degenerative disc disease: a literature review of in vivo animal and clinical data. Global Spine J. 2016;6(5):497–518.
18. Wu T, Song HX, Dong Y, Li JH. Cell-based therapies for lumbar discogenic low back pain: systematic review and single-arm meta-analysis. Spine (Phila Pa 1976). 2018;43:49–57.
19. Pirvu TN, Schroeder JE, Peroglio M, et al. Platelet-rich plasma induces annulus fibrosus cell proliferation and matrix production. Eur Spine J. 2014;23(4):745–53.
20. Kim H, Yeom JS, Koh Y, Yeo J, Kang K, Kang Y, Chang B, Lee C. Anti-inflammatory effect of platelet-rich plasma on nucleus pulposus cells with response of TNF-α and IL-1. J Orthop Res. 2014;32:551–6.

21. Akeda K, An HS, Pichika R, Attawia M, Thonar EJ, Lenz ME, Uchida A, Masuda K. Platelet-rich plasma (PRP) stimulates the extracellular matrix metabolism of porcine nucleus pulposus and anulus fibrosus cells cultured in alginate beads. Spine (Phila Pa 1976). 2006;31(9):959–66.
22. Wang SZ, Jin JY, Guo YD, et al. Intervertebral disc regeneration using platelet-rich plasma-containing bone marrow-derived mesenchymal stem cells: a preliminary investigation. Mol Med Rep. 2016;13(4):3475–81.
23. Xu X, Hu J, Lu H, Zhao C. Histological observation of a gelatin sponge transplant loaded with bone marrow-derived mesenchymal stem cells combined with platelet-rich plasma in repairing an annulus defect. PLoS One. 2017;12(2):0171500.
24. Hou Y, Shi G, Shi J, Xu G, Guo Y, Xu P. Study design: in vitro and in vivo assessment of bone morphogenic protein 2 combined with platelet-rich plasma on treatment of disc degeneration. Int Orthop. 2016;40(6):1143–55.
25. Gui K, Ren W, Yu Y, Li X, Dong J, Yin W. Inhibitory effects of platelet-rich plasma on intervertebral disc degeneration: a preclinical study in a rabbit model. Med Sci Monit. 2015;21:1368–75. Published 2015 May 12. https://doi.org/10.12659/MSM.892510.
26. Gullung GB, Woodall JW, Tucci MA, James J, Black DA, McGuire RA. Platelet-rich plasma effects on degenerative disc disease: analysis of histology and imaging in an animal model. Evid Based Spine Care J. 2011;2(4):13–8.
27. Miller MR, Mathews RS, Reeves KD. Treatment of painful advanced internal lumbar disc derangement with intradiscal injection of hypertonic dextrose. Pain Physician. 2006;9(2):115–21.
28. Akeda K, Ohishi K, Masuda K, et al. Intradiscal injection of autologous platelet-rich plasma releasate to treat discogenic low back pain: a preliminary clinical trial. Asian Spine J. 2017;11(3):380–9.
29. Levi D, Horn S, Tyszko S, Levin J, Hecht-Leavitt C, Walko E. Intradiscal platelet-rich plasma injection for chronic discogenic low back pain: preliminary results from a prospective trial. Pain Med. 2016;17(6):1010–22.
30. Tuakli-Wosornu YA, Terry A, Boachie-Adjei K, et al. Lumbar intradiscal platelet-rich plasma (prp) injections: a prospective, double-blind, randomized controlled study. PM R. 2016;8(1):1–10.
31. Sys J, Weyler J, Van Der Zijden T, Parizel P, Michielsen J. Platelet-rich plasma in mono-segmental posterior lumbar interbody fusion. Eur Spine J. 2011;20(10):1650–7.
32. Mohammed S, Yu J. Platelet-rich plasma injections: an emerging therapy for chronic discogenic low back pain. J Spine Surg. 2018;4(1):115–22.
33. Orozco L, Soler R, Morera C, Alberca M, Sanchez A, Garcia-Sancho J. Intervertebral disc repair by autologous mesenchymal bone marrow cells: a pilot study. Transplantation. 2011;92:822–8.
34. Elabd C, Centeno CJ, Schultz JR, Lutz G, Ichim T, Silva FJ. Intra-discal injection of autologous, hypoxic cultured bone marrow-derived mesenchymal stem cells in five patients with chronic lower back pain: a long-term safety and feasibility study. J Transl Med. 2016;14(1):253. Published 2016 Sep 1.
35. Pettine K, Suzuki R, Sand T, Murphy M. Treatment of discogenic back pain with autologous bone marrow concentrate injection with minimum two year follow-up. Int Orthop. 2016;40:135–40.
36. Centeno C, Markle J, Dodson E, et al. Treatment of lumbar degenerative disc disease-associated radicular pain with culture-expanded autologous mesenchymal stem cells: a pilot study on safety and efficacy. J Transl Med. 2017;15(1):197. Published 2017 Sep 22. https://doi.org/10.1186/s12967-017-1300-y.
37. Noriega DC, Ardura F, Hernández-Ramajo R, Martín-Ferrero MÁ, Sánchez-Lite I, Toribio B, Alberca M, García V, Moraleda JM, Sánchez A, García-Sancho J. Intervertebral disc repair by allogeneic mesenchymal bone marrow cells: a randomized controlled trial. Transplantation. 2017;101(8):1945–51.

38. Bae HW, Amirdelfan K, Coric D, McJunkin TL, Pettine KA, Hong HJ, DePalma MJ, Kim KD, Beckworth WJ, et al. A phase II study demonstrating efficacy and safety of mesenchymal precursor cells in low back pain due to disc degeneration. Spine J. 2014;14:S31–2.
39. Mochida J, Sakai D, Nakamura Y, Watanabe T, Yamamoto Y, Kato S. Intervertebral disc repair with activated nucleus pulposus cell transplantation: a three-year, prospective clinical study of its safety. Eur Cell Mater. 2015;29:202–12.
40. Kumar H, Ha DH, Lee EJ, et al. Safety and tolerability of intradiscal implantation of combined autologous adipose-derived mesenchymal stem cells and hyaluronic acid in patients with chronic discogenic low back pain: 1-year follow-up of a phase I study. Stem Cell Res Ther. 2017;8(1):262. Published 2017 Nov 15.
41. Comella K, Silbert R, Parlo M. Effects of the intradiscal implantation of stromal vascular fraction plus platelet rich plasma in patients with degenerative disc disease. J Transl Med. 2017;15(1):12.
42. Pang X, Yang H, Peng B. Human umbilical cord mesenchymal stem cell transplantation for the treatment of chronic discogenic low back pain. Pain Physician. 2014;17(4):E525–30.
43. Haufe S. Intradiscal injection of hematopoietic stem cells in an attempt to rejuvenate the intervertebral discs. Stem Cells Dev. 2006;12(1):136.
44. Yin W, Pauza K, Olan W, Doerzbacher J, Thorne K. Intradiscal injection of fibrin sealant for the treatment of symptomatic lumbar internal disc disruption: results of a prospective multicenter pilot study with 24-month follow-up. Pain Med. 2014;15(1):16–31.
45. Peng B, Pang X, Wu U, Zhao C, Song X. A randomized placebo-controlled trial of intradiscal methylene blue injection for the treatment of chronic discogenic low back pain. Pain. 2010;149(1):124–9.
46. Adams M, Stefanakis M, Dolan P. Healing of a painful intervertebral disc should not be confused with reversing disc degeneration: implications for physical therapies for discogenic back pain. Clin Biomech (Bristol, Avon). 2010;25:961–71. https://doi.org/10.1016/j.clinbiomech.2010.07.016.
47. Bhatia R, Chopra G. Efficacy of platelet rich plasma via lumbar epidural route in chronic prolapsed intervertebral disc patients-a pilot study. J Clin Diagn Res. 2016;10(9):UC05–7.
48. Cameron JA, Thielen KM. Autologous platelet rich plasma for neck and lower back pain secondary to spinal disc herniation: midterm results. Spine Res. 2017;3(2):10.
49. Centeno C, Markle J, Dodson E, et al. The use of lumbar epidural injection of platelet lysate for treatment of radicular pain. J Exp Orthop. 2017;4(1):38. Published 2017 Nov 25. https://doi.org/10.1186/s40634-017-0113-5.
50. Maniquis-Smigel L, Dean Reeves K, Jeffrey Rosen H, et al. Short term analgesic effects of 5% dextrose epidural injections for chronic low back pain: a randomized controlled trial. Anesth Pain Med. 2016;7(1):e42550. Published 2016 Dec 6.
51. Bertagnoli R, et al. EuroDisc study – assessment of efficacy and safety of sequestrectomy plus autologous disc chondrocytes – second analysis of a subgroup. Spine J. 2007;7(Suppl 5):56S–7.
52. Wu J, et al. A new technique for the treatment of lumbar facet joint syndrome using intraarticular injection with autologous platelet rich plasma. Pain Pract. 2016;19(8):617–25.
53. Wu J, et al. A prospective study comparing platelet-rich plasma and local anesthetic (LA)/corticosteroid in intra-articular injection for the treatment of lumbar facet joint syndrome. Pain Pract. 2017;17(7):914–24.
54. Hooper RA, Ding M. Retrospective case series on patients with chronic spinal pain treated with dextrose prolotherapy. J Altern Complement Med. 2004;10(4):670–4.
55. Hooper RA, Frizzell JB, et al. Case series on chronic whiplash related chronic neck pain treated with intraarticular zygapophyseal joint regeneration injection therapy. Pain Physician. 2007;10(2):313–8.
56. Cleary M, Keating C, Poynton AR. Viscosupplementation in lumbar facet joint arthropathy: a pilot study. J Spinal Disord Tech. 2008;21(1):29–32.

57. DePalma MJ, Ketchum JM, Queler ED, Trussell BS. Prospective pilot study of painful lumbar facet joint arthropathy after intra-articular injection of hylan G-F 20. PM R. 2009;1(10):908–15.
58. Fuchs S, Erbe T, Fischer HL, Tibesku CO. Intraarticular hyaluronic acid versus glucocorticoid injections for nonradicular pain in the lumbar spine. J Vasc Interv Radiol. 2005;16(11):1493–8.
59. Annaswamy TM, Bierner SM, Avraham R, Armstead C, Carlson L. Triamcinolone vs. hyaluronate injections for lumbar facet arthropathy: a pragmatic, double blind randomized controlled trial. PM&R: Supplement. 2015;7(9):91. https://doi.org/10.1016/j.pmrj.2015.06.040.
60. Srejic U, Calvillo O, Kabakibou K. Viscosupplementation: a new concept in the treatment of sacroiliac joint syndrome: a preliminary report of four cases. Reg Anesth Pain Med. 1999;24(1):84–8.
61. Hoffman MD, Agnish V. Functional outcome from sacroiliac joint prolotherapy in patients with sacroiliac joint instability. Complement Ther Med. 2018;37:64–8. https://doi.org/10.1016/j.ctim.2018.01.014.
62. Mitchell RR, Barnard A. Efficacy of prolotherapy treatment for sacroiliac joint instability and pain. J Sci Med Sport. 2015;19:70. https://doi.org/10.1016/j.jsams.2015.12.170.
63. Kim W, Lee H, Jeong C, Kim C, Yoon M. A randomized controlled trial of intra-articular prolotherapy versus steroid injection for sacroiliac joint pain. J Altern Complement Med. 2010;16(12):1285–90.
64. Khan SA, Kumar A, Varshney MK, Trikha V, Yadav CS. Dextrose prolotherapy for recalcitrant coccygodynia. J Orthop Surg. 2008;16(1):27–9.
65. Ko GD, et al. Case series of ultrasound-guided platelet-rich plasma injections for sacroiliac joint dysfunction. J Back Musculoskelet Rehabil. 2017;30:363–70.
66. Singla V, Batra YK, Bharti N, Goni VG, Marwaha N. Steroid vs. platelet-rich plasma in ultrasound-guided sacroiliac ioint injection for chronic low back pain. Pain Pract. 2017;17(6):782–91.
67. Saunders J, Cusi M, et al. A comparison of ultrasound guided PRP injection and prolotherapy for mechanical dysfunction of the sacroiliac joint. J Prolotherapy. 2018;10:e992–9.
68. Hussein M, Hussein T. Effect of autologous platelet leukocyte rich plasma injections on atrophied lumbar multifidus muscle in low back pain patients with monosegmental degenerative disc disease. SICOT J. 2016;2:12. Published 2016 Mar 22.
69. Dechow E. A randomized, double-blind, placebo-controlled trial of sclerosing injections in patients with chronic low back pain. Rheumatology. 1999;38(12):1255–9.
70. Hauser R, Hauser M. Dextrose prolotherapy for unresolved low back pain: a retrospective case series study. J Prolotherapy. 2009;1(3):145–55.
71. Klein RG, et al. A randomized double-blind trial of dextrose-glycerine-phenol injections for chronic, low back pain. J Spinal Disord. 1993;6(1):23–33.
72. Yelland MJ, Glasziou PP, Bogduk N, Schluter PJ, McKernon M. Prolotherapy injections, saline injections, and exercises for chronic low-back pain: a randomized trial. Spine. 2004;29(1):9–16.
73. Manchikanti L, Hirsch JA, Cohen SP, Heavner JE, Falco FJ, Diwan S, Boswell MV, Candido KD, Onyewu CO, Zhu J, Sehgal N. Assessment of methodologic quality of randomized trials of interventional techniques: development of an interventional pain management specific instrument. Pain Physician. 2014;17(3):E263–90.
74. Berkowitz AL, Miller MB, Mir SA, et al. Correspondence: glioproliferative lesion of the spinal cord as a complication of "stem-cell tourism". N Engl J Med. 2016; Epub 2016 Jun 22.
75. From bench to FDA to bedside: US regulatory trends for new stem cell therapies. Adv Drug Deliv Rev. 2014;82-83:192–6.
76. Park KM, Shin YM, Kim K, Shin H. Tissue engineering part B: reviews. New Rochelle: Mary Ann Liebert, Inc; 2018.
77. Chang YH, Wu KC, Harn HJ, Lin SZ, Ding DC. Exosomes and stem cells in degenerative disease diagnosis and therapy. Cell Transplant. 2018;27(3):349–63.

Chapter 8
Regenerative Medicine for the Shoulder

Eliana Cardozo and Jonathan Ramin

Tendinopathy in the Shoulder: The Rotator Cuff and Proximal Biceps Tendon

The rotator cuff (RTC) is a group of scapulohumeral muscles primarily involved in shoulder motion and stabilization. It is comprised of the supraspinatus, infraspinatus, teres minor, and subscapularis. Injury to one or more of the RTC muscles can be both painful and a cause significant impairment in daily functions and overhead tasks.

Rotator Cuff Tendinopathy

When evaluating RTC tendinopathies, it is important to be able to differentiate between the underlying subtypes in order to best manage the injury. Historically, RTC tendinopathies have often been referred to as "RTC tendonitis," although this term remains controversial as most histopathological studies have shown little to no evidence for inflammatory cells in the tendon of people who have underdone arthroscopic tendon repair [1]. Rotator cuff tendinosis on the other hand is thought to stem from the repetitive overuse of a previously injured tendon that had not had adequate time to heal [2]. Calcific tendinopathy of the RTC refers to an unexplained buildup of calcium deposits on one or more of the RTC tendons, resulting in pain and limitations with range of motion [3].

Identifying which muscle of the RTC is injured begins with a proper physical examination of the shoulder. After evaluating active and passive range of motion

E. Cardozo (✉) · J. Ramin
Sports Medicine and Interventional Spine, Department of Rehabilitation Medicine and Human Performance, Icahn School of Medicine at Mount Sinai, New York, NY, USA
e-mail: eliana.cardozo@mountsinai.org

© Springer Nature Switzerland AG 2020
G. Cooper et al. (eds.), *Regenerative Medicine for Spine and Joint Pain*,
https://doi.org/10.1007/978-3-030-42771-9_8

of the shoulder, provocative testing can help decipher which muscle of the RTC is affected. The goal of each test is to isolate the muscle and assess for pain and/or weakness. The provocative tests have varying sensitivities and specificities but collectively allow for a more accurate assessment and diagnosis.

The supraspinatus muscle is primarily a shoulder abductor and can be tested for pathology using multiple provocative tests in order to increase overall sensitivity and specificity. The gold standard test, however, is the "empty can" test which evaluates for pain and weakness during shoulder abduction [4].

The infraspinatus muscle is the primary external rotator of the shoulder and is best tested with the patient's elbow flexed to 90 degrees, adducted against the patient's waist, and the humerus medially rotated 45 degrees. A positive test would be pain and/or weakness with resisted external rotation of the shoulder in this position [5].

The teres minor muscle is also an external rotator and is best isolated with the patient's arm raised to 90 degrees in the scapular plane and the forearm flexed to 90 degrees. A positive test would be pain and/or weakness with resisted external rotation of the shoulder. This is known as a positive Hornblower's sign [6].

The subscapularis muscle is primarily an internal rotator of the shoulder. Gerber's "lift off" test will assess the subscapularis by placing the patient's arm in internal rotation behind the patient's back and having the patient to push off posteriorly against resistance. Pain or weakness is a sign of subscapularis pathology [5].

Rotator Cuff Tears

The prevalence of RTC tears increases with age and are present in about 20.7% of the population, many of whom may be asymptomatic [7]. Tears can be classified based on their size, location, and attachment of the tendon relative to the humeral head. If there is a "through and through" tear of a RTC tendon but the tendon is still well attached to the humeral head, it is considered a "full-thickness" tear. When the tendon tear involves complete detachment from the humeral head, the tear is more serious and is considered a "complete" tear [4]. A RTC tear is considered "partial thickness" when the tear does not involve the entire tendon. Partial-thickness tears are graded based on the percentage of the tendon which is torn. Grade I <25%; Grade II 25% to <50%; Grade III >50% [7]. Partial-thickness tears are further classified as either bursal-sided (outer portion of tendon) or articular-sided (inner portion of tendon) based on tear location. If the tear is located in the middle layers of the tendon and does not involve the inner/outer layers, then the tear is considered an intrasubstance tear [7].

Treatment of RTC tendinopathies often depends on the severity and chronicity of the injury. While strong evidence is lacking for the treatment of RTC tendinopathies, approach to treatment generally begins conservatively. In addition to rest after an acute injury, cryotherapy is one of the first recommended treatments followed by a period of rest and 7–10-day course of nonsteroidal anti-inflammatory drugs (NSAIDs). If cryotherapy is not available, ice may also be used in the early stages. Efficacy and evidence for the use of NSAIDs in acute injuries are controversial but generally remain a part of the initial standard of care used by most physicians. Both acute and chronic RTC tendinopathies can benefit from a comprehensive rehabilitation program that focuses on the shoulder girdle, emphasizing strength, range of motion, and coordination training [8].

Chronic RTC injuries or those that did not respond to acute therapies may benefit from glucocorticoid-analgesic mixed injections. Evidence is limited in support of glucocorticoid injections, but few studies show some benefit of glucocorticoid injections over placebo and often equally but not more effective than NSAIDs. There have been studies, however, that show that a single subacromial glucocorticoid injection prior to initiation of physical therapy is superior to that of physical therapy alone, as it reduces acute pain and allows for more aggressive range of motion exercises [2, 9]. Another treatment option for patients with chronic RTC tendinopathies is topical nitrates. One double-blinded, placebo-controlled study showed a significant improvement in patients with chronic RTC tendinopathies treated with topical nitrates [10].

Surgical options are considered when conservative treatment has failed or if the RTC injury is an acute complete tear in an athlete or patient whose work requires a significant amount of overhead use. Lack of consistent improvement in the current treatment options has led to multiple new innovative measures in the treatment of RTC tendinopathies including topical NSAIDs, shockwave therapy, and regenerative techniques [11].

Biceps Tendinopathy

Biceps tendinopathies encompass a broad range of pathology most often involving the long head of the biceps tendon. They are generally known to be "overuse" injuries and over time tend to progress to a degenerative, thickened tendon that becomes entrapped in the bicipital groove causing significant discomfort and pain. Biceps tendinopathies typically occur in conjunction with other injuries to the shoulder girdle, particularly the RTC [12].

The biceps brachii muscles are primarily elbow flexors and forearm supinators. Provocative testing is performed to isolate these motions and aid in the diagnosis of biceps tendinopathy. The two commonly performed provocative maneuvers are the Speed's and Yergason's test which assess for pain in resisted elbow flexion and forearm supination, respectively [12].

Treatment of biceps tendinopathy usually begins conservatively with ice, rest, and a short 5–7-day course of NSAIDs. Topical NSAIDs are also often used in the early treatment phase, although their efficacy is not yet well established. Management continues with a comprehensive rehabilitation program focused on strengthening the muscles of the shoulder girdle, range of motion exercises, and proper stretching techniques. If ineffective, glucocorticoid injections into the biceps tendon sheath are tried next and should be done with ultrasound guidance for accuracy and to prevent intratendinous injection [12–14].

Surgical management of biceps tendon injuries includes biceps tenotomy and biceps tenodesis. These are generally performed after conservative management has failed in complete tendon rupture and when the patient is an athlete or does work requiring significant upper extremity strength. Although surgery is often performed, there is limited evidence in its efficacy and in overall patient satisfaction [15].

Tendinopathy in the Shoulder: Regenerative Medicine Applications

Lack of consistent improvement using current standard of care treatments in patients with shoulder dysfunction has led to the exploration of alternative means of therapy, particularly through regenerative medicine. Although relatively novel, regenerative therapies such as application of platelet-rich plasma (PRP) or mesenchymal stem cells are rapidly evolving and being experimented in the treatment of a variety of shoulder pathologies.

Rotator Cuff Tendinopathies and Tears

The majority of therapies using PRP or autologous stem cells to treat RTC tendinopathies involve injection into the subacromial space, with few studies published about injecting directly into the tendon.

The subacromial space can be accessed using ultrasound guidance. The patient is seated with the affected arm hanging down and ultrasound transducer placed in the coronal view over the lateral end of the acromion (Fig. 8.1a). Using sterile technique, use a 25-gauge, 1.5-inch needle to enter in plane with the transducer aiming for the anechoic space between the peribursal fat which represents the subacromial bursa (Fig. 8.1b). Once the needle tip is visualized within the subacromial bursa, aspirate and inject [16].

When injecting the tendon directly, identify the target tendon, specifically the site of pathology (tendon tear or area of tendinopathy). A 25-gauge needle is then inserted in-plane with the transducer aiming for the lesion. It is provider preference whether to use lidocaine first. Once the needle tip is visualized within the lesion, aspirate and inject directly into the lesion. If difficult to inject directly into the lesion itself, then the injectate is infiltrated around the lesion [17].

Kesikburun et al. performed a randomized study comparing the efficacy of PRP to saline when injected into the subacromial space in patients with chronic RTC tendinopathy. While both groups showed significant improvement in pain and functional measures at each point throughout the 2-year time course, there were no significant differences found between PRP and saline [18].

Fig. 8.1 (a) Transducer and needle placement for ultrasound guided subacromial injection. (b) Ultrasound image of subacromial space with patient seated and affected arm hanging

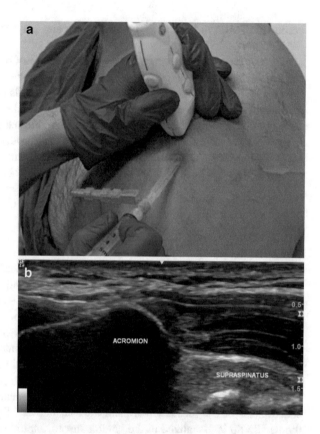

Rha et al. performed a randomized controlled trial comparing the effects of PRP versus dry needling directly into an RTC tendon that either had tendinosis or a partial tear. Their study showed that while both groups had symptomatic relief and functional improvements at 6 months, the PRP group had significantly more relief and functional improvement than the dry-needling group [17].

Von Wehren et al. performed a randomized study comparing treatment of partial RTC tears using a subacromial PRP injection with that of a subacromial corticosteroid injection. While both groups showed significant improvements in shoulder score outcomes in the 6 months they were monitored, the PRP group showed a significantly greater improvement in all shoulder score outcomes at each measured time point. MRI findings improved in both groups as well, but no significant differences were found between the two groups. Shams et al. replicated this study with similar results [19, 20]. These results are significant as they provide a potentially safer alternative treatment to corticosteroid injections which have been shown to weaken tendons and increase the risk of tendon rupture [21].

Several studies have also been published comparing the use of regenerative techniques in conjunction with arthroscopic rotator cuff repairs. While evidence is scarce and sometimes conflicting, the current research suggests that use of PRP in conjunction with arthroscopic rotator cuff repairs may decrease the retear rate of the tendon [22–25].

There is paucity of literature that evaluates the use of bone marrow-derived stem cells in the treatment of RTC repairs. Gomes et al. complemented conventional RTC repair with the use of mononuclear autologous stem cells in 14 patients and found a significant improvement in overall functional scores and tissue integrity when compared to conventional RTC repair alone [26]. Additional studies by Gullota et al. have evaluated the effects of autologous stem cells transduced with helix-loop-helix transcription factor in rat model repairs of supraspinatus tears. Early studies have revealed enhanced healing in the first 2–4 weeks post-RTC tendon repair [27].

Biceps Tendinopathy

At this time there is limited evidence evaluating the efficacy of platelet-rich plasma or other regenerative techniques for proximal biceps tendinopathies.

The biceps tendon sheath should be injected using a sterile technique with ultrasound guidance. With the axial-in-plane technique, the patient should be seated with the elbow flexed and hand supinated (Fig. 8.2a). The ultrasound transducer will then be placed in the axial plane on the proximal humerus, centering the biceps tendon in the bicipital groove (Fig. 8.2b). The circumflex humeral artery should be identified in this groove using Doppler imaging. Avoiding the artery, a 25-gauge needle is then inserted in-plane with the transducer from lateral to medial aiming for the tendon sheath between the biceps tendon and the transhumeral ligament (Fig. 8.2c). Once the needle tip is visualized in the tendon sheath, aspirate and inject, observing for injectate flowing around the tendon [16].

Osteoarthritis in the Shoulder, Glenoid Labral Tears, and Adhesive Capsulitis

Glenohumeral Osteoarthritis

Osteoarthritis is a multifactorial process characterized by degeneration of joint cartilage. There are morphologic changes in the joint including cartilage degeneration, synovial inflammation, subchondral sclerosis, and osteophyte formation which can be seen on radiological studies [28]. Osteoarthritis (OA) becomes clinically significant when it causes symptoms; in the glenohumeral joint, these usually manifest as shoulder pain and eventually loss of range of motion (ROM). Shoulder pain is usually gradual and progressive; ROM is decreased, usually with a decrease in external rotation first. On physical exam the person may have tenderness to palpation in the anterior, lateral, and/or posterior compartments of the shoulder. The workup

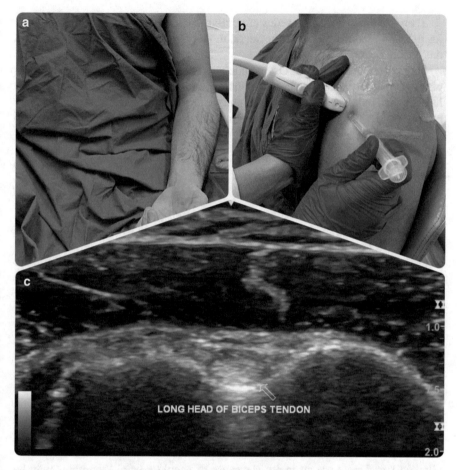

Fig. 8.2 (**a**) Patient positioning for ultrasound guided biceps tendon injection. (**b**) Transducer and needle placement for ultrasound guided injection. (**c**) Ultrasound image of biceps tendon with patient seated with elbow flexed and hand supinated

for suspected GH OA includes shoulder X-rays, including anterior posterior (AP), axillary, and scapular in Y views. Common X-ray findings include joint space narrowing, subchondral sclerosis, and osteophyte formation [28].

Current treatment for glenohumeral OA includes activity modification, analgesic medication including acetaminophen and nonsteroidal anti-inflammatories (NSAIDs), physical therapy, and injections, usually of a steroid solution or viscosupplementation [29]. There is limited evidence-based literature on the efficacy of intra-articular glenohumeral steroid and viscosupplementation for GH OA. Merolla et al. found improvements in the visual analog pain scale for both intra-articular steroid injection of methylprednisolone (for 1 month posttreatment) and intra-articular Hylan G-F 20 (for 3 months posttreatment) although the results were not as favorable in severe OA or in patients with concomitant large rotator cuff tears [30].

There have also been case series of intra-articular GH botulinum toxin injections for the pain modulation effect; however, more research works need to be done in this area to assess efficacy [31].

Surgical treatments for GH OA include surgical debridement and shoulder arthroplasty (hemiarthroplasty versus total shoulder arthroplasty). Most of the evidence is level IV, and in some studies, patients undergoing total shoulder arthroplasty show better shoulder function compared to hemiarthroplasty [32, 33].

Acromioclavicular Osteoarthritis

Acromioclavicular (AC) osteoarthritis (OA) often presents as pain in the deltoid region. On physical exam there may be tenderness over the AC joint and pain with horizontal adduction movements of the shoulder. Diagnostic imaging for AC OA includes shoulder X-rays, specifically the Zanca view. Arthritic changes include joint space narrowing, subchondral sclerosis, and other findings discussed previously. Conservative treatment usually begins with activity modification and oral analgesics such as acetaminophen and NSAIDs. Steroid injections in the AC joint, either palpation guided or ultrasound guided are also common practice [34]. Efficacy of intra-articular AC joint steroid injections in the literature is controversial, but most studies show short-term (<2 mo) relief [34].

Glenoid Labral Tears

Glenoid labral tears are an important cause of shoulder pain. Symptoms may be nonspecific, but usually patients will complain of shoulder pain which worsens with abduction and external rotation (ABER). Special physical exam tests include pain with ABER as well as with a positive O'Brien test. The O'Brien test is performed with the patient flexing their arm at the shoulder with their thumb facing down, with the shoulder slightly adducted and elevating against resistance; pain in that position which improves when changing the arm to the supinated position is considered positive [35]. Traditionally, a MR arthrogram with contrast injected intra-articularly is obtained to confirm a suspected labral tear in the shoulder. Now, some physicians are also evaluating for posterior superior labral tears with arthrosonography [36]. Treatment for symptomatic glenoid labral tears includes activity modification, physical therapy, NSAIDs, and glenohumeral steroid injections. Studies show that for glenoid labral tears this conservative treatment may improve function and pain [37].

Adhesive Capsulitis

Adhesive capsulitis presents as shoulder pain accompanied with progressive loss of range of motion, initially of external rotation. It is due to shoulder capsular thickening and contracture. It may be divided into four stages: (1) pre-freezing: limited ROM and start of symptoms; (2) freezing: severely limited ROM and pain; (3) frozen: severely limited ROM, pain subsides; and (4) thawing: improving ROM and minimal pain [38]. It can take 1 year or more for the four stages to advance. Conservative treatment includes activity modification, physical therapy, NSAIDs, and glenohumeral steroid injections, including glenohumeral capsular distention. This involves injecting the GH joint with a high volume of injectate, usually a combination of a steroid, anesthetic, and saline.

Osteoarthritis in the Shoulder, Glenoid Labral Tears, and Adhesive Capsulitis: *Regenerative Medicine Applications*

Many regenerative treatments, including platelet-rich plasma, bone marrow aspirate, adipose-derived stem cells, and viscosupplementation, are being used to treat different shoulder pathologies. We will discuss injection techniques as well as available evidence for these treatments in different causes of shoulder pain.

Glenohumeral Osteoarthritis (GH OA)

The glenohumeral joint may be injected using ultrasound or fluoroscopic guidance. When using ultrasound guidance, a posterior approach is utilized. The author finds that the best position is to have the patient side-lying with the affected shoulder up and the patient facing the physician (Fig. 8.3a). The posterior glenohumeral joint is identified by placing the transducer axially, below the spine of the scapula (Fig. 8.3b, c). Once the joint is identified it can be reached using a lateral to medial, in-plane approach (Fig. 8.3b). Using sterile technique, the area of entry is anesthetized with a 25-gauge, 1.5-inch needle with about 2 mL of 1% lidocaine. A 22-gauge, 3.5-inch needle is then used to enter the joint space, and after negative aspiration, the injectate is administered [39].

Using fluoroscopic guidance for the glenohumeral joint can be performed both from an anterior and from a posterior approach. Here we will describe a posterior approach. The patient lies prone with their arm lying on their side. Using sterile technique the area overlying the superior lateral humeral head is marked with a

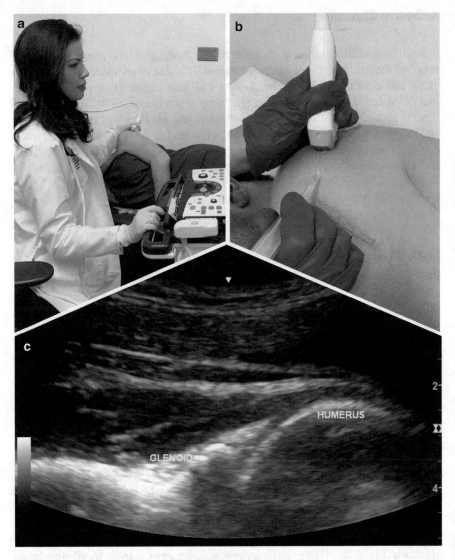

Fig. 8.3 (**a**) Patient position for ultrasound guided glenohumeral injection. (**b**) Ultrasound transducer and needle alignment for glenohumeral injection. (**c**) Ultrasound image of glenohumeral joint with patient sidelying

skin marker. When the desired area is confirmed, the skin is anesthetized using a 25-gauge, 1.5-inch needle with about 2 mL of 1% lidocaine. A 22-gauge, 3.5-inch needle is then used to enter the joint space; when a bony endpoint is felt, 2 mL of contrast dye is injected to confirm joint placement and nonvascular flow. After this is confirmed and negative aspiration, the injectate is administered [40].

Research on platelet-rich plasma for GH OA is limited to case reports. In a case report by Freitag, a 62-year-old woman with GH OA underwent three ultrasound-guided glenohumeral PRP injections, each 1 week apart [41]. Her pain improved substantially on the numerical pain rating scale and stayed between 0 and 1 out of 10 at 42 weeks post-procedure; she also improved functionally. More research is needed in regenerative medicine applications for GH OA. This case report used photoactivated PRP, but the author did not note if it was leukocyte rich or leukocyte poor. Extrapolating from research on knee osteoarthritis, leukocyte-poor PRP seems to be better for joint osteoarthritis than leukocyte-rich PRP, but more research is needed. There is also limited evidence to recommend a series of three injections versus one.

Glenohumeral injections of platelet-rich plasma for adhesive capsulitis have shown benefits in some studies. Kothari et al. randomized 162 patients with adhesive capsulitis to a single GH PRP injection, a corticosteroid injection, or ultrasonic therapy (7 sessions). They found statistically significant improvements in active and passive shoulder ROM and visual analog pain scores in the PRP group compared to the other two groups [42].

The benefits of viscosupplementation for glenohumeral osteoarthritis have been investigated. Kwon et al. compared a series of three sodium hyaluronate injections to saline injections in a randomized controlled trial on subjects with glenohumeral OA. In a subset analysis, they found improvements in pain in the hyaluronate group who did not have concomitant shoulder pathologies; however their initial analysis did not show any statistically significant differences in pain between both groups [43]. Other studies have not found statistically significant differences in viscosupplementation versus placebo (saline injections) for GH OA. More studies are needed.

Glenoid Labral Tears

Literature on outcomes of platelet-rich plasma and other regenerative treatments for glenoid labral tears is scarce. The labrum can be targeted by injecting the glenohumeral joint itself as described above.

Acromioclavicular Osteoarthritis

At this time there is limited evidence evaluating the efficacy of viscosupplementation, platelet-rich plasma, or other regenerative techniques for acromioclavicular osteoarthritis (AC OA).

The AC joint may be accessed for injection using ultrasound guidance. Here we will describe an axial, out of plane approach. Start with the patient in a sitting position with their arm resting at their side. Place the transducer over the acromioclavicular joint in the coronal plane (Fig. 8.4a, b). Using the center marker on the

Fig. 8.4 (a) Ultrasound transducer placement in the coronal plane for acromioclavicular joint injection. (b) Ultrasound image of the acromioclavicular joint with patient in sitting position and arm resting at the side

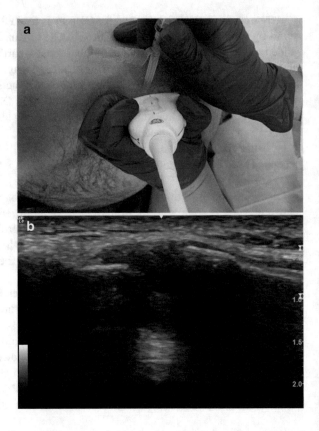

transducer and corresponding marker on the screen, place the target entry point of the AC joint at this point. Using sterile technique with a transducer cover and sterile gel, use a 25-gauge, 1.5-inch needle to enter; then using a step-down approach, enter the joint. Once your needle tip is visualized within the joint, aspirate and inject [44].

References

1. Khan KM, Cook JL, Bonar F, et al. Histopathology of common tendinopathies. Update and implications for clinical management. Sports Med. 1999;27:393.
2. Dela Rosa TL, Wang AW, Zheng MH. Tendinosis of the rotator cuff: a review. J Musculoskel Res. 2001;5:143.
3. Uhthoff HK, Loehr JW. Calcific tendinopathy of the rotator cuff: pathogenesis, diagnosis, and management. J Am Acad Orthop Surg. 1997;5:183.
4. Itoi E, Kido T, Sano A, et al. Which is more useful, the "full can test" or the "empty can test," in detecting the torn supraspinatus tendon? Am J Sports Med. 1999;27:65–8.
5. Jain NB, Luz J, Higgins LD, et al. The diagnostic accuracy of special tests for rotator cuff tear: the ROW Cohort Study. Am J Phys Med Rehabil. 2017;96:176.
6. Walch G, Boulahia A, Calderone S, Robinson AH. The 'dropping' and 'hornblower's' signs in evaluation of rotator-cuff tears. J Bone Joint Surg Br. 1998;80:624.

7. Sambandam SN, Khanna V, et al. Rotator cuff tears: an evidence based approach. World J Orthop. 2015;6(11):902–18.
8. Kibler WB. Rehabilitation of rotator cuff tendinopathy. Clin Sports Med. 2003;22:837.
9. Green S, Buchbinder R, Hetrick S. Physiotherapy interventions for shoulder pain. Cochrane Database Syst Rev. 2003:CD004258.
10. Paoloni JA, Appleyard RC, Nelson J, Murrell GA. Topical glyceryl trinitrate application in the treatment of chronic supraspinatus tendinopathy: a randomized, double-blinded, placebo-controlled clinical trial. Am J Sports Med. 2005;33:806.
11. Giombini A, Di Cesare A, Safran MR, et al. Short-term effectiveness of hyperthermia for supraspinatus tendinopathy in athletes: a short-term randomized controlled study. Am J Sports Med. 2006;34:1247.
12. Nho SJ, Strauss EJ, Lenart BA, et al. Long head of the biceps tendinopathy: diagnosis and management. J Am Acad Orthop Surg. 2010;18:645.
13. Schickendantz M, King D. Nonoperative management (including ultrasound-guided injections) of proximal biceps disorders. Clin Sports Med. 2016;35:57.
14. Hashiuchi T, Sakurai G, Morimoto M, et al. Accuracy of the biceps tendon sheath injection: ultrasound-guided or unguided injection? A randomized controlled trial. J Shoulder Elbow Surg. 2011;20:1069.
15. Virk MS, Nicholson GP. Complications of proximal biceps tenotomy and tenodesis. Clin Sports Med. 2016;35:181.
16. Baxi N, Spinner DA. Shoulder. In: Spinner D, Kirschner J, Herrera J, editors. Atlas of ultrasound guided musculoskeletal injections. Musculoskeletal medicine. New York, NY: Springer; 2014.
17. Rha DW, Park GY. Comparison of the therapeutic effects of ultrasound-guided platelet-rich plasma injection and dry needling in rotator cuff disease: a randomized controlled trial. Clin. Rehabil. 2012;27(2).
18. Kesikburun S, Tan AK, et al. Platelet-rich plasma injections in the treatment of chronic rotator cuff tendinopathy: a randomized controlled trial with 1-year follow-up. Am J Sports Med. 2013;41:2609–16.
19. Von Wehren L, Blanke F, et al. The effect of subacromial injections of autologous conditioned plasma versus cortisone for the treatment of symptomatic partial rotator cuff tears. Knee Surg Sports Traumatol Arthrosc. 2016;24:3787.
20. Shams A, El-Sayed M, et al. Subacromial injection of autologous platelet-rich plasma versus corticosteroid for the treatment of symptomatic partial rotator cuff tears. Eur J Orthop Surg Traumatol. 2016;26:837.
21. Kennedy JC, Baxter WR. The effects of local steroid injections on tendons: a biomechanical and microscopic correlative study. Am J Sports Med. 1976;4:1.
22. Vavken P, Sadoghi P, Palmer M, Rosso C, Mueller AM, Szoelloesy G, et al. Platelet-rich plasma reduces retear rates after arthroscopic repair of small- and medium-sized rotator cuff tears but is not cost-effective. Am J Sports Med. 2015;43:3071–6.
23. Saltzman BM, Jain A, Campbell KA, Mascarenhas R, Romeo AA, Verma NN, et al. Does the use of platelet-rich plasma at the time of surgery improve clinical outcomes in arthroscopic rotator cuff repair when compared with control cohorts? A systematic review of meta-analyses. Arthroscopy. 2016;32:906–18.
24. Jo CH, Shin JS, Shin WH, Lee SY, Yoon KS, Shin S. Platelet-rich plasma for arthroscopic repair of medium to large rotator cuff tears: a randomized controlled trial. Am J Sports Med. 2015;43:2102–10.
25. Pandey V, Bandi A, Madi S, Agarwal L, Acharya KKV, Maddukuri S, et al. Does application of moderately concentrated platelet-rich plasma improve clinical and structural outcome after arthroscopic repair of medium-sized to large rotator cuff tear? A randomized controlled trial. J Shoulder Elb Surg. 2016;25:1312–22.
26. Ellera Gomes JL, da Silva RC, Silla LMR. Conventional rotator cuff repair complemented by the aid of mononuclear autologous stem cells. Knee Surg Sports Traumatol Arthrosc. 2012;20(2):373–7.

27. Gulotta LV, Kovacevic D, Packer JD. Bone marrow-derived mesenchymal stem cells transduced with scleraxis improve rotator cuff healing in a rat model. Am J Sports Med. 2011;39(6):1282–9.
28. Bijlsma JW, Berenbaum F, Lafeber FP. Osteoarthritis: an update with relevance for clinical practice. Lancet. 2011;377:2115–26.
29. Macías-Hernández SI, Morones-Alba JD, Miranda-Duarte A. Glenohumeral osteoarthritis: overview, therapy, and rehabilitation. Disabil Rehabil. 2017;39(16):1674–82.
30. Merolla G, Sperling JW, Paladini P, Porcellini G. Efficacy of Hylan G-F 20 versus 6-methylprednisolone acetate in painful shoulder osteoarthritis: a retrospective controlled trial. Musculoskelet Surg. 2011;95(03):215–24.
31. Cinone N, Letizia S, Santoro L, Gravina M. Intra-articular injection of botulinum toxin type A for shoulder pain in glenohumeral osteoarthritis: a case series summary and review of the literature. J Pain Res. 2018;11:1239–45.
32. Singh JA, Sperling J, Buchbinder R, McMaken K. Surgery for shoulder osteoarthritis. Cochrane Database Syst Rev. 2010(10):CD008089. https://doi.org/10.1002/14651858.CD008089.pub2
33. Sayegh ET, Mascarenhas R, Chalmers PN, Cole BJ, Romeo AA, Verma NN. Surgical treatment options for glenohumeral arthritis in young patients: a systematic review and meta-analysis. Arthroscopy. 2015;31:1156–1166.e8.
34. Buttaci CJ, Stitik TP, Yonclas PP, Foye PM. Osteoarthritis of the acromioclavicular joint: a review of anatomy, biomechanics, diagnosis, and treatment. Am J Phys Med Rehabil. 2004;83:791–7.
35. Guanche CA, Jones DC. Clinical testing for tears of the glenoid labrum. Arthroscopy. 2003;19(5):517–23.
36. Park D. Clinical characteristics of patients with posterosuperior labral tear: a comparison with patients with other shoulder disorders. J Pain Res. 2018;11:1795–802.
37. Shin SJ, Lee J, Jeon YS, Ko YW, Kim RG. Clinical outcomes of non-operative treatment for patients presenting SLAP lesions in diagnostic provocative tests and MR arthrography. Knee Surg Sports Traumatol Arthrosc. 2016;(June):24.
38. Fields BKK, Skalski MR, Patel DB, et al. Adhesive capsulitis: review of imaging findings, pathophysiology, clinical presentation, and treatment options. Skeletal Radiol. 2019. https://doi.org/10.1007/s00256-018-3139-6
39. Spinner DA, Kirschner JS, Herrera JE, editors. Atlas of ultrasound guided musculoskeletal injections. New York, NY: Springer; 2014. https://doi.org/10.1007/978-1-4614-8936-8.
40. Farmer KD, Hughes PM. MR arthrography of the shoulder: fluoroscopically guided technique using a posterior approach. AJR Am J Roentgenol. 2002;178:433–4.
41. Freitag J. The effect of photoactivated platelet-rich plasma injections in the novel treatment of shoulder osteoarthritis. Int J Case Rep Imag. 2014;5:546.
42. Kothari SY, Srikumar V, Singh N. Comparative efficacy of platelet rich plasma injection, corticosteroid injection and ultrasonic therapy in the treatment of periarthritis shoulder. J Clin Diagn Res. 2017;11:RC15–8.
43. Kwon YW, Eisenberg G, Zuckerman JD. Sodium hyaluronate for the treatment of chronic shoulder pain associated with glenohumeral osteoarthritis: a multicenter, randomized, double-blind, placebo-controlled trial. J Shoulder Elbow Surg. 2013;22:584–94.
44. Furman MB, Berkwits L, editors. Atlas of image-guided spinal procedures. 2nd ed. Philadelphia, PA: Elsevier; 2018.

Chapter 9
Regenerative Medicine for the Elbow

Allison N. Schroeder, Michael Guthrie, Stephen Schaaf, and Kentaro Onishi

Bones/Joints

The elbow joint consists of articulations between the humerus proximally and radius and ulna distally. The distal humerus fans out to form the medial and lateral epicondyles, which serve as an attachment point for ligaments and tendons. The trochlea of the humerus (medial condyle) articulates with the ulna forming the ulnohumeral joint, and the capitellum of the humerus (lateral condyle) articulates with the radial head forming the radiocapitellar joint. The proximal radioulnar joint is formed between the radius and the ulna. Conditions affecting the elbow joint include arthritis, which is more common in older adults, and osteochondritis dissecans, which is more common in adolescents.

Arthritis

Arthritis of the elbow joint can result from rheumatoid arthritis, primary osteoarthritis, or post-traumatic arthritis but is less common than arthritis of other joints [1]. Osteoarthritis commonly presents with pain, swelling, stiffness, and sometimes loss of passive ROM in an older individual who often has a history indicative of traumatic elbow injury or rheumatological disease.

A. N. Schroeder · M. Guthrie · S. Schaaf
University of Pittsburgh Medical Center, Department of PM&R, Pittsburgh, PA, USA

K. Onishi (✉)
University of Pittsburgh School of Medicine, Department of PM&R, Department of Orthopaedic Surgery, Pittsburgh, PA, USA

© Springer Nature Switzerland AG 2020
G. Cooper et al. (eds.), *Regenerative Medicine for Spine and Joint Pain*,
https://doi.org/10.1007/978-3-030-42771-9_9

Osteochondritis Dissecans (OCD)

OCD is a disease process that results in separation of a focal lesion of cartilage from subchondral bone and is most commonly seen on the capitellum of male adolescent throwing athletes [2, 3]. OCD typically presents with progressively worsening activity-related pain and stiffness in the dominant arm of an overhead throwing athlete [4]. Patients often lack 15–30 degrees of full extension, which should point to the need for further evaluation with X-rays and subsequent MRI if X-rays are normal [4].

Ligaments

All ligaments about the elbow are extra-articular and provide the main source of stability. These include ulnar (medial) collateral ligamentous complex, radial (lateral) collateral ligamentous complex, anterior ligament, posterior ligament, and the joint capsule.

Ulnar Collateral Ligament (UCL)

The UCL originates from the medial condyle of the humerus and inserts on the sublime tubercle on the ulna. It consists of three distinct bands: the anterior bundle, posterior bundle, and transverse ligaments [5]. The anterior bundle runs from the medial humeral epicondyle to the sublime tubercle on the medial side of the coronoid process of the ulna and is thought to be the most clinically relevant as these fibers provide resistance to valgus instability, especially during the late cocking phase of throwing, and are most commonly injured with repetitive overhead throwing [5, 6]. Injury to the UCL commonly presents with pain and improved throwing performance, and acute injury may be associated with a "pop." Physical exam is notable for laxity with valgus stress.

Lateral Collateral Ligamentous Complex

The lateral collateral (radial) ligamentous complex consists of the annular ligament which surrounds the radial head, the radial collateral ligament (RCL) that spans from the lateral epicondyle to the annular ligament in a fan shape, and the lateral ulnar collateral ligament (LUCL) that runs from the lateral humeral epicondyle to the supinator crest. This complex plays a key role in preventing posterolateral and varus instability and is most commonly injured in overhead athletes with repeated varus stress or traumatic elbow dislocations [5, 7]. Injury to this complex commonly presents with pain and may result in mechanical symptoms with laxity to varus stress seen on physical examination.

Tendons

Tendons about the elbow at highest risk of injury include the proximal common extensor tendons (extensor carpi radialis brevis and extensor digitorum) and common flexor/pronator tendons (flexor carpi radialis and pronator teres), as well as the distal biceps and triceps tendons. Injury to these tendons results in tendinopathy that encompasses a spectrum of acute inflammation (tendinitis) to chronic inflammation and degeneration (tendinosis) to partial- or full-thickness tear. Most patients present with sustained pain and functional impairment with tendinosis due to repetitive microtrauma resulting in collagen disarray, necrotic tenocytes, and neovascularization that ultimately results in impaired healing and fibrotic scarring that is difficult to treat with conventional modalities. Acute rupture results in tendon defect.

Common Extensor Tendon

The extensor carpi radialis brevis, extensor digitorum, extensor carpi ulnaris, and extensor digiti minimi originate from the lateral epicondyle of the humerus and make up the common extensor tendon. Tendinopathy of the common extensor tendon at the lateral elbow is one of the most common tendon injuries in the upper extremity and occurs in 1–3% of the general population from repetitive contraction and micro-tearing of the tendon with pain most commonly located about 1–2 centimeters distal to the lateral epicondyle in the dominant extremity of middle-aged adults; it worsens with resisted wrist extension or passive stretch on the tendons [8–10].

Common Flexor/Pronator Tendon

The pronator teres, flexor carpi radialis, palmaris longus, flexor carpi ulnaris, and flexor digitorum superficialis originate from the medial epicondyle of the humerus and from the common flexor/pronator tendon. Tendinopathy of the common flexor/pronator tendon also occurs in middle-aged adults from an overuse mechanism but is less common, occurring in only 0.4% of the general population, and presents as pain over the medial epicondyle that worsens with resisted wrist flexion or passive stretch on the tendons [8].

Distal Biceps Tendon

The distal biceps tendon inserts on the radial tuberosity. Tendinopathy of the distal biceps is thought to be rare but typically occurs from repetitive microtraumas in those between the ages of 40 and 50 years that perform a large eccentric load, resulting in anterior elbow pain that worsens with resisted elbow flexion and supination [11].

Distal Triceps Tendon

The distal triceps tendon attaches on the olecranon process of the ulna. Distal triceps tendon injury is less commonly observed but can occur with overuse or trauma, resulting in partial avulsion of the medial portion of the tendon or complete rupture at the osteotendinous junction [12].

Treatment: The Standard of Care and Evidence

A thorough diagnostic evaluation must precede treatment. Making an accurate diagnosis is the most important step in the treatment process. All patients should be screened for alarm symptoms that would prompt consideration for further workup or imaging evaluation. Traumatic injury, history of dislocation, joint swelling without trauma, and mechanical symptoms should be considered, and, if present, further workup should be pursued.

In general, the standard of care for treatment of nontraumatic injuries at the elbow begins with rest, ice, nonsteroidal anti-inflammatory drugs (NSAIDs), activity modification, and physical therapy to address the underlying pathology. The use of corticosteroid injections is controversial, as they typically result in improved short-term outcomes but have similar or worse outcomes at 1year and may negatively affect long-term tendon health or lead to rupture [13–15]. Typical surgical indications include displaced or intra-articular fractures, tendon or ligament ruptures, unstable or complete osteochondral lesions, or failure of injuries to respond to conservative treatment after 6–12 months.

Bone/Joint

Arthritis

Elbow osteoarthritis is typically treated conservatively with rest, nonsteroidal anti-inflammatory drugs, activity modification, and dynamic hinged or static splinting along with physical therapy [1]. Intra-articular steroid injections can also be considered [16]. Injections should be performed under ultrasound guidance (100% accuracy), which has been shown to be more accurate than use of landmark guidance (77.5% accuracy) [17]. Injection of hyaluronic acid has not been shown to be effective in the elbow albeit the small sample size in one study [18]. Surgery is reserved for those that fail conservative management, with total elbow arthroplasty as a last resort since it is associated with complications in 11–38% of cases, including persistent minor infection, persistent contracture, and transient nerve palsies [1, 19, 20].

OCD

Stable OCD lesions can be treated conservatively, but unstable lesions require surgical repair [21]. Conservative treatment involves an initial period of rest with avoidance of aggravating activities (throwing, weightlifting, gymnastics), with or without the use of a hinged elbow brace, followed by progression to strengthening exercises when patients are pain free [22]. Typically, athletes can start gentle overhead throwing at 3–4 months if they remain pain free, and 84.2% of patients return to play at 6 months if they are compliant with conservative management [22, 23]. Operative treatment is necessary in patients who fail conservative management, have unstable lesions, or have loose bodies associated with mechanical symptoms [22]. Surgical options vary and depend on several factors (lesion size, cartilage cap presence, etc.) and include loose body removal/chondroplasty [24], microfracture/retrograde drilling [22, 24], fixation (with wires, screws, bone pegs) [4, 25], or osteochondral allograft transplantation system [26]. Despite complications being rare, reported rates of return to sport in throwing athletes are less than 50% [27]. A detailed discussion of surgical management is beyond the scope of this chapter.

Ligaments

UCL

Nonoperative treatment is often first line and includes rest (for 6 weeks) followed by initial physical therapy for flexor/pronator strengthening and then a progressive throwing program, but only 42% of athletes returned to sport after nonoperative treatment [28]. Surgery is indicated in complete tears and partial tears that are not responsive to conservative management. Reconstruction using a palmaris longus autograft is typically preferred over repair. Eighty-three percent of athletes were able to return to sport at the same or a higher level at an average of 11.6 months after surgery [29]. Repair is typically reserved for partial tears near the UCL origin or insertion in young athletes and consists of direct suture repair of the injured ligament with placement of an augmentation device with 87% of patients returning to sport [30].

Tendons

Common Extensor Tendon

Common extensor tendinopathy, commonly known as "tennis elbow" or lateral epicondylosis, is typically self-limiting with 90% of patients recovering by 1 year with conservative multimodal treatment consisting of physical therapy with modalities, use of counterforce brace or wrist splint, nonsteroidal anti-inflammatory drugs (NSAIDs), topical nitroglycerin, and extracorporeal shock wave therapy, though there is no consensus treatment algorithm [31–36]. Nitroglycerin patches have been shown to significantly reduce activity-related elbow pain and epicondylar tenderness and improve long-term functional outcomes but have side effects including headaches, facial flushing, and contact dermatitis [37, 38]. Corticosteroid injections are still commonly used to address pain associated with common extensor tendinopathy and show short-term benefits and functional improvements, but tenotoxic effects and increased incidence of recurrence have been reported [13, 39]. Percutaneous needle tenotomy (PNT) is an office-based procedure where a needle is used to repeatedly fenestrate the diseased portions of tendon under sonographic guidance with local anesthesia [40]. In a case series, subjects were treated using PNT, and 80% of these subjects reported good to excellent results at an average follow-up duration of 28 months, and a subsequent corticosteroid injection was not necessary [41]. PNT is also referred to as a "peppering" technique and is sometimes performed in conjunction with regenerative medicine procedures, as discussed later in this chapter. Other studies point to efficacy of dry needling or acupuncture to treat common extensor tendinopathy [42, 43].

Surgery is typically reserved for those who do not improve with conservative therapy by 6 months or those who have complete tendon rupture. Several surgical techniques (open, arthroscopic, and percutaneous microtenotomy) have been described with no differences in postoperative pain, recurrence rate, or procedural failure among the different surgical techniques [44, 45]. The general surgical principle consists of first identifying the affected portion of the tendon which is excised to further facilitate a biologic response and is then usually repaired. Those undergoing arthroscopic treatment have greater functional outcomes or more rapid return to work with utilization of less postoperative physical therapy compared to those undergoing an open procedure [46, 47]. Those more likely to have residual symptoms after surgery are those with a high level of baseline symptoms, acute occurrence of symptoms, or long duration of symptoms [48]. Patients typically recover in 4–12 weeks with 95% achieving good to excellent results and only about 1.5% of patients requiring surgical revision surgery, which is usually successful [49].

Common Flexor/Pronator Tendon

Common flexor/pronator tendinopathy, commonly known as "golfer's elbow" or medial epicondylosis, is often treated in a similar manner to common extensor tendinopathy, as described above.

Distal Biceps Tendon

For distal biceps tendinopathy or partial tear, nonoperative management consists of rest, analgesia as needed, and a rehabilitation program. Studies have shown that patients with complete rupture that are treated using the above options can have continued pain and up to 40% loss of supination strength and 30% loss of range of motion strength compared to their normal side [50]. Corticosteroid injections are rarely used. A cadaveric investigation has shown that sonographically guided distal biceps tendon injections are feasible and can be done through multiple approaches, with the posterior approach being technically easiest, safest, and most accurate [51]. Accuracy and safety are unclear for landmark-guided injections to this tendon. Case series report success of surgical repair for symptomatic refractory distal biceps tendon complete tears [52, 53], but surgical fixation has been shown to be associated with complications, most commonly nerve dysfunction and radioulnar synostosis in up to 27% of patients [54].

Distal Triceps Tendon

The treatment of triceps tendinopathy or partial distal triceps tears is somewhat controversial, and conservative treatment consisting of an initial period of immobilization can be attempted based on the patient's tear severity (<50%), functional demands (low demands), and improvement with conservative management [12, 55]. Complete distal triceps tendon tears require immediate surgical repair in healthy patients, but postoperative range of motion restrictions and rehabilitation is variable [56]. Injury to the ulnar nerve is a reported complication [56].

Regenerative Treatments

Regenerative treatments are currently considered for refractory symptoms of tendinopathy or partial tears of the tendon, partial symptomatic tears of the ligaments, or refractory osseous or chondral pathologies about the elbow, particularly in patients who are poor surgical candidates or wish to avoid surgery.

Bone/Joint

Arthritis

There are no studies that have investigated the use of regenerative therapies to treat elbow osteoarthritis, but regenerative therapies have shown promise in other joints (as discussed in other chapters in the book).

OCD

One small surgical study examined the use of regenerative therapies to treat OCD. In this case series, three adolescent boys (ages 12, 15, and 17) with MRI diagnosis of osteochondral lesions of the elbow (stage not described) were treated with arthroscopy or arthroscopy plus a mini-open procedure augmented with autologous platelet gel and bone marrow aspirate concentrate [57]. After progression through a rehabilitation protocol beginning with passive range of motion and ending with sports-specific drills, all three subjects returned to sport pain free by 9 months [57]. There are no studies examining the use of regenerative medicine therapies without arthroscopy, and it is difficult to draw a conclusion from this small surgical study.

Ligament

Elbow Ulnar Collateral Ligament (UCL)

With the advancement of ultrasound technology, the ability to visualize partial tears of the ulnar collateral ligament, especially dynamically, has drastically improved, and there is increasing interest in nonoperative management with the use of regenerative medicine. A survey of American elbow and shoulder surgeons showed that 36.3% of responders currently use PRP to treat UCL injuries where 43.9% of those using PRP prefer leukocyte-poor PRP, 16.6% prefer leukocyte-rich PRP, and the remaining 39.9% had no preference [58]. In the same survey, 8% reported using stem cell therapies with bone marrow lipoaspirate concentrate being most commonly used (31.3%) [58].

Two case series of a combined 78 athletes with UCL partial tears who failed conservative management and who were treated with sonographically guided leukocyte-poor PRP injection(s) showed improvement in pain and function with a mean return to play of 12 weeks [10, 59]. An additional small case series showed more rapid return to play (mean 36 days) in non-throwing professional athletes (hockey players) who sustained a mid- to high-grade traumatic UCL injury that was treated with two sonographically guided injections of leukocyte-poor PRP a mean of 9 days apart and resulted in improved pain and decreased laxity on follow-up sonographic imaging [60]. Despite showing promise in case series, the use of PRP to treat UCL injuries in 133 major and minor league baseball players who had failed conservative management showed a significantly more rapid return to play in those treated conservatively than those that received PRP injection (51 vs. 64 days), but this study did not mention the use of sonographic guidance, which may improve the efficacy of an injection if it is accurately placed [61]. With proper patient selection, treatment of partial UCL injuries with sonographically guided PRP injection offers a viable treatment option with a more rapid return to play than surgical reconstruction, though RCTs are lacking.

The use of other regenerative treatments for UCL injury has not been studied.

Annular Ligament and Radial Collateral Ligament

Isolated annular ligament and radial collateral ligament tears are very rare, and there are no studies on regenerative medicine to treat injuries to these structures in isolation. Two RCTs studying prolotherapy for the common extensor tendon also involved injection into the annular ligament or the annular ligament and radial collateral ligament and are described later in this chapter [62, 63].

Tendon

Common Extensor Tendon

The use of regenerative treatments for elbow injuries has been most extensively studied in patients with common extensor tendinopathy.

Platelet-Rich Plasma (PRP)

Initial uncontrolled studies have shown promising benefits and safety of PRP used to treat common extensor tendinopathy which inspired level 1 studies comparing PRP to corticosteroids, percutaneous needle tenotomy, saline, and surgery that will be discussed here. It is important to note that the formulation of PRP (leukocyte rich vs. leukocyte poor, platelet count and use of an activating agent), use of additional procedures (percutaneous needle tenotomy), use of sonographic guidance, and postinjection rehabilitation protocol varied across studies [64]. In general, leukocyte-rich PRP is preferred over leukocyte-poor PRP in the treatment of tendon injury [65], but when compared directly to treat common extensor tendinopathy, no difference was found between the two [66]. Though the optimum rehabilitation protocol has yet to be determined, animal studies show improved efficacy when PPR injections are combined with mechanical loading of the tendon, indicating that rehabilitation should be performed after injection [67]. Specific discussion of the details of the methods of each RCT is beyond the scope of this chapter.

In randomized control trials (RCTs) that compare one injection of leukocyte-poor PRP to corticosteroids, similar improvement in pain and function was noted in the short term (2 weeks–6 months) [68–70], but leukocyte-rich or leukocyte-poor PRP tends to provide continued improvement in pain and function leading to superiority in the intermediate to long term (6 months–2 years) [71–73] with sonographic structural improvements in tendinosis seen in those treated with leukocyte-poor PRP at 6 months [74]. When used in isolation, PRP has been shown to have slightly superior outcomes to PNT (5–10 passages with a 22- to 27-gauge needle is most commonly used) at up to 1 year, but the two treatments are complementary, leading to greatest improvement in pain and function when used in combination in RCTs [75–78]. RCTs comparing PRP to autologous blood injection (ABI) with associated

PNT have shown clinically equal efficacy at up to 1 year [79–82]. Although retrospective studies show equality or superiority of PRP injections to surgery to treat common extensor tendinopathy at 1 month–1 year follow-up [83, 84], the only RCT comparing PRP to surgery notes significantly better overall pain, night pain, and functional scores at 2 years after surgery, despite more similar outcomes in efficacy in the short and midterm [64]. It should also be noted that in this study, only the surgical group received physical therapy while the PRP injection group did not, negating the direct comparison between the two groups. Overall, PRP is safe and can be an effective treatment for common extensor tendinopathy and should be considered in the appropriate clinical context.

Autologous Blood Injection (ABI)

There are several case series and prospective clinical studies that have indicated that ABI is a safe and effective treatment for recalcitrant common extensor tendinopathy [80, 85–91], but the evidence in RCTs does not show superiority when compared to other treatments, including PRP [80–82], extracorporeal shockwave therapy (received once a week for 3 weeks) [92], and saline injection [93]. When comparing corticosteroid and ABI, small RCTs have shown superiority of corticosteroid at 1 month [92] with better results using ABI at 6 months [93] and up to 2 years [92]. Though high-level evidence is lacking, ABI seems to be a safe and effective treatment for common extensor tendinopathy.

Prolotherapy

A few studies examining prolotherapy for the treatment of common extensor tendinopathy have shown promising results, but small sample sizes, variability in contents of the "prolotherapy" mixture, number of injections given, and lack of sonographic guidance for the injections limit our ability to draw definitive conclusions on an optimum protocol. Two RCTs compared multiple injections of different formulations of prolotherapy (consisting of sodium morrhuate, dextrose, lidocaine, Sensorcaine, and normal saline or phenol 1.2%, glycerine 12.5%, dextrose 12.5% in sterile water, and sodium morrhuate) to normal saline [94] or corticosteroid [62] into the tendon near the lateral epicondyle and surrounding structures, including the annular ligament, with prolotherapy showing superiority to normal saline from 8 weeks to 52 weeks but non-superiority to corticosteroids at up to 6 months, though the shorter follow-up in this study limits the ability to draw conclusions. In an attempt to directly compare prolotherapy formulations, there was no difference in functional improvement between prolotherapy consisting of dextrose and prolotherapy consisting of dextrose morrhuate, but both were superior to "watchful waiting" from 4 to 16 weeks [63]. Treatment with prolotherapy can be considered given the low risks of use of an inert substance but may require multiple injections; the duration of follow-up to see clinical efficacy and the optimum formulation are still not known.

Autologous Tenocyte Injection

Autologous tenocyte injection (ATI) is a novel therapy that has been studied to treat chronic, refractory common extensor tendinopathy. One case series of 17 patients examined the use of culturally expanded patellar-tendon-derived autologous tenocytes that were injected under sonographic guidance and showed improvement in pain, self-reported function, grip strength, and level of tendinosis seen on MRI at 12 months. Clinical measures also remained significantly improved at final follow-up at a mean of 4.5 years [95, 96]. Notably, no adverse events were observed, and only one patient progressed to surgery after a subsequent work-related injury [95, 96]. In another small case series, laboratory-prepared collagen-producing cells derived from dermal fibroblasts were injected under sonographic guidance into the site of intrasubstance tears of the common extensor tendon which resulted in improvement in patient-reported function and tendinosis severity on ultrasound at 6 weeks, 3 months, and 6 months with only one patient proceeding to surgery at 3 months [97]. In these small case series, ATI shows promise, but larger studies are needed to better determine its safety and efficacy and to gain FDA approval.

Mesenchymal Stem Cells (MSCs)

Bone marrow aspirate concentrate (BMAC) and allogenic adipose-derived mesenchymal stem cells are promising procedures that involve injection of MSCs into the area of disease/disrepair and have been examined in pilot studies. A case series of 30 patients with refractory common extensor tendinopathy who received landmark-guided injection of BMAC showed a highly significant improvement in self-reported functional outcomes at 2, 6, and 12 weeks of follow-up [98]. In another case series, 12 subjects underwent sonographically guided injection of enzymatically digested culturally expanded adipose-derived cells and reported improvement in pain and function with sonographic evidence of improvement in tendon defects at up to 52 weeks without significant adverse events [99]. Though treatment with MSCs shows promise, it is important to note that treatments that contain tissue that has been "more than minimally manipulated" are not currently approved by the FDA outside of the research setting.

Amniotic Membrane Injection

Amniotic membrane allograft injection has shown benefit in small case series, but FDA homologous use guidelines pose a barrier to future use of this injection clinically. A retrospective case series of 10 patients with common extensor tendinopathy treated with micronized dehydrated human amniotic chorionic membrane allograft showed improvement in self-reported function, with a 77% improvement of pain at 24–36 weeks [100]. In a case series of 40 patients with joint or tendon pathology treated with dehydrated human amnion/chorion membrane allograft injection under ultrasound guidance, 7 patients with lateral epicondylitis were treated [101]. There was no subgroup analysis that examined only those with lateral epicondylitis, but treatment of all conditions resulted in improved pain and function in all patients without significant adverse events at up to 3 months [101]. Utility of amniotic membrane allograft is still up for debate.

Percutaneous Ultrasonic Tenotomy

Percutaneous ultrasonic tenotomy is a device that uses a rapidly vibrating needle tip to emulsify diseased tendon and promote tendon fiber growth and reorganization that is performed under ultrasound guidance and is a promising treatment for tendinopathy at the elbow. A case series of 12 patients with common extensor tendinopathy and 7 patients with common flexor tendinopathy showed improvement in pain and function at 6 weeks that continued at 12 months without adverse events [102]. When retrospectively compared to PRP, patients who received percutaneous ultrasonic tenotomy for common flexor and extensor tendinopathy had equally significant improvements in pain, function, and patient satisfaction [103]. Percutaneous ultrasonic tenotomy shows promise though higher-level studies are needed and, theoretically, patients may benefit from percutaneous ultrasonic tenotomy in combination with other regenerative procedures such as PRP.

Common Flexor/Pronator Tendon

Clinical use of regenerative therapies to treat common flexor/pronator tendinopathy is primarily translated from studies on common extensor tendinopathy. Nevertheless, there are a few studies that specifically examine the use of regenerative medicine therapies to treat common flexor/pronator tendinopathy. A small case series showed that 1–2 injections of leukocyte-poor PRP showed overall functional improvement in the group that received a single injection (8 patients), but there was no functional improvement noted in the group that received two injections (6 patients) [104]. An earlier study showed that two injections with autologous blood injection (ABI) under sonographic guidance and combined with percutaneous needle tenotomy showed a significant reduction in pain and function, as well as a reduction in the amount of hypoechoic tendon and neovascularity seen on ultrasound at 10 months post-procedure [87]. Percutaneous ultrasonic tenotomy has been shown to be effective for treatment of medial elbow tendinosis, as stated above [102, 103]. These studies suggest that the use of regenerative therapies combined with a mechanical debridement of the tendon (percutaneous needle tenotomy or percutaneous ultrasonic tenotomy) may be beneficial, but subsequent injections without mechanical debridement may not be efficacious in treating common flexor/ pronator tendinopathy.

Use of other regenerative therapies has not been described for treatment of common flexor/pronator tendinopathy.

Distal Biceps Tendon

Ultrasound-guided PRP injection to treat biceps tendinopathy (confirmed on imaging) has been described in a cohort and case series study of 18 total patients and may be an alternative to traditional conservative nonoperative treatment for refractory tendinopathy [105, 106]. In the cohort study, a single sonographically guided injection of leukocyte-rich PRP (10 patients) or leukocyte-reduced PRP (2 patients) resulted in significant improvement in pain at rest and with activity, function, and biceps strength at median final follow-up of 47 months [105]. In a small case series, 6 patients with distal biceps tendinopathy confirmed by MRI or ultrasound that was refractory to conservative management were treated with needle tenotomy and leukocyte-rich nonactivated PRP with platelet concentration < 5 times serum concentration [106]. With the use of sonographic guidance to accurately evaluate the location of the tendon and target the area of injury [51], regenerative treatments have shown promise for the treatment of distal biceps tendon injury.

Use of other regenerative therapies has not been described for treatment of distal biceps tendon injury.

Distal Triceps Tendon

Only one case reports on the use of regenerative medicine to treat triceps tendon injury in a 47-year-old male weight lifter who suffered an acute partial rupture of the distal triceps tendon with MRI confirmation of the injury [107]. After failure to improve with physical therapy 5 weeks after the injury, the patient was treated with a landmark-guided leukocyte-poor PRP injection followed by physical therapy at 2 weeks postinjection; he was pain free at rest and able to return to weight lifting with minimal pain at 4 weeks postinjection [107].

Conclusion

Regenerative treatments for injuries about the elbow are best supported by many RCTs that examine outcomes in the treatment of common extensor tendinopathy. Studies suggest that PRP injections have long-term therapeutic benefit when compared to corticosteroid injection, local anesthetic injections, and conservative management alone, but the efficacy of PRP compared to mechanical debridement with percutaneous ultrasonic tenotomy or surgery has not been described in well-controlled studies. There is variability in the literature in the formulation of PRP, inconsistent use of additional procedures (percutaneous needle tenotomy) and sonographic guidance to perform the injection, as well as varied postinjection rehabilitation protocols across studies. There is limited evidence for the use of ABI, prolotherapy, ATI, BMAC, adipose tissue, amniotic membrane, and PUT with none of these treatments consistently showing superiority to other management options. Beyond treatment for common extensor tendinopathy, the data is limited by small sample sizes and case series or case studies but suggest that regenerative treatments such as PRP, prolotherapy, and BMAC might have promise in treating other injuries involving the elbow including common flexor/pronator tendinopathy, UCL injury, distal biceps tendinopathy, and distal triceps tendinopathy. There is limited evidence for the use of regenerative therapies to treat elbow arthritis, but based on our knowledge of the use of PRP to treat arthritis of other joints, it may also show efficacy in the elbow. Lastly, regenerative therapies have only been used to augment surgery for OCD and are less likely to be beneficial when injected in the setting of stable OCD.

References

1. Papatheodorou LK, Baratz ME, Sotereanos DG. Elbow arthritis: current concepts. J Hand Surg Am. 2013;38(3):605–13.
2. Schenck RC Jr, Athanasiou KA, Constantinides G, Gomez E. A biomechanical analysis of articular cartilage of the human elbow and a potential relationship to osteochondritis dissecans. Clin Orthop Relat Res. 1994;299:305–12.
3. Takahara M, Mura N, Sasaki J, Harada M, Ogino T. Classification, treatment, and outcome of osteochondritis dissecans of the humeral capitellum. J Bone Joint Surg Am. 2007;89(6):1205–14.
4. Baker CL 3rd, Romeo AA, Baker CL Jr. Osteochondritis dissecans of the capitellum. Am J Sports Med. 2010;38(9):1917–28.
5. Morrey BF, An KN. Functional anatomy of the ligaments of the elbow. Clin Orthop Relat Res. 1985;201:84–90.
6. Jackson TJ, Jarrell SE, Adamson GJ, Chung KC, Lee TQ. Biomechanical differences of the anterior and posterior bands of the ulnar collateral ligament of the elbow. Knee Surg Sports Traumatol Arthrosc. 2016;24(7):2319–23.
7. O'Driscoll SW, Bell DF, Morrey BF. Posterolateral rotatory instability of the elbow. J Bone Joint Surg Am. 1991;73(3):440–6.
8. Shiri R, Viikari-Juntura E, Varonen H, Heliovaara M. Prevalence and determinants of lateral and medial epicondylitis: a population study. Am J Epidemiol. 2006;164(11):1065–74.
9. Ruiz-Ruiz B, Fernandez-de-Las-Penas C, Ortega-Santiago R, Arendt-Nielsen L, Madeleine P. Topographical pressure and thermal pain sensitivity mapping in patients with unilateral lateral epicondylalgia. J Pain. 2011;12(10):1040–8.
10. Podesta L, Crow SA, Volkmer D, Bert T, Yocum LA. Treatment of partial ulnar collateral ligament tears in the elbow with platelet-rich plasma. Am J Sports Med. 2013;41(7):1689–94.
11. Stucken C, Ciccotti MG. Distal biceps and triceps injuries in athletes. Sports Med Arthrosc Rev. 2014;22(3):153–63.
12. Keener JD, Sethi PM. Distal triceps tendon injuries. Hand Clin. 2015;31(4):641–50.
13. Coombes BK, Bisset L, Brooks P, Khan A, Vicenzino B. Effect of corticosteroid injection, physiotherapy, or both on clinical outcomes in patients with unilateral lateral epicondylalgia: a randomized controlled trial. JAMA. 2013;309(5):461–9.
14. Smidt N, van der Windt DA, Assendelft WJ, Deville WL, Korthals-de Bos IB, Bouter LM. Corticosteroid injections, physiotherapy, or a wait-and-see policy for lateral epicondylitis: a randomised controlled trial. Lancet (London, England). 2002;359(9307):657–62.
15. Lambert MI, St Clair Gibson A, Noakes TD. Rupture of the triceps tendon associated with steroid injections. Am J Sports Med. 1995;23(6):778.
16. Soojian MG, Kwon YW. Elbow arthritis. Bull NYU Hosp Jt Dis. 2007;65(1):61–71.

17. Kim TK, Lee JH, Park KD, Lee SC, Ahn J, Park Y. Ultrasound versus palpation guidance for intra-articular injections in patients with degenerative osteoarthritis of the elbow. J Clin Ultrasound. 2013;41(8):479–85.
18. van Brakel RW, Eygendaal D. Intra-articular injection of hyaluronic acid is not effective for the treatment of post-traumatic osteoarthritis of the elbow. Arthroscopy. 2006;22(11):1199–203.
19. Welsink CL, Lambers KTA, van Deurzen DFP, Eygendaal D, van den Bekerom MPJ. Total elbow arthroplasty: a systematic review. JBJS Reviews. 2017;5(7):e4.
20. Kelly EW, Morrey BF, O'Driscoll SW. Complications of elbow arthroscopy. J Bone Joint Surgery Am Volume. 2001;83-a(1):25–34.
21. Maruyama M, Takahara M, Satake H. Diagnosis and treatment of osteochondritis dissecans of the humeral capitellum. J Orthop Sci. 2018;23(2):213–9.
22. Ahmad CS, Vitale MA, ElAttrache NS. Elbow arthroscopy: capitellar osteochondritis dissecans and radiocapitellar plica. Instr Course Lect. 2011;60:181–90.
23. Matsuura T, Kashiwaguchi S, Iwase T, Takeda Y, Yasui N. Conservative treatment for osteochondrosis of the humeral capitellum. Am J Sports Med. 2008;36(5):868–72.
24. Tis JE, Edmonds EW, Bastrom T, Chambers HG. Short-term results of arthroscopic treatment of osteochondritis dissecans in skeletally immature patients. J Pediatr Orthop. 2012;32(3):226–31.
25. Hennrikus WP, Miller PE, Micheli LJ, Waters PM, Bae DS. Internal fixation of unstable in situ osteochondritis dissecans lesions of the capitellum. J Pediatr Orthop. 2015;35(5):467–73.
26. Shimada K, Tanaka H, Matsumoto T, Miyake J, Higuchi H, Gamo K, et al. Cylindrical costal osteochondral autograft for reconstruction of large defects of the capitellum due to osteochondritis dissecans. J Bone Joint Surg Am. 2012;94(11):992–1002.
27. Byrd JW, Jones KS. Arthroscopic surgery for isolated capitellar osteochondritis dissecans in adolescent baseball players: minimum three-year follow-up. Am J Sports Med. 2002;30(4):474–8.
28. Rettig AC, Sherrill C, Snead DS, Mendler JC, Mieling P. Nonoperative treatment of ulnar collateral ligament injuries in throwing athletes. Am J Sports Med. 2001;29(1):15–7.
29. Cain EL Jr, Andrews JR, Dugas JR, Wilk KE, McMichael CS, Walter JC 2nd, et al. Outcome of ulnar collateral ligament reconstruction of the elbow in 1281 athletes: results in 743 athletes with minimum 2-year follow-up. Am J Sports Med. 2010;38(12):2426–34.
30. Erickson BJ, Bach BR Jr, Verma NN, Bush-Joseph CA, Romeo AA. Treatment of ulnar collateral ligament tears of the elbow: is repair a viable option? Orthop J Sports Med. 2017;5(1):2325967116682211.
31. Svernlov B, Adolfsson L. Non-operative treatment regime including eccentric training for lateral humeral epicondylalgia. Scand J Med Sci Sports. 2001;11(6):328–34.
32. Garg R, Adamson GJ, Dawson PA, Shankwiler JA, Pink MM. A prospective randomized study comparing a forearm strap brace versus a wrist splint for the treatment of lateral epicondylitis. J Shoulder Elb Surg. 2010;19(4):508–12.
33. Labelle H, Guibert R, Joncas J, Newman N, Fallaha M, Rivard CH. Lack of scientific evidence for the treatment of lateral epicondylitis of the elbow. An attempted meta-analysis. J Bone Joint Surg. 1992;74(5):646–51.
34. Niedermeier SR, Crouser N, Speeckaert A, Goyal KS. A survey of fellowship-trained upper extremity surgeons on treatment of lateral epicondylitis. Hand (New York, NY). 2018:1558944718770212.
35. Pettrone FA, McCall BR. Extracorporeal shock wave therapy without local anesthesia for chronic lateral epicondylitis. J Bone Joint Surg Am. 2005;87(6):1297–304.
36. Rompe JD, Decking J, Schoellner C, Theis C. Repetitive low-energy shock wave treatment for chronic lateral epicondylitis in tennis players. Am J Sports Med. 2004;32(3):734–43.
37. Paoloni JA, Appleyard RC, Nelson J, Murrell GA. Topical nitric oxide application in the treatment of chronic extensor tendinosis at the elbow: a randomized, double-blinded, placebo-controlled clinical trial. Am J Sports Med. 2003;31(6):915–20.

38. McCallum SD, Paoloni JA, Murrell GA. Five-year prospective comparison study of topical glyceryl trinitrate treatment of chronic lateral epicondylosis at the elbow. Br J Sports Med. 2011;45(5):416–20.
39. Claessen FM, Heesters BA, Chan JJ, Kachooei AR, Ring D, et al. J Hand Surg. 2016;41(10):988–98.e2.
40. McShane JM, Nazarian LN, Harwood MI. Sonographically guided percutaneous needle tenotomy for treatment of common extensor tendinosis in the elbow. J Ultrasound Med. 2006;25(10):1281–9.
41. McShane JM, Shah VN, Nazarian LN. Sonographically guided percutaneous needle tenotomy for treatment of common extensor tendinosis in the elbow: is a corticosteroid necessary? J Ultrasound Med. 2008;27(8):1137–44.
42. Uygur E, Aktas B, Ozkut A, Erinc S, Yilmazoglu EG. Dry needling in lateral epicondylitis: a prospective controlled study. Int Orthop. 2017;41(11):2321–5.
43. Ural FG, Ozturk GT, Boluk H, Akkus S. Ultrasonographic evaluation of acupuncture effect on common extensor tendon thickness in patients with lateral epicondylitis: a randomized controlled study. J Altern Complement Med (New York, NY). 2017;23(10):819–22.
44. Szabo SJ, Savoie FH 3rd, Field LD, Ramsey JR, Hosemann CD. Tendinosis of the extensor carpi radialis brevis: an evaluation of three methods of operative treatment. J Shoulder Elb Surg. 2006;15(6):721–7.
45. Gregory BP, Wysocki RW, Cohen MS. Controversies in surgical management of recalcitrant enthesopathy of the extensor carpi radialis brevis. J Hand Surg Am. 2016;41(8):856–9.
46. Solheim E, Hegna J, Oyen J. Arthroscopic versus open tennis elbow release: 3- to 6-year results of a case-control series of 305 elbows. Arthroscopy. 2013;29(5):854–9.
47. Peart RE, Strickler SS, Schweitzer KM Jr. Lateral epicondylitis: a comparative study of open and arthroscopic lateral release. Am J Orthop (Belle Mead, NJ). 2004;33(11):565–7.
48. Solheim E, Hegna J, Oyen J. Extensor tendon release in tennis elbow: results and prognostic factors in 80 elbows. Knee Surg Sports Traumatol Arthrosc. 2011;19(6):1023–7.
49. Degen RM, Cancienne JM, Camp CL, Altchek DW, Dines JS, Werner BC. Three or more preoperative injections is the most significant risk factor for revision surgery after operative treatment of lateral epicondylitis: an analysis of 3863 patients. J Shoulder Elb Surg. 2017;26(4):704–9.
50. Geaney LE, Brenneman DJ, Cote MP, Arciero RA, Mazzocca AD. Outcomes and practical information for patients choosing nonoperative treatment for distal biceps ruptures. Orthopedics. 2010;33(6):391.
51. Sellon JL, Wempe MK, Smith J. Sonographically guided distal biceps tendon injections: techniques and validation. J Ultrasound Med. 2014;33(8):1461–74.
52. Kelly EW, Steinmann S, O'Driscoll SW. Surgical treatment of partial distal biceps tendon ruptures through a single posterior incision. J Shoulder Elb Surg. 2003;12(5):456–61.
53. Vardakas DG, Musgrave DS, Varitimidis SE, Goebel F, Sotereanos DG. Partial rupture of the distal biceps tendon. J Shoulder Elb Surg. 2001;10(4):377–9.
54. Bisson L, Moyer M, Lanighan K, Marzo J. Complications associated with repair of a distal biceps rupture using the modified two-incision technique. J Shoulder Elb Surg. 2008;17(1 Suppl):67s–71s.
55. Vidal AF, Drakos MC, Allen AA. Biceps tendon and triceps tendon injuries. Clin Sports Med. 2004;23(4):707–22. xi.
56. van Riet RP, Morrey BF, Ho E, O'Driscoll SW. Surgical treatment of distal triceps ruptures. J Bone Joint Surg Am Vol. 2003;85-a(10):1961–7.
57. Guerra E, Fabbri D, Cavallo M, Marinelli A, Rotini R. Treatment of capitellar osteochondritis dissecans with a novel regenerative technique: case report of 3 patients after 4 years. Orthop J Sports Med. 2018;6(9):2325967118795831.
58. Hurwit DJ, Garcia GH, Liu J, Altchek DW, Romeo A, Dines J. Management of ulnar collateral ligament injury in throwing athletes: a survey of the American Shoulder and Elbow Surgeons. J Shoulder Elb Surg. 2017;26(11):2023–8.

59. Dines JS, Williams PN, ElAttrache N, Conte S, Tomczyk T, Osbahr DC, et al. Platelet-rich plasma can be used to successfully treat elbow ulnar collateral ligament insufficiency in high-level throwers. Am J Orthop (Belle Mead, NJ). 2016;45(5):296–300.
60. McCrum CL, Costello J, Onishi K, Stewart C, Vyas D. Return to play after PRP and rehabilitation of 3 elite ice hockey players with ulnar collateral ligament injuries of the elbow. Orthop J Sports Med. 2018;6(8):2325967118790760.
61. McQueen PD, Camp CL, Chauhan A, Erickson BJ, Potter HG, D'Angelo, J, Fealy S, Ciccotti MG, Fronek J. Comparative analysis of the nonoperative treatment of elbow ulnar collateral ligament injuries in professional baseball players with and without platelet-rich plasma. Orthop J Sports Med. 2018;6(7_suppl4).
62. Carayannopoulos A, Borg-Stein J, Sokolof J, Meleger A, Rosenberg D. Prolotherapy versus corticosteroid injections for the treatment of lateral epicondylosis: a randomized controlled trial. PM R. 2011;3(8):706–15.
63. Rabago D, Lee KS, Ryan M, Chourasia AO, Sesto ME, Zgierska A, et al. Hypertonic dextrose and morrhuate sodium injections (prolotherapy) for lateral epicondylosis (tennis elbow): results of a single-blind, pilot-level, randomized controlled trial. Am J Phys Med Rehabil. 2013;92(7):587–96.
64. Merolla G, Dellabiancia F, Ricci A, Mussoni MP, Nucci S, Zanoli G, et al. Arthroscopic debridement versus platelet-rich plasma injection: a prospective, randomized, comparative study of chronic lateral epicondylitis with a nearly 2-year follow-up. Arthroscopy. 2017;33(7):1320–9.
65. Fitzpatrick J, Bulsara M, Zheng MH. The effectiveness of platelet-rich plasma in the treatment of tendinopathy: a meta-analysis of randomized controlled clinical trials. Am J Sports Med. 2017;45(1):226–33.
66. Yerlikaya M, Talay Calis H, Tomruk Sutbeyaz S, Sayan H, Ibis N, Koc A, et al. Comparison of effects of leukocyte-rich and leukocyte-poor platelet-rich plasma on pain and functionality in patients with lateral epicondylitis. Arch Rheumatol. 2018;33(1):73–9.
67. Virchenko O, Aspenberg P. How can one platelet injection after tendon injury lead to a stronger tendon after 4 weeks? Interplay between early regeneration and mechanical stimulation. Acta Orthop. 2006;77(5):806–12.
68. Krogh TP, Fredberg U, Stengaard-Pedersen K, Christensen R, Jensen P, Ellingsen T. Treatment of lateral epicondylitis with platelet-rich plasma, glucocorticoid, or saline: a randomized, double-blind, placebo-controlled trial. Am J Sports Med. 2013;41(3):625–35.
69. Palacio EP, Schiavetti RR, Kanematsu M, Ikeda TM, Mizobuchi RR, Galbiatti JA. Effects of platelet-rich plasma on lateral epicondylitis of the elbow: prospective randomized controlled trial. Rev Bras Ortop. 2016;51(1):90–5.
70. Yadav R, Kothari SY, Borah D. Comparison of local injection of platelet rich plasma and corticosteroids in the treatment of lateral epicondylitis of humerus. J Clin Diagn Res: JCDR. 2015;9(7):Rc05–7.
71. Gosens T, Peerbooms JC, van Laar W, den Oudsten BL. Ongoing positive effect of platelet-rich plasma versus corticosteroid injection in lateral epicondylitis: a double-blind randomized controlled trial with 2-year follow-up. Am J Sports Med. 2011;39(6):1200–8.
72. Peerbooms JC, Sluimer J, Bruijn DJ, Gosens T. Positive effect of an autologous platelet concentrate in lateral epicondylitis in a double-blind randomized controlled trial: platelet-rich plasma versus corticosteroid injection with a 1-year follow-up. Am J Sports Med. 2010;38(2):255–62.
73. Lebiedzinski R, Synder M, Buchcic P, Polguj M, Grzegorzewski A, Sibinski M. A randomized study of autologous conditioned plasma and steroid injections in the treatment of lateral epicondylitis. Int Orthop. 2015;39(11):2199–203.
74. Gautam VK, Verma S, Batra S, Bhatnagar N, Arora S. Platelet-rich plasma versus corticosteroid injection for recalcitrant lateral epicondylitis: clinical and ultrasonographic evaluation. J Orthop Surg (Hong Kong). 2015;23(1):1–5.

75. Behera P, Dhillon M, Aggarwal S, Marwaha N, Prakash M. Leukocyte-poor platelet-rich plasma versus bupivacaine for recalcitrant lateral epicondylar tendinopathy. J Orthop Surg (Hong Kong). 2015;23(1):6–10.
76. Mishra A, Pavelko T. Treatment of chronic elbow tendinosis with buffered platelet-rich plasma. Am J Sports Med. 2006;34(11):1774–8.
77. Mishra AK, Skrepnik NV, Edwards SG, Jones GL, Sampson S, Vermillion DA, et al. Efficacy of platelet-rich plasma for chronic tennis elbow: a double-blind, prospective, multicenter, randomized controlled trial of 230 patients. Am J Sports Med. 2014;42(2):463–71.
78. Stenhouse G, Sookur P, Watson M. Do blood growth factors offer additional benefit in refractory lateral epicondylitis? A prospective, randomized pilot trial of dry needling as a standalone procedure versus dry needling and autologous conditioned plasma. Skelet Radiol. 2013;42(11):1515–20.
79. Raeissadat SA, Rayegani SM, Hassanabadi H, Rahimi R, Sedighipour L, Rostami K. Is Platelet-rich plasma superior to whole blood in the management of chronic tennis elbow: one year randomized clinical trial. BMC Sports Sci Med Rehabil. 2014;6:12.
80. Raeissadat SA, Sedighipour L, Rayegani SM, Bahrami MH, Bayat M, Rahimi R. Effect of platelet-rich plasma (PRP) versus autologous whole blood on pain and function improvement in tennis elbow: a randomized clinical trial. Pain Res Treat. 2014;2014:191525.
81. Thanasas C, Papadimitriou G, Charalambidis C, Paraskevopoulos I, Papanikolaou A. Platelet-rich plasma versus autologous whole blood for the treatment of chronic lateral elbow epicondylitis: a randomized controlled clinical trial. Am J Sports Med. 2011;39(10):2130–4.
82. Creaney L, Wallace A, Curtis M, Connell D. Growth factor-based therapies provide additional benefit beyond physical therapy in resistant elbow tendinopathy: a prospective, single-blind, randomised trial of autologous blood injections versus platelet-rich plasma injections. Br J Sports Med. 2011;45(12):966–71.
83. Karaduman M, Okkaoglu MC, Sesen H, Taskesen A, Ozdemir M, Altay M. Platelet-rich plasma versus open surgical release in chronic tennis elbow: a retrospective comparative study. J Orthop. 2016;13(1):10–4.
84. Tetschke E, Rudolf M, Lohmann CH, Starke C. Autologous proliferative therapies in recalcitrant lateral epicondylitis. Am J Phys Med Rehabil. 2015;94(9):696–706.
85. Massy-Westropp N, Simmonds S, Caragianis S, Potter A. Autologous blood injection and wrist immobilisation for chronic lateral epicondylitis. Adv Orthop. 2012;2012:387829.
86. Edwards SG, Calandruccio JH. Autologous blood injections for refractory lateral epicondylitis. J Hand Surg Am. 2003;28(2):272–8.
87. Suresh SP, Ali KE, Jones H, Connell DA. Medial epicondylitis: is ultrasound guided autologous blood injection an effective treatment? Br J Sports Med. 2006;40(11):935–9; discussion 9.
88. Bostan B, Balta O, Asci M, Aytekin K, Eser E. Autologous blood injection works for recalcitrant lateral epicondylitis. Balkan Med J. 2016;33(2):216–20.
89. Sung CM, Hah YS, Kim JS, Nam JB, Kim RJ, Lee SJ, et al. Cytotoxic effects of ropivacaine, bupivacaine, and lidocaine on rotator cuff tenofibroblasts. Am J Sports Med. 2014;42(12):2888–96.
90. Karimi Mobarakeh M, Nemati A, Fazli A, Fallahi A, Safari S. Autologous blood injection for treatment of tennis elbow. Trauma Mon. 2013;17(4):393–5.
91. Jindal N, Gaury Y, Banshiwal RC, Lamoria R, Bachhal V. Comparison of short term results of single injection of autologous blood and steroid injection in tennis elbow: a prospective study. J Orthop Surg Res. 2013;8:10.
92. Ozturan KE, Yucel I, Cakici H, Guven M, Sungur I. Autologous blood and corticosteroid injection and extracoporeal shock wave therapy in the treatment of lateral epicondylitis. Orthopedics. 2010;33(2):84–91.
93. Wolf JM, Ozer K, Scott F, Gordon MJ, Williams AE. Comparison of autologous blood, corticosteroid, and saline injection in the treatment of lateral epicondylitis: a prospective, randomized, controlled multicenter study. J Hand Surg Am. 2011;36(8):1269–72.

94. Scarpone M, Rabago DP, Zgierska A, Arbogast G, Snell E. The efficacy of prolotherapy for lateral epicondylosis: a pilot study. Clin J Sport Med. 2008;18(3):248–54.
95. Zhang J, Keenan C, Wang JH. The effects of dexamethasone on human patellar tendon stem cells: implications for dexamethasone treatment of tendon injury. J Orthop Res. 2013;31(1):105–10.
96. Zhou Y, Zhang J, Wu H, Hogan MV, Wang JH. The differential effects of leukocyte-containing and pure platelet-rich plasma (PRP) on tendon stem/progenitor cells – implications of PRP application for the clinical treatment of tendon injuries. Stem Cell Res Ther. 2015;6:173.
97. Connell D, Datir A, Alyas F, Curtis M. Treatment of lateral epicondylitis using skin-derived tenocyte-like cells. Br J Sports Med. 2009;43(4):293–8.
98. Singh A, Gangwar DS, Singh S. Bone marrow injection: a novel treatment for tennis elbow. J Nat Sci Biol Med. 2014;5(2):389–91.
99. Lee SY, Kim W, Lim C, Chung SG. Treatment of lateral epicondylosis by using allogeneic adipose-derived mesenchymal stem cells: a pilot study. Stem Cells (Dayton, Ohio). 2015;33(10):2995–3005.
100. Aufiero DSS, Onishi K, Botto van Bemden A. Treatment of medial and lateral elbow tendinosis with an injectable amniotic membrane allograft: a retrospective case series. J Pain Relief. 2016;5(242):3.
101. Gellhorn AC, Han A. The use of dehydrated human amnion/chorion membrane allograft injection for the treatment of tendinopathy or arthritis: a case series involving 40 patients. PM R. 2017;9(12):1236–43.
102. Barnes DE, Beckley JM, Smith J. Percutaneous ultrasonic tenotomy for chronic elbow tendinosis: a prospective study. J Shoulder Elb Surg. 2015;24(1):67–73.
103. Boden AL, Scott MT, Dalwadi PP, Mautner K, Mason RA, Gottschalk MB. Platelet-rich plasma versus Tenex in the treatment of medial and lateral epicondylitis. J Shoulder Elb Surg. 2019;28(1):112–9.
104. Glanzmann MC, Audige L. Efficacy of platelet-rich plasma injections for chronic medial epicondylitis. J Hand Surg Eur Vol. 2015;40(7):744–5.
105. Sanli I, Morgan B, van Tilborg F, Funk L, Gosens T. Single injection of platelet-rich plasma (PRP) for the treatment of refractory distal biceps tendonitis: long-term results of a prospective multicenter cohort study. Knee Surg Sports Traumatol Arthrosc. 2016;24(7):2308–12.
106. Barker SL, Bell SN, Connell D, Coghlan JA. Ultrasound-guided platelet-rich plasma injection for distal biceps tendinopathy. Shoulder Elbow. 2015;7(2):110–4.
107. Cheatham SW, Kolber MJ, Salamh PA, Hanney WJ. Rehabilitation of a partially torn distal triceps tendon after platelet rich plasma injection: a case report. Int J Sports Phys Ther. 2013;8(3):290–9.

Chapter 10
Regenerative Medicine for Hand and Wrist Pain

Anokhi Mehta and Gerardo Miranda-Comas

Osteoarthritis

Osteoarthritis (OA), or degenerative joint disease (DJD), just as it can affect any other joint in the body, can affect the hand and wrist. Currently, the treatments typically performed are palliative and analgesic and range from conservative to surgical management. Nonpharmacologic interventions include joint protection techniques, use of splints, assistive devices to perform ADLs, and physical modalities. Pharmacological interventions include topical or oral medications [1]. Although the American College of Rheumatology (ACR) does not recommend intra-articular injections [1], they are often used in patients refractory to other treatments.

The prevalence of carpometacarpal (CMC) joint arthritis in men is 21–27% and in women 24–29% [2]. CMC arthritis can result in pain, weakness, and deformity [3]. Nonpharmacologic and pharmacologic treatments should be attempted first, including a thumb spica splint and/or hand therapy [4]. Modalities such as heat, ice, transcutaneous electrical stimulation, and therapeutic ultrasound can be used. If nonpharmacologic treatment fails, then pharmacologic treatment can be attempted.

Pharmacologic treatment consists of oral or topical medications and injections. Oral medications include acetaminophen or paracetamol, various anti-inflammatories (NSAIDs, steroids), neuropathic agents (gabapentin, pregabalin), SSRIs (duloxetine), and glucosamine chondroitin. Topical medications available include capsaicin, lidocaine, and diclofenac. These agents are available in various preparations like patches, gels, or ointments. Injections that are available are steroid and viscosupplementation injections, although evidence of their effectiveness is lacking [4].

A. Mehta · G. Miranda-Comas (✉)
Department of Rehabilitation and Human Performance,
Icahn School of Medicine at Mount Sinai, New York, NY, USA
e-mail: Gerardo.Miranda-comas@mountsinai.org

© Springer Nature Switzerland AG 2020
G. Cooper et al. (eds.), *Regenerative Medicine for Spine and Joint Pain*,
https://doi.org/10.1007/978-3-030-42771-9_10

If these nonpharmacologic and pharmacologic treatments fail, surgery remains an option. Per Vermeulen et al., there are eight common surgical procedures performed for CMC arthritis, but one has not been demonstrated to be superior to the others [3].

With the advent of regenerative medicine techniques, there is treatment available that can potentially regenerate or heal arthritic cartilage and bone. At this time, no studies have been carried out on the effects of platelet-rich plasma (PRP) or stem cell therapy on hand or wrist OA. However, there are studies looking at the effects of stem cell therapy and PRP on hip and knee OA.

Intra-articular PRP injections have been shown to be efficacious for knee arthritis; therefore, intra-articular PRP injections for CMC joint arthritis could be efficacious as well. Dai et al. performed a meta-analysis that included ten studies looking at PRP for knee osteoarthritis versus saline or viscosupplementation [5]. Thus study showed that PRP and viscosupplementation had similar outcomes regarding pain relief and functional improvement at 6 months postinjection. However, at 12 months postinjection, PRP demonstrated greater pain relief and functional improvement. Furthermore, PRP demonstrated greater pain relief and functional improvement when compared to saline at 6 and 12 months postinjection [5].

Similarly, stem cell use has demonstrated positive outcomes in several studies for knee OA; therefore, its use for wrist/hand OA may be beneficious as well. Jayaram et al. reviewed studies that looked at the efficacy of bone marrow-derived stem cells (BMSC) and adipose-derived stem cells (ADSC) on knee OA in animal and human models [6]. Several studies demonstrated regeneration and improvement in knee joint cartilage quality after intra-articular injection with BMSCs; this was determined by magnetic resonance imaging, gross examination, and histologic examination. Along with improvement in cartilage quality, BMSC decreased the rate of joint damage and cartilage degeneration. Pain improvement after injection with BMSC was seen in individuals as well [6]. Intra-articular injection with ADSCs was also shown to slow knee OA progression by slowing the rate of cartilage degeneration. Pain and function improved after ADSC treatment as well [6].

Mesenchymal stem cells, such as BMSCs and ADSCs, and PRP injections have consistently demonstrated a high safety profile when used for musculoskeletal conditions, such as OA. Additionally, studies on knee OA have demonstrated efficacy; therefore, these interventions, with the right protocol, could potentially be applied to CMC joint arthritis as well.

Tendinopathies

In addition to being beneficial for OA in the hand and wrist, regenerative medicine can be of benefit when treating different tendinopathies in the hand and wrist. Common tendinopathies in the hand and wrist are De Quervain's, intersection syndrome, extensor carpi ulnaris tendon injury, and trigger finger or stenosing tenosynovitis.

De Quervain's tenosynovitis is due to overuse and is the result of thickening of the first extensor retinaculum at the wrist. It occurs due to repetitive movement of the abductor pollicis longus (APL) and extensor pollicis brevis (EPB) tendons as they pass through the first dorsal compartment of the wrist under the first extensor retinaculum [7]. On physical examination, one will find tenderness to palpation in the first dorsal compartment with possibly local swelling. Finkelstein's test is performed by placing the thumb inside a clenched fist and ulnar deviation at the wrist. The test is considered positive if it reproduces pain over the radial styloid. Currently, conservative management consists of oral anti-inflammatories, topical cream, thumb spica splint, occupational therapy, and sono-guided steroid injection to the first dorsal compartment if pain and functional impairment is severe enough. If conservative management fails, surgical opening of the first dorsal compartment is an option [7].

Intersection syndrome is another overuse disorder of the wrist and another cause of pain. This disorder results in pain in the dorsal forearm approximately 4–8 centimeters proximal to Lister's tubercle [8]. Friction between the APL and EPB tendons and the extensor carpi radialis brevis and longus (ECRB and ECRL) tendons results in inflammation and pain. Swelling and pain can be seen at the site of intersection between these tendons. Crepitus at the site has been described, along with pain that worsens with activity and use. It is a clinical diagnosis, but ultrasound and/or MRI can be performed for confirmation. Conservative management should be attempted first with rest, analgesia, and immobilization. In some cases, this may not be enough to reduce the inflammation, and a sono-guided tendon sheath steroid injection is warranted. Saline hydrodissection to reduce the adhesions has been described as an interventional treatment as well [9].

Another common overuse injury in the hand/wrist is extensor carpi ulnaris (ECU) tendinopathy. This pathology is commonly found in athletes who use sticks, bats, or clubs [10]. The ECU is in the sixth extensor compartment of the wrist. Unlike the other five compartments, the sixth compartment is found along the ulna, not the radius. Another unusual characteristic of the ECU is that it is not housed exclusively by the extensor retinaculum; there is also an ECU tendon sub-sheath. There are two types of ECU tendinopathy that can occur. One is a constrained tendinopathy – the ECU is being compressed within the ECU tendon sub-sheath. The other type is an unconstrained tendinopathy; this involves subluxation or dislocation of the tendon [10].

Clinically, on exam, one will find weakness of the ECU and tenderness to palpation over the dorsal-ulnar aspect of the wrist. Many individuals describe the pain as a burning sensation. There is rarely a history of trauma or specific injury to the wrist for individuals with a constrained tendinopathy. Those who have an unconstrained tendinopathy will typically have a history of a hypersupination injury with ulnar deviation and flexion of the wrist. Swelling can be seen along the sixth dorsal compartment of the wrist. The diagnosis of an ECU injury is made clinically, but often concomitant injuries such as triangular fibrocartilage (TFCC) tears occur as well. Therefore, ordering an MRI to further delineate any concomitant injuries and to assess the status of the tendon is advisable [10]. Management of an

ECU tendinopathy is dependent upon the type of tendinopathy – constrained versus unconstrained. In constrained tendinopathies, the goal of treatment is to avoid rupture of the tendon and further deterioration of the ECU tendon. In unconstrained tendinopathies, the goal of treatment is to stabilize the ECU tendon and to re-establish normal, anatomical alignment. Immobilization with a splint for 2–3 weeks, oral or topical anti-inflammatories, and occupational therapy are the initial treatment for constrained tendinopathies. The splint should hold the forearm in pronation with the wrist extended and in slight ulnar deviation. If indicated, a sono-guided steroid injection to the tendon sub-sheath can be performed. If all of the above treatments fail, one can consider surgical release of the tendon. In unconstrained ECU tendinopathies, open reduction and reconstruction are typically advised [10].

Trigger finger, or stenosing tenosynovitis, is another common tendinopathy of the hand. It has a prevalence of 2–3% of the population. Individuals present with locking and pain of the involved digit. A palpable nodule can be felt as well. Individuals can have trigger finger of just one to several fingers, and it can appear unilaterally or bilaterally. Management begins with conservative treatment with occupational therapy and hand use (occupational and ADLs) modification if needed. If symptoms persist, a sono-guided steroid injection into the tendon sheath under the A1 pulley can be performed. If symptoms persist after a steroid injection, surgical release of the A1 pulley can be considered [11].

Although regenerative medicine in the treatment of overuse injuries in the wrist and hand has not been substantially documented at the time of writing this text, there is literature regarding the use of PRP specifically in other overuse injuries. The use of PRP to treat patellar tendinopathy has been documented in case series and small randomized controlled trials [12]. Mainly due to lack of protocol standardization for aspirate preparation or injection technique (infiltration with or without needle tenotomy), there is still controversy in the use of PRP for soft tissue injuries [13]. Nevertheless, Mautner et al. did a retrospective study on the efficacy of sono-guided tenotomy and PRP injection in patients with chronic tendinopathy: lateral and medial epicondylitis, patellar tendonitis, Achilles tendonitis, rotator cuff tendonitis, hamstring tendonitis, and gluteus medius tendonitis [14]. They demonstrated a moderate (>50%) improvement in pain after ultrasound-guided PRP injections for chronic tendinopathy. The pathology of tendinosis is similar regardless of location. Therefore, it can be reasonably expected that PRP will be efficacious in chronic tendinopathies in the hand, but more research is warranted. Additionally, stem cell use for tendinopathies has not been studied, and its use in other more common tendinopathies like rotator cuff injury is currently not advised [15].

Ligamentous Injuries

Two important ligamentous injuries that can occur in the hand and wrist are scapholunate ligament and ulnar collateral ligament (UCL) injuries. The scapholunate ligament is one of the interosseous membranes of the wrist. Scapholunate ligament injuries typically occur with a fall onto an outstretched hand. These injuries are commonly seen concomitantly with a distal radius fracture, perilunate dislocation, or a scaphoid fracture. Alternatively, they can be seen as an isolated injury [16]. Acute scapholunate injuries present with acute swelling over the anatomical snuffbox and radiocarpal joint. Individuals with a scapholunate injury will experience weakness and pain, as well as instability. Treatment of acute static scapholunate ligament dissociation is surgical, with closed reduction and pinning or with open reduction and repair of the ligament. Acute partial ligaments injuries without any of the collapse deformities are best treated in a short-arm thumb spica cast for at least 6 weeks [16, 17].

Similarly, UCL injury, Skier's thumb, or Gamekeeper's thumb is an injury that affects the stability of the medial aspect of the first MCP joint where first- and second-degree tears can be treated with immobilization with a short-arm thumb spica cast for 4 weeks. After 2 weeks, the cast can be changed, and if the patient is pain free, a removable splint can be used and ROM exercises started. A non-displaced avulsion fracture can be treated with a cast for 4–6 weeks. Operative treatment should be considered if the avulsion fracture is greater than 10–15% of the articular surface, if displacement is more than 2–3 millimeters, or if angulation is present [18, 19]. There are no studies or case reports on the use of regenerative interventions for this type of injuries, but theoretically they might be beneficial, especially in partial tears where nonsurgical treatment is preferred.

Other Soft Tissue Injuries

A common wrist pathology is carpal tunnel syndrome (CTS) or median neuropathy at the wrist. CTS can lead to paresthesia in the thumb, index finger, middle finger, and radial side of the fourth finger. In extreme cases, individuals can have thenar weakness [20]. Conservative management consists of nighttime splinting, oral medications, and occupational therapy. If these treatments fail, then a sono-guided steroid injection can be attempted. Cases refractory to conservative management or those with evidence of axonal injury can be referred for surgical decompression.

Now, with the advent of regenerative medicine, there is an additional option for individuals suffering from CTS. The scientific evidence has demonstrated mixed results on the efficacy of PRP as treatment for CTS. Malahias et al. and Özçakar et al. demonstrated additional benefit from a single PRP injection into the carpal tunnel when compared to night splints and activity modification-only group [21, 22]. On the other hand, Raeissadat et al. found that although safe, in short term, PRP plus splint is not more effective than splint in reducing pain, symptom severity, and functional status in mild and moderate carpal tunnel syndrome [23]. As previously seen in other pathologies, PRP seems to be safe, but its efficacy in treating most MSK conditions is still questionable; however, it is still a viable treatment option before having to consider surgery in conditions such as CTS.

Another common wrist pathology is triangular fibrocartilage complex (TFCC) injury. The TFCC stabilizes the distal radioulnar joint. It consists of the ulnotriquetral ligament, meniscal homologue, articular disc, dorsal radioulnar ligament, volar radioulnar ligament, ulnolunate ligament, and ulnar collateral ligament. Injury to the complex results in ulnar-sided pain and instability to the distal radioulnar joint [24]. It is commonly seen in athletes who use bats, clubs, or rackets. Individuals report a deep aching pain, a clicking with pronation-supination of the forearm, and pain with gripping. MRI should be obtained if TFCC injury is suspected to delineate extent of injury and to look for any concomitant injuries. As previously mentioned, ECU injuries can be seen with TFCC injuries. Nevertheless, the gold standard for diagnosis is wrist arthroscopy. Active individuals with suspected TFCC tears should undergo wrist arthroscopy for possible debridement of central tears or repair of peripheral tears [25]. Like in other pathologies in the hand and wrist, there is no evidence in the literature for the use of regenerative medicine interventions on TFCC injuries, but it is a possible alternative to surgery.

Conclusion

There is very limited scientific evidence of efficacy of regenerative medicine interventions for the treatment of hand and wrist injuries. The main reason for this is lack of studies focused in this anatomic area. Nevertheless, there is some evidence for PRP and stem cells for similar pathology, OA, tendinopathy, and ligamentous injury, in other areas of the body that has consistently demonstrated a high safety profile but mixed results on positive outcomes. These procedures seem to be safe; therefore they can be recommended as an alternative to patients refractory to proven conservative modalities who do not want to undergo surgery.

References

1. Hochberg MC, Altman RD, April KT, Benkhalti M, Guyatt G, McGowan J, et al. American College of Rheumatology 2012 recommendations for the use of nonpharmacologic and pharmacologic therapies in osteoarthritis of the hand, hip, and knee. Arthritis Care Res. 2012;64(4):465–74.
2. Haugen IK, Englund M, Aliabadi P, Niu J, Clancy M, Kvien TK, et al. Prevalence, incidence and progression of hand osteoarthritis in the general population: the Framingham Osteoarthritis Study. Ann Rheum Dis. 2011;70(9):1581–6.
3. Vermeulen GM, Slijper H, Feitz R, Hovius SER, Moojen TM, Selles RW. Surgical management of primary thumb carpometacarpal osteoarthritis: a systematic review. J Hand Surg Am. 2011;36(1):156–69.
4. Kroon FPB, Carmona L, Schoones JW, Kloppenburg M. Efficacy and safety of non-pharmacological, pharmacological and surgical treatment for hand osteoarthritis: a systematic literature review informing the 2018 update of the EULAR recommendations for the manage-

ment of hand osteoarthritis. RMD Open [Internet]. 2018;4(2):e000734. Available from: http://rmdopen.bmj.com/content/4/2/e000734.abstract.

5. Dai WL, Zhou AG, Zhang H, Zhang J. Efficacy of platelet-rich plasma in the treatment of knee osteoarthritis: a meta-analysis of randomized controlled trials. Arthroscopy. 2017;33(3):659–70.

6. Jayaram P, Ikpeama U, Rothenberg JB, Malanga GA. Bone marrow–derived and adipose-derived mesenchymal stem cell therapy in primary knee osteoarthritis: a narrative review. PM R. 2019;11:177–91.

7. Goel R, Abzug JM. de Quervain's tenosynovitis: a review of the rehabilitative options. Hand. 2015;10(1):1–5.

8. Chatterjee R, Vyas J. Diagnosis and management of intersection syndrome as a cause of overuse wrist pain. BMJ Case Rep [Internet]. 2016;2016:bcr2016216988. Available from: http://casereports.bmj.com/content/2016/bcr-2016-216988.abstract.

9. Skinner TM. Intersection syndrome: the subtle squeak of an overused wrist. J Am Board Fam Med. 2017;30(4):547–51.

10. Garcia-Elias M. Tendinopathies of the extensor carpi ulnaris. Handchir Mikrochir Plast Chir. 2015;47(5):281–9.

11. Giugale JM, Fowler JR. Trigger finger: adult and pediatric treatment strategies. Orthop Clin North Am. 2015;46(4):561–9.

12. Andia I, Maffulli N. Use of platelet-rich plasma for patellar tendon and medial collateral ligament injuries: best current clinical practice. J Knee Surg. 2015;28(1):11–8.

13. Moraes VY, Lenza M, Tamaoki MJ, Faloppa F, Belloti JC. Platelet-rich therapies for musculoskeletal soft tissue injuries. Cochrane Database Syst Rev. 2014;4:CD010071.

14. Mautner K, Colberg RE, Malanga G, Borg-Stein JP, Harmon KG, Dharamsi AS, et al. Outcomes after ultrasound-guided platelet-rich plasma injections for chronic tendinopathy: a multicenter, retrospective review. PM R. 2013;5(3):169–75.

15. Pas HIMFL, Moen MH, Haisma HJ, Winters M. No evidence for the use of stem cell therapy for tendon disorders: a systematic review. Br J Sports Med. 2017;51(13):996–1002.

16. Chim H, Moran SL. Wrist essentials: the diagnosis and management of scapholunate ligament injuries. Plast Reconstr Surg. 2014;134(2):312e–22e.

17. Lewis DM, Lee Osterman A. Scapholunate instability in athletes. Clin Sports Med. 2001;20:131–40.

18. Schroeder NS, Goldfarb CA. Thumb ulnar collateral and radial collateral ligament injuries. Clin Sports Med. 2015;34(1):117–26.

19. Rettig AC. Athletic injuries of the wrist and hand. Part I: traumatic injuries of the wrist. Am J Sports Med. 2003;31(6):1038–48.

20. Kuo YC, Lee CC, Hsieh LF. Ultrasound-guided perineural injection with platelet-rich plasma improved the neurophysiological parameters of carpal tunnel syndrome: a case report. J Clin Neurosci. 2017;44:234–6.

21. Malahias MA, Johnson EO, Babis GC, Nikolaou VS. Single injection of platelet-rich plasma as a novel treatment of carpal tunnel syndrome. Neural Regen Res. 2015;10(11):1856–9.

22. Özçakar L, Kaymak B, Kara M, Akinci A, Güven SC. Short term effectiveness of platelet-rich plasma in carpal tunnel syndrome: a controlled study. J Tissue Eng Regen Med. 2019;13(5):709–14.

23. Raeissadat SA, Karimzadeh A, Hashemi M, Bagherzadeh L. Safety and efficacy of platelet-rich plasma in treatment of carpal tunnel syndrome; a randomized controlled trial. BMC Musculoskelet Disord. 2018;19(1):49.

24. Avery DM, Rodner CM, Edgar CM. Sports-related wrist and hand injuries: a review. J Orthop Surg Res. 2016;11(1):99.

25. Pulos N, Kakar S. Hand and wrist injuries common problems and solutions. Clin Sports Med. 2019;37(2018):217–43.

Chapter 11
Regenerative Medicine for the Hip

Walter Alomar-Jimenez and Gerardo Miranda-Comas

Introduction

The hip is a common source of pain not only in the adult and elderly population but also in our competitive athletes. Hip pathology can be found in newborns (developmental hip dysplasia), childhood (Legg-Calve-Perthes disease), adolescence (slipped femoral epiphysis), and adulthood (osteoarthritis, labral tears, tendinopathies, etc.). With adavancement in imaging studies and surgical techniques, we have gained insight into the incidence of labral tear pathologies, for example, and anatomical variants that can contribute to hip and groin pain. However, much work is still needed to search for new techniques that will improve our patient's clinical outcomes and quality of life. The goal of this chapter is to review the role of regenerative medicine techniques, including viscosupplementation, platelet-rich plasma, and stem cells in the management of hip pathologies. We will discuss the most common causes of hip pain, the current standard of care for management, and the evidence for the use of regenerative medicine in those pathologies.

Osteoarthritis (OA)

Hip osteoarthritis (OA), also known as degenerative joint disease, is the most common pathologic finding of the hip. The age-adjusted prevalence of radiographic and symptomatic hip osteoarthritis is 19.6% and 4.2%, respectively [1]. The etiology of hip OA is cartilage breakdown. The most common form is primary, due to the wear and tear occurring over time. Unlike rheumatoid arthritis, osteoarthritis is relatively

W. Alomar-Jimenez · G. Miranda-Comas (✉)
Department of Rehabilitation and Human Performance,
Icahn School of Medicine at Mount Sinai, New York, NY, USA
e-mail: Gerardo.Miranda-comas@mountsinai.org

© Springer Nature Switzerland AG 2020
G. Cooper et al. (eds.), *Regenerative Medicine for Spine and Joint Pain*,
https://doi.org/10.1007/978-3-030-42771-9_11

noninflammatory during most stages of the disease process [2]. The treatment goals for hip OA are to decrease pain, improve function, and prevent subsequent joint damage. Current treatment options involve non-pharmacologic, pharmacologic, intra-articular injections, and surgery.

The American College of Rheumatology (ACR) 2012 guidelines for the management of hand, hip, and knee osteoarthritis strongly recommend that all patients with symptomatic hip osteoarthritis be enrolled in an exercise program that includes range of motion, muscle strengthening, and aerobic conditioning [3].

Pharmacologic therapy should be initiated when patients fail to respond to non-pharmacologic treatment. Pharmacologic recommendations for the initial treatment of symptomatic hip osteoarthritis include using one of the following: acetaminophen or paracetamol, oral nonsteroidal anti-inflammatory drugs (NSAIDs), and/or tramadol [3].

A detailed patient medical history and comorbidities should be addressed when prescribing pain medications. Acetaminophen or paracetamol is associated with hepatic side effects; NSAIDs are associated with gastrointestinal, renal, and cardiovascular side effects; and tramadol may cause sedation and dizziness.

The most common nonsurgical procedure for hip OA is an intra-articular injection. The most widely used among these are corticosteroids, and the ACR conditionally recommends their use for hip OA [3].

The evidence suggest that corticosteroid injections are effective improving range of motion, function, and pain at least short term. Studies have compared the effect of corticosteroid versus anesthetic injections [4] or simply normal saline [5] with sustained effects only seen for up to 3 months. Therefore, their utility for long-term relief has been questioned. There is also a wide variation in degree of response, and it has been difficult to identify specific characteristics such as age, BMI, gender, and even radiologic severity that will help select those who will respond to the intervention [6]. Nevertheless, due to their accessibility and cost-effectiveness, they are still a reasonable option, particularly for nonsurgical candidates.

Ultimately, there are concerns regarding their local as well as systemic side effects [7]. There is no clear consensus on the safe total number of injections, total volume, or frequency of corticosteroids that can be injected in a given timeframe. Therefore, the demand for other effective and safer therapies increased.

Hyaluronic acid, also known as viscosupplementation, was approved by the Food and Drug Administration (FDA) in 1997 for the treatment of knee OA. The regenerative effects are thought to be mediated by restoration of elastic and viscous properties of synovial fluid and hyaluronan synthesis by synoviocytes [8]. However, the medication is not currently approved for hip OA even when the evidence suggests that viscosupplementation for the hip is as effective as it has been shown for the knee [8]. In addition, it appears to be a safe and reasonable alternative to NSAIDs and intra-articular corticosteroids. In Mulvaney et al. literature review, they concluded that viscosupplementation of the hip may delay the need for hip replacement surgery and appears to work best in patients with fewer radiographic changes of osteoarthritis [8].

Among the emerging regenerative techniques, platelet-rich plasma (PRP) has been the one that has gained more popularity in part due to cost and ease of preparation. In contrast to HA, it has been widely applied, not only for arthritis but also soft tissue pathologies (muscle, tendon, and ligaments). The proposed mechanism of action involves the stimulation of release of growth factors that are responsible for inducing tissue healing and interfering with catabolic processes [9].

Since the first randomized clinical trial of PRP in 2012, most of the studies have compared the effectiveness and safety of PRP to another intra-articular injection. Sanchez et al. in 2012 showed a significant benefit of PRP in patients with hip OA [10]. They studied 40 patients with unilateral severe osteoarthritis prospectively to assess the safety and effectiveness of intra-articular PRP [10]. They demonstrated a statistically significant reduction in hip pain at 7 weeks and 6 months and negligible side effects limited to a sensation of heaviness at the injection site. Notably, this study specifically used leukocyte-poor PRP preparation.

Recently, Ye et al. conducted a meta-analysis of randomized controlled trials comparing PRP versus HA in patients with hip osteoarthritis [11]. The authors concluded that PRP was associated with a significant reduction in pain at 2 months compared with HA. However, it did not show significantly better outcomes at 6 and 12 months. Again, no increased risk of adverse effects was observed.

The evidence suggests that intra-articular PRP injections for hip OA are safe and seem to be effective in pain reduction. In addition, studies have shown that PRP has a greater initial effect in pain reduction compared to HA. However, this effect is not sustained over time. An important aspect to consider when interpreting the available evidence is the inconsistency in preparation methods of PRP samples, particularly, leukocyte-rich versus leukocyte-poor, as it has been identified as a critical aspect for the outcomes among different pathologies. A call for standardization of regenerative medicine techniques has been advocated to minimize conflicting results [12].

The evidence for stem cell use and effectiveness in hip OA is lacking. To our knowledge there are no randomized clinical trials evaluating the use of stem cells in hip OA. However, there are randomized controlled trials evaluating stem cells in knee OA. Shapiro et al. [13] studied 25 patients with bilateral knee osteoarthritis who received bone marrow aspirate concentration (BMAC) plus PRP in one knee and saline placebo into the other knee. Pain scores in both knees decreased significantly from baseline at 1 week, 3 months, and 6 months; however there was no significant difference in pain reduction between the two groups. There were no serious adverse events from the BMAC procedure. There are cohort studies and case series demonstrating pain improvement. In 2017, Mardones et al. [14] investigated the safety and efficacy of the intra-articular infusion of bone marrow-derived mesenchymal stem cells (BM-MSC) in a cohort of ten patients with functional and radiological evidences of hip OA. Patients were evaluated, before and after completion of the cell infusion. Authors concluded that BM-MSC injections were safe and improved pain and function. Interestingly, the radiographic scores of the hip joint remained without variation in nine out of ten patients, therefore apparently halting the progression of hip OA. In 2018, Darrow et al. [15] reported a case series of four patients treated with bone marrow concentrate (BMC) for hip OA, who underwent four BMC injections and experienced decreased pain at rest and when active when compared with baseline.

Also in 2018, Rodriguez-Fontan et al. [16] conducted a cohort study evaluating BMAC for early hip and knee OA. A total of 25 joints (10 knees, 15 hips) were treated with intra-articular BMAC. They concluded that intra-articular injections of BMAC for the treatment of early knee or hip osteoarthritis were safe and demonstrated satisfactory results in 63.2% of patients.

Currently, there is limited evidence to support the use of stem cells in the treatment of hip OA. Initial studies of stem cells have not reported significant side effects, suggesting that they might be safe. Further high-level quality studies are needed to evaluate its effectiveness and to continue evaluating their safety profile.

Tendinopathies

Tendon pathologies include tears (partial and complete) and acute and chronic tendinopathies. Tendonitis is often used to describe acute tendinopathies, whereas chronic tendinopathy refers to a chronic overload injury with possible tendon degeneration. Tendinopathies were initially described as tendonitis, as there was a belief that inflammation contributed to the pathology, but histopathological studies in the 1990s showed little to no evidence of inflammation. Tendon pathologies are considered to be a continuum, as described by Cook and Purdam model [17], where tendons that receive an excessive load and do not adapt properly are predisposed to have pathology, described in 3 stages: stage 1, reactive tendinopathy; stage 2, tendon disrepair; and stage 3, degenerative tendinopathy. This model served to establish targeted muscle therapies for tendon rehabilitation with the main goal to decrease pain, restore function, and improve tendon capacity with progressive loads. This model can be applied to the hip joint tendon rehabilitation as well.

Greater trochanteric pain syndrome (GTPS) is a common cause of lateral hip pain that affects 10–25% of people in developed countries [18]. Historically, it was thought that symptoms were caused by an isolated trochanteric bursitis. However, the underlying etiology for GTPS is most commonly a tendon tear or tendinopathy of the gluteus medius, minimus, or both at their insertion on the greater trochanter with or without a bursitis. Additionally, the greater trochanter serves as the insertion site for the piriformis and obturator internus muscles. The gluteus medius and minimus muscles are involved in stabilizing and externally rotating the hip. Similar to its counterparts at the shoulder rotator cuff, the hip rotator cuff concept has gained more attention in the last years.

The standard of care for GTPS includes activity modification, avoiding pressure over the lateral hip, ice, and physical therapy. Exercises focus on the core muscles, hip abductors, extensors, and external rotators. In addition, eccentric loading exercises of the gluteal muscles are recommended in cases of tendinopathy. Analgesic medications such as acetaminophen and NSAIDs can be used for pain management in the acute phase.

Patients not improving with conservative treatment may undergo a sono-guided corticosteroid injection into the bursa. Labrosse et al. [19] evaluated the effectiveness of these for the treatment GTPS associated with gluteus medius tendinopathy in 54 patients, with 72% of patients showing significant improvement in pain level at 1 month. However, the effect was only short term.

Regenerative interventions, mainly PRP, have been studied as treatment of GTPS. One of the first studies that included hip pathology was a collaborative multicentered retrospective study by Mautner and colleagues that evaluated the use of PRP to treat chronic tendinopathies [20]. From a total of 180 patients who received ultrasound-guided PRP injections, 16 were to the gluteus medius tendon. Of these, 13 (82%) of the patients reported moderate to complete resolution of symptoms postinjection at an average follow-up of 15 months. In 2018, Fitzpatrick et al. compared the effects of PRP versus corticosteroid injection for the treatment of chronic gluteal tendinopathy [21]. This was a double-blind randomized controlled trial that included 80 patients, with follow-up up to 12 weeks. No difference was observed within 2 or 6 weeks. However, significant clinical improvement in pain and function was observed at 12 weeks for 82% of the patients on the PRP arm when compared to 56.7% on the corticosteroid arm. In 2018, Ali et al. [22] performed a systematic literature review that included three randomized controlled trials and two case series for a total of 209 patients. It showed that PRP is an effective alternative for GTPS with improvements observed during the first 3 months and sustained up to 12 months.

While this evidence shows promising results for GTPS, controversy exists around the direct contribution of PRP among the different injection techniques. It is a common practice to perform tendon fenestration along with PRP injections. Some authors hypothesized that the tendon fenestration alone might be as effective as the PRP injections. This is highlighted by Jacobson et al. [23] where they compared PRP versus simple percutaneous tendon fenestration for treatment of GTPS. The study included a total of 30 patients; half were treated with fenestration and the other half were treated with PRP. While both groups showed significant pain score reduction, there was no difference between the two groups at 3 months. This suggests that tendon fenestration alone could be an effective treatment for GTPS. Further studies are needed to standardize these procedures along with PRP preparations.

Psoas tendinopathy, which may present as internal snapping hip syndrome, is a common cause of hip pain. It is usually caused by friction of the iliopsoas tendon sheath over the iliopectineal ridge or the iliacus tendon [24]. Iliopsoas tendinopathy typically responds within a few weeks of activity modification, physical therapy, acetaminophen, and/or NSAIDs. Patients unresponsive to initial treatment may undergo a sono-guided steroid injection into the bursa. However, there is limited evidence for its efficacy and long-term effect. Agten et al. [25] reported that fluoroscopic-guided injections into the iliopsoas bursa with corticosteroids were an effective treatment for suspected iliopsoas tendinopathy, with 49% reported clinically relevant improvement at 1 month. Additionally, Han et al. [26] showed that regardless of coexisting intra-articular hip pathology, corticosteroid injections are effective for iliopsoas tendinopathy, for at least 6 weeks. On the other hand, Garala et al. [24] carried out a 14-year retrospective case-control study showing that image-guided corticosteroid injection into both the iliopsoas tendon sheath and the bursa was an effective treatment for reducing pain long term for only 8 out the 23 patients on the study. It is also suggested that in those patients who experienced temporary relief from the injection, psoas tenotomy might be a treatment with long-term efficacy [24].

Moreover, patients who remained symptomatic after a steroid injection may resort to surgical psoas release. To our knowledge, no study has evaluated the efficacy of regenerative medicine on iliopsoas tendinopathy.

The adductor muscles of the hip include sartorius, gracilis, pectineus, adductor longus, and adductor brevis. Groin pain over the adductor musculature is most commonly associated with the adductor longus muscle insertion site; therefore an entity that must be considered is athletic pubalgia, which will not be covered in this chapter. The standard of care is physical therapy, focused on Holmich's exercise protocol [27], which has showed its long-term effectiveness for adductor-related groin pain in athletes [28]. In patients not responding to physical therapy, injections can be considered. Lidocaine injections could help to confirm the diagnosis [29]. Corticosteroids has been used, however, due to the potential risk for tendon damage, has fallen in disuse. There is very limited evidence available to support the use of regenerative medicine techniques. Dallaudiere et al. [30] retrospectively evaluated the effectiveness of a single ultrasound-guided PRP injection for upper- and lower-extremity tendinopathies in 408 subjects that included 40 patients with adductor/hamstring tendinopathy. Those patients demonstrated significant functional and pain improvement at 6 weeks and at a mean of 20.2 months following injection. Like previously stated, standardized protocols need to be established in order to compare therapeutic interventions and reliably evaluate efficacy.

The hamstring muscles include the semimembranosus, semitendinosus, and biceps femoris. Hamstring tendinopathy can occur proximal at the ischial tuberosity or distally at the medial or lateral hamstring tendons. Imbalance between quadriceps and hamstring muscles predisposes injuries to the latter. Standard care consists of ice, NSAIDs, and physical therapy. Physical therapy should focus on hamstring stretching, strengthening with eccentric lengthening exercises, and correcting errors in the kinetic chain. In addition, there is evidence that shockwave therapy, another regenerative medicine modality not often discussed, is effective in the treatment of chronic proximal hamstring tendinopathy. Evidence comes from a randomized controlled clinical trial, consisting of 40 patients, which showed that the shockwave therapy group had significant difference in pain reduction compared to traditional exercise program for hamstring muscles [31]. Peritendinous injections with lidocaine and/or steroids can be effective short term. PRP injections have also been used in the treatment of hamstring tendinopathy. A study involving 17 patients, demonstrated that patients refractory to conservative treatment responded well to one PRP injection and returned to sport at average of 4.5 months [32]. Other studies with shorter follow-ups have not necessarily report benefits of PRP. Levy et al. [33] evaluated 29 patients up to 8 weeks postinjection and did not observe statistically significant difference of a single PRP injection for proximal hamstring tendinopathy. However, a level 1 systematic review by Miller et al. in 2017 suggested that PRP injections are superior to other injections in patients with symptomatic tendinopathy [34]. They included a total of 16 randomized controlled trials of PRP versus control in different tendinopathies.

Stem cells theoretically have potential characteristics that may benefit injured multiple musculoskeletal structures, including tendon disorders. However, a systematic review in 2017 by Pas et al. concluded that there is no evidence to support the use of stem cells in tendinopathies [35].

Ligament Injuries

The main hip joint ligaments (iliofemoral, pubofemoral, and ischiofemoral ligament) are very strong and stable, therefore requiring a great amount of force to cause a ligament sprain or rupture. Typically, the mechanism of injury involves twisting and/ or overstretching. The standard of care for any ligament injury involves protecting the injured area, rest, ice, compression, and elevation. Analgesics might be used as needed. In addition, clinical studies have also demonstrated that early mobilization improves ligament healing and strength. Temporary bracing might be needed; however, casting and prolonged brace should be avoided. Lastly, rehabilitation should focus in decreasing pain and swelling and improving range of motion and strength.

PRP in Ligament Injuries

To our knowledge there is no report of platelet-rich plasma on hip ligaments. The evidence in the knee suggests that PRP injections to the MCL in chronic injuries and the ACL intraoperative during reconstruction may accelerate healing and decrease pain post-reconstruction, respectively [36, 37].

Hip Labral Injury

The hip labrum is a fibrocartilaginous structure that attaches to the margin of the acetabulum and provides stability and support. Labral tears are the most common reasons to undergo a hip arthroscopy [38]. Hip labral tears are usually associated with traumatic injury such as a hip dislocation or bony abnormality like a hip dysplasia or femoroacetabular impingement (FAI). The standard of care for hip labral tears include activity modification, unloading the damaged labrum, gait retraining to minimize excessive hip extension, physical modalities, and analgesics as needed. Physical therapy is recommended focusing in core muscles, hip girdle, and proprioceptive exercises. Sono-guided corticosteroid hip injections seem to have limited therapeutic effect in patients with labral tears and FAI [39]. However, an anesthetic only injection might be a good diagnostic tool for possible hip arthroscopy candidates [39].

PRP has been used intraoperatively in patients undergoing hip arthroscopy for labral treatment. However, *Redmond* et al. did not observe significant difference between groups receiving anesthetic versus PRP at a minimum of a 2-year follow-up [40]. There is no evidence to support platelet-rich plasma as an effective treatment of hip labral tears.

Conclusion

Hip pain is one of the most common complaints in a musculoskeletal practice. However, due to its intrinsic anatomic and functional complexity, pain can arise secondary to multiple etiologies. In many occasions the current standard of care does not improve the patient's symptoms. Therefore, there is increasing demand for new approaches that can effectively and safely target these pathologies. Among these, regenerative medicine techniques have become an attractive approach, especially with the widespread use of sports ultrasound to guide such procedures. We found evidence that among these, PRP is a reasonable alternative for hip tendinopathy. For hip osteoarthritis, PRP also appears to be superior to hyaluronic acid, at least for the first 2 months, however with similar effectiveness thereafter. Evidence for stem cells' role in hip pathology is still deficient, with available data not supporting its use for other tendinopathies. When making clinical decisions, we should evaluate the included patient population and specific pathology targeted in these studies, to establish their applicability to our specific patient population.

References

1. Allen KD, Golightly YM. State of the evidence. Curr Opin Rheumatol. 2015;27(3):276–83.
2. Foye P, Todd S, Shah V. Hip osteoarthritis. In: WR Frontera, Silver J, editors. Essentials of physical medicine and rehabilitation. 4th ed. Philadelphia: Hanley & Belfus; 2018. p. 307.
3. Hochberg MC, Altman RD, April KT, Benkhalti M, Guyatt G, McGowan J, et al. American College of Rheumatology 2012 recommendations for the use of nonpharmacologic and pharmacologic therapies in osteoarthritis of the hand, hip, and knee. Arthritis Care Res. 2012;64(4):465–74.
4. Kullenberg B, Runesson R, Tuvhag R, Olsson C, Resch S. Intraarticular corticosteroid injection: pain relief in osteoarthritis of the hip? J Rheumatol. 2004;31(11):2265–8.
5. Qvistgaard E, Christensen R, Torp-Pedersen S, Bliddal H. Intra-articular treatment of hip osteoarthritis: a randomized trial of hyaluronic acid, corticosteroid, and isotonic saline. Osteoarthr Cartil. 2006;14(2):163–70.
6. Lai WC, Arshi A, Wang D, Seeger LL, Motamedi K, Levine BD, et al. Efficacy of intraarticular corticosteroid hip injections for osteoarthritis and subsequent surgery. Skelet Radiol. 2018;47(12):1635–40.
7. Freire V, Bureau NJ. Injectable corticosteroids: take precautions and use caution. Semin Musculoskelet Radiol. 2016;20(5):401–8.

8. Mulvaney SW. A review of viscosupplementation for osteoarthritis of the hip and a description of an ultrasound-guided hip injection technique. Curr Sports Med Rep. 2009;8(6):291–4.
9. Bennell KL, Hunter DJ, Paterson KL. Platelet-rich plasma for the management of hip and kee osteoarthritis. Curr Rheumatol Rep. 2017;19(5):24.
10. Sánchez M, Guadilla J, Fiz N, Andia I. Ultrasound-guided platelet-rich plasma injections for the treatment of osteoarthritis of the hip. Rheumatology. 2012;51(1):144–50.
11. Ye Y, Zhou X, Mao S, Zhang J, Lin B. Platelet rich plasma versus hyaluronic acid in patients with hip osteoarthritis: a meta-analysis of randomized controlled trials. Int J Surg. 2018;53:279–87.
12. Mautner K, Malanga GA, Smith J, Shiple B, Ibrahim V, Sampson S, et al. A call for a standard classification system for future biologic research: the rationale for new PRP nomenclature. PM R. 2015;7(4 suppl):s53–9.
13. Shapiro SA, Kazmerchak SE, Heckman MG, Zubair AC, O'Connor MI. A prospective, single-blind, placebo-controlled trial of bone marrow aspirate concentrate for knee osteoarthritis. Am J Sports Med. 2017;45(1):82–90.
14. Mardones R, Jofré CM, Tobar L, Minguell JJ. Mesenchymal stem cell therapy in the treatment of hip osteoarthritis. J Hip Preserv Surg. 2017;4(2):159–63.
15. Darrow M, Shaw B, Darrow B, Wisz S. Short-term outcomes of treatment of hip osteoarthritis with 4 bone marrow concentrate injections: a case series. Clin Med Insights Case Rep. 2018;11. https://doi.org/10.1177/1179547618791574.
16. Rodriguez-Fontan F, Piuzzi NS, Kraeutler MJ, Pascual-Garrido C. Early clinical outcomes of intra-articular injections of bone marrow aspirate concentrate for the treatment of early osteoarthritis of the hip and knee: a cohort study. PM R. 2018;10(12):1353–9.
17. Cook JL, Rio E, Purdam CR, Docking SI. Revisiting the continuum model of tendon pathology: what is its merit in clinical practice and research? Br J Sports Med. 2016;43(6):409–16.
18. Torres A, Fernández-Fairen M, Sueiro-Fernández J. Greater trochanteric pain syndrome and gluteus medius and minimus tendinosis: nonsurgical treatment. Pain Manag. 2018;8(1):45–55.
19. Labrosse JM, Cardinal É, Leduc BE, Duranceau J, Rémillard J, Bureau NJ, et al. Effectiveness of ultrasound-guided corticosteroid injection for the treatment of gluteus medius tendinopathy. Am J Roentgenol. 2010;194(1):202–6.
20. Mautner K, Colberg RE, Malanga G, Borg-Stein JP, Harmon KG, Dharamsi AS, et al. Outcomes after ultrasound-guided platelet-rich plasma injections for chronic tendinopathy: a multicenter, retrospective review. PM R. 2013;5(3):169–75.
21. Fitzpatrick J, Bulsara MK, O'Donnell J, McCrory PR, Zheng MH. The effectiveness of platelet-rich plasma injections in gluteal tendinopathy: a randomized, double-blind controlled trial comparing a single platelet-rich plasma injection with a single corticosteroid injection. Am J Sports Med. 2018;46:933.
22. Ali M, Oderuth E, Atchia I, Malviya A. The use of platelet-rich plasma in the treatment of greater trochanteric pain syndrome: a systematic literature review. J Hip Preserv Surg. 2018;5(3):209–19.
23. Jacobson JA, Yablon CM, Henning PT, Kazmers IS, Urquhart A, Hallstrom B, et al. Greater trochanteric pain syndrome: percutaneous tendon fenestration versus platelet-rich plasma injection for treatment of gluteal tendinosis. J Ultrasound Med. 2016;35(11):2413–20.
24. Garala K, Prasad V, Jeyapalan K, Power RA. Medium-term and long-term outcomes of interventions for primary psoas tendinopathy. Clin J Sport Med. 2014;24(3):205–10.
25. Agten CA, Rosskopf AB, Zingg PO, Peterson CK, Pfirrmann CWA. Outcomes after fluoroscopy-guided iliopsoas bursa injection for suspected iliopsoas tendinopathy. Eur Radiol. 2015;25(3):865–71.
26. McKee-Proctor MH, Sugimoto D, Han JS, Stracciolini A, D'Hemecourt PA. Short-term effect of ultrasound-guided iliopsoas peritendinous corticosteroid injection. J Ultrasound Med. 2018. https://doi.org/10.1002/jum.14841.
27. Hölmich P, Uhrskou P, Ulnits L, Kanstrup IL, Bachmann Nielsen M, Bjerg AM, et al. Effectiveness of active physical training as treatment for long-standing adductor-related groin pain in athletes: randomised trial. Lancet. 1999;353(151):439–43.

28. Hölmich P, Nyvold P, Larsen K. Continued significant effect of physical training as treatment for overuse injury: 8- to 12-year outcome of a randomized clinical trial. Am J Sports Med. 2011;39(11):2447–51.
29. Gill TJ, Carroll KM, Makani A, Wall AJ, Dumont GD, Cohn RM. Surgical technique for treatment of recalcitrant adductor longus tendinopathy. Arthrosc Tech. 2014;3(2):e293–7.
30. Dallaudière B, Pesquer L, Meyer P, Silvestre A, Perozziello A, Peuchant A, et al. Intratendinous injection of platelet-rich plasma under US guidance to treat tendinopathy: a long-term pilot study. J Vasc Interv Radiol. 2014;25:717.
31. Cacchio A, Rompe JD, Furia JP, Susi P, Santilli V, De Paulis F. Shockwave therapy for the treatment of chronic proximal hamstring tendinopathy in professional athletes. Am J Sports Med. 2011;39(1):146–53.
32. Wetzel RJ, Patel RM, Terry MA. Platelet-rich plasma as an effective treatment for proximal hamstring injuries. Orthopedics. 2012;36(1):e64–70.
33. Levy GM, Lucas P, Hope N. Efficacy of a platelet-rich plasma injection for the treatment of proximal hamstring tendinopathy: a pilot study. J Sci Med Sport. 2019;22:247.
34. Miller LE, Parrish WR, Roides B, Bhattacharyya S. Efficacy of platelet-rich plasma injections for symptomatic tendinopathy: systematic review and meta-analysis of randomised injection-controlled trials. BMJ Open Sport Exerc Med. 2017;3(1):e000237.
35. Pas HIMFL, Moen MH, Haisma HJ, Winters M. No evidence for the use of stem cell therapy for tendon disorders: a systematic review. Br J Sports Med. 2017;51(13):996–1002.
36. Yoshida M, Marumo K. An autologous leukocyte-reduced platelet-rich plasma therapy for chronic injury of the medial collateral ligament in the knee: a report of 3 successful cases. Clin J Sport Med. 2019;29(1):e4–6.
37. Seijas R, Cuscó X, Sallent A, Serra I, Ares O, Cugat R. Pain in donor site after BTB-ACL reconstruction with PRGF: a randomized trial. Arch Orthop Trauma Surg. 2016;136(6):829–35.
38. Safran MR. The acetabular labrum: anatomic and functional characteristics and rationale for surgical intervention. J Am Acad Orthop Surg. 2010;18(6):338–45.
39. Krych AJ, Griffith TB, Hudgens JL, Kuzma SA, Sierra RJ, Levy BA. Limited therapeutic benefits of intra-articular cortisone injection for patients with femoro-acetabular impingement and labral tear. Knee Surg Sport Traumatol Arthrosc. 2014;22(4):750–5.
40. Redmond JM, Gupta A, Stake CE, Hammarstedt JE, Finch NA, Domb BG. Clinical results of hip arthroscopy for labral tears: a comparison between intraoperative platelet-rich plasma and bupivacaine injection. Arthrosc – J Arthrosc Relat Surg. 2015;31(3):445–53.

Chapter 12
Regenerative Medicine for the Knee

Mariam Zakhary and Gerardo Miranda-Comas

Knee Osteoarthritis

The two joints within the knee that are susceptible to osteoarthritis (OA) are the tibiofemoral joint and the patellofemoral joint. The tibiofemoral joint consisting of the femur proximally and the tibia distally is the major weight-bearing joint of the two. The patellofemoral joint consists of the patella and the femur, more specifically the patellar groove of which the patella would glide through.

Knee osteoarthritis is the most common OA in the lower extremities. The severity of knee OA ranges from mild to severe and usually classified using X-rays. For this reason, many approaches to treating this major joint have been described. The American College of Rheumatology (ACR) recommends several non-pharmacological interventions like aerobic and resistance exercise, aquatic therapy, weight loss for those overweight, psychosocial intervention, lateral or medial wedged insoles for medial or lateral compartment OA, respectively, walking aids, thermal agents, Tai chi programs, acupuncture, and transcutaneous electrical stimulation [1]. Pharmacological treatment can also be recommended. The ACR strongly recommended in 2012 the use acetaminophen or paracetamol, oral or topical nonsteroidal anti-inflammatory drugs (NSAIDs), tramadol, and intra-articular glucocorticoids injections [1]. In one meta-analysis, Gregori et al. looked at several classes of medications that are now used to treat the condition which included a long list consisting of analgesics, antioxidants, bone-acting agents, NSAIDs, intra-articular injection medications such as hyaluronic acid (HA) and corticosteroids, symptomatic slow-acting drugs in osteoarthritis, and putative disease-modifying agents [2]. In the advent of systemic medication control and individuals wanting

M. Zakhary · G. Miranda-Comas (✉)
Department of Rehabilitation and Human Performance,
Icahn School of Medicine at Mount Sinai, New York, NY, USA
e-mail: Gerardo.Miranda-comas@mountsinai.org

© Springer Nature Switzerland AG 2020
G. Cooper et al. (eds.), *Regenerative Medicine for Spine and Joint Pain*,
https://doi.org/10.1007/978-3-030-42771-9_12

to remain active and avoid surgery, regenerative medicine has been proven to be an option worth exploring.

The use of regenerative medicine in the knee has certainly been described in the literature, but strong evidence is still lacking. Though first described in 2008 to be used in the treatment of knee osteoarthritis, platelet-rich plasma (PRP) continues to have contradicting literature on its efficacy as a treatment modality. In 2017, Bennell et al. published a paper reviewing randomized control trials done between the years 2012 through 2017 [3]. Though, ultimately, the paper concludes that, due to methodological variability, much research have to be done before a true conclusion is to be made, it does report that there is evidence, though not strong, that PRP is promising in the treatment of knee osteoarthritis [3]. The evidence of the PRP being efficacious seems to be more promising in younger participants with less structural changes and also when put head to head with HA injections. In a meta-analysis done by Laudy et al., 10 RCTs which included 1069 subjects concluded that at 6-month follow-up, pain relief and improvement in function in subjects injected with PRP and those injected with HA were comparable. However, at 12-month follow-up, it appears that those who received PRP did significantly better than those who received HA [4]. Importantly, this paper concluded that there was no noted increase in adverse events with PRP when compared to HA and saline injections. In a systematic review, Xing et al. looked even closer at risks associated with PRP injections and also concluded that there was no increased risk with the proposed procedure [5].

Another regenerative medicine modality with "therapeutic potential" is stem cell therapy. Mesenchymal stem cells possess the theoretical potential to promote tissue growth and regeneration. In one prospective, single-blinded, placebo-controlled trial, individuals with bilateral knee OA were injected with bone marrow aspirate concentrate (BMAC) in one knee and saline in the other knee. There was significant pain relief with BMAC; however, there was no statistical significance in the difference of symptoms between the BMAC knee and placebo control knee [6]. A promising study done by Gobbi and Whyte showed significant improvement in pain and function in subjects who had HA injection + BMAC versus microfracture procedure [7]. Significant improvements in outcome scores were achieved in both treatment groups at 2 years ($P < 0.001$). In the microfracture group, 64% were classified as normal or nearly normal according to the International Knee Documentation Committee (IKDC) objective score at 2 years, compared with 100% of those treated with HA + BMAC ($P < 0.001$). Normal or nearly normal objective assessments in the microfracture group declined significantly after 5 years to 28% of patients ($P = 0.004$). All patients treated with HA + BMAC maintained improvement at 5 years according to IKDC subjective scores. Lysholm and IKDC subjective scores were similar between treatment groups at 5 years [7]. Several other similar studies were done with similar results; however, it is hard to give definitive recommendations as there is no standardized approach to BMAC preparation and injection technique, therefore making the evidence harder to correlate and apply. Another study that looked at the effect of peripheral blood stem cells (PBSC) and their effect on cartilage growth investigated histological effect of using them postoperatively after arthroscopic subchondral drilling. Results showed that after arthroscopic sub-chondral drilling into grade 3 and 4 chondral lesions, postoperative intra-articular injections of autologous PBSC in combination with HA resulted in an improvement of the quality of articular cartilage repair over the same treatment without PBSC, as shown by histologic and MRI evaluation [8].

Prolotherapy is another modality with potential benefit in treating knee OA. A meta-analysis looked at the role of prolotherapy in knee pain, and it showed promis-ing results in the treatment of knee osteoarthritis [9]. Studies used subjective scales such as the WOMAC that were used to assess posttreatment pain. Results showed that prolotherapy yielded higher score difference (decrease in pain and symptoms) when compared to the control group who performed exercise alone. Another study discussed in this meta-analysis showed that prolotherapy with exercise yielded a greater decrease in WOMAC score than placebo saline injection with exercise [9].

Tendinopathies

Bony structures in the knee serve as attachment sites for several tendons. These tendons include the quadriceps, patellar, popliteus, as well as distal hamstrings. Tendons are susceptible to multiple modes of injuries from acute or chronic ten-dinopathies to partial and complete ruptures. These injuries are quite often seen in not only the athletic setting, with an estimated 40–50% of athletes getting tendon injuries, but also in the aging population and in some occupational settings [10].

Similar to degenerative disease in the knee, different modalities for treating tendinopathies have been studied and include both interventional procedures and physical therapy and modalities. A focus on eccentric strengthening of the muscles to promote healing has been the standard of care when treating tendinopathies with physical therapy and exercise. Treating pain is accomplished by the use of oral analgesics, topicals to the area (more effective for superficial tendons), and more recently described interventional regenerative techniques.

The evidence for use of regenerative medicine in soft tissue injuries was found to be insufficient by a large Cochrane review performed by Moraes et al. [11]. The main reason is the lack of standardization of PRP and aspirate preparation. There has been literature on the composition of the injectate, most popularly stating that leukocyte-rich PRP is recommended for tendons, while leukocyte poor for intra-articular appli-cations. The key components of leukocytes are neutrophils and monocytes, which may also release many bioactive factors and proteins. Neutrophils mainly release myeloperoxidase, bactericidal phagocytins, collagenase, gelatinase, and proteases. Monocytes secrete platelet-activating factor, TGF-β, VEGF, FGF, and EGF. Many of these factors have been shown to influence tendon healing [12]. One double-blinded randomized control trial looking at patellar tendinopathy compared con-comitant ultrasound-guided dry needling with the injection of leukocyte-rich PRP (PRP group) versus dry needling alone (DN group), both groups receiving physi-cal therapy adjunctively. Exercises consisted of eccentric strengthening routines which are currently widely accepted for the treatment of tendinopathy. The Victorian Institute of Sports Assessment (VISA) score for patellar tendinopathy improved at 12 weeks significantly more in the PRP group, but this difference was not significant at 26 weeks. Of note, no adverse events were reported on either group [13].

Though the literature remains promising, there is a lot in the way of standardizing preparation and administration of PRP into the tendons of the knee. The majority of the literature looks at the patellar tendon, presented mostly in case series and smaller randomized control trials [14]. Further investigation is needed before definitive recommendations are given concerning PRP in musculoskeletal soft tissue, especially the surrounding knee tendons not mentioned in many studies. On the opposite side of the coin, it appears that knowing the proposed mechanism of leukocyte-rich PRP and the evidence strongly against any adverse events, it is a safe and reasonable option to use in the treatment of tendinopathy. Of the regenerative medicine modalities, PRP seems to be the most described in treating tendon injuries in the knee. Prolotherapy has been described in treating tendons in the ankle, such as the Achilles, and also in the shoulder, such as the rotator cuff. The literature on prolotherapy for the knee is more for treating intra-articular pathologies, namely, knee OA, as previously discussed.

Ligamentous Injuries

Common injuries that can cause significant pain and instability in the knees are ligamentous injuries. The more commonly discussed ligaments of the knee include the cruciate ligaments (ACL and PCL), medial collateral and lateral (fibular) collateral ligaments (MCL and LCL), as well as the medial patellofemoral ligament (MPFL). Injury to these structures includes sprains and complete or partial tears and can cause significant mechanical symptoms and subsequently pain. Treatment of such pathology includes both surgical and nonsurgical management. Most cases with severe instability, intractable pain, and failed conservative measures become surgical. However, in a clinically stable knee and also in a patient without intricate demand on the knee, nonoperative management is preferred. To date, the most common management would be physical rehabilitation to strengthen the secondary stabilizers of the knees which are dynamic muscles to compensate for the loss of the static ligament stabilization. Pain is managed similarly to the above pathologies with the use of oral analgesics and intra-articular injections of corticosteroids to reduce the local inflammatory effects of injury.

As previously mentioned, evidence is still lacking when it comes to the application of regenerative techniques with soft tissue injuries. Several studies observed the use of regenerative medicine (PRP, stem cells) as an adjunct to ACL reconstructive surgery. The earlier studies investigated the effect in animal models (rabbits) using adipose-derived regenerative cells (ADRC). Rabbits were divided into two groups, both receiving allograft ACLs; one group had the tissue coated with ADRC while the other group did not. Though histological patterns were improved and appeared to be more favorable toward healing, the failure load was higher in the treated group. However, this was not statistically significant. It seemed that local administration of ADRCs promoted the early healing process at the tendon-bone junction, both histologically and mechanically, in a rabbit ACL reconstruction model [15]. With promising results in these animal model studies, further investigation was done on treating ACL injuries nonsurgical or surgical with allografts to determine whether it would enhance biological healing [16].

Though the literature is stronger for prolotherapy in knee OA and tendons involved in other joints, there is case study-level evidence for the use of prolotherapy in ACL injury. In one case study, an 18-year-old female skier suffered a complete rupture of her ACL and deferred surgical management. At 21 weeks post-injury, she was having pain with ambulation and was unable to negotiate stairs and had a 1 cm positive anterior drawer test. She agreed to and had seven prolotherapy sessions over 15 weeks and exercise program that started after her third injection. The patient showed improvement with walking on flat ground, which improved 4 weeks after initiation of prolotherapy. She was also able to ride a stationary bicycle for 30 minutes by week 12. By 15 weeks, the patient had no reported instability climbing and descending stairs, the anterior drawer test was negative, and MRI showed an intact ACL with fibrosis. Subsequently, she returned to full sport activity [17].

References

1. Hochberg MC, Altman RD, April KT, Benkhalti M, Guyatt G, McGowan J, et al. American College of Rheumatology 2012 recommendations for the use of nonpharmacologic and pharmacologic therapies in osteoarthritis of the hand, hip, and knee. Arthritis Care Res. 2012;64(4):465–74.
2. Gregori D, Rovati LC, Giacovelli G, Barbetta B, Azzolina D, Gualtieri F, et al. Association of pharmacological treatments with long-term pain control in patients with knee osteoarthritis. JAMA. 2018;320(24):2564–79.
3. Bennell KL, Hunter DJ, Paterson KL. Platelet-rich plasma for the management of hip and knee osteoarthritis. Curr Rheumatol Rep. 2017;19(5):24.
4. Laudy ABM, Bakker EWP, Rekers M, Moen MH. Efficacy of platelet-rich plasma injections in osteoarthritis of the knee: a systematic review and meta-analysis. Br J Sports Med. 2015;49(10):657–72.
5. Xing D, Wang B, Zhang W, Yang Z, Hou Y, Chen Y, et al. Intra-articular platelet-rich plasma injections for knee osteoarthritis: an overview of systematic reviews and risk of bias considerations. Int J Rheum Dis. 2017;20(11):1612–30.
6. Shapiro SA, Kazmerchak SE, Heckman MG, Zubair AC, O'Connor MI. A prospective, single-blind, placebo-controlled trial of bone marrow aspirate concentrate for knee osteoarthritis. Am J Sports Med. 2017;45(1):82–90.
7. Gobbi A, Whyte GP. One-stage cartilage repair using a hyaluronic acid-based scaffold with activated bone marrow-derived mesenchymal stem cells compared with microfracture. Am J Sports Med. 2016;44(11):2846–54.
8. Saw KY, Anz A, Siew-Yoke Jee C, Merican S, Ching-Soong Ng R, Roohi SA, et al. Articular cartilage regeneration with autologous peripheral blood stem cells versus hyaluronic acid: a randomized controlled trial. Arthrosc – J Arthrosc Relat Surg. 2013;29(4):684–94.
9. Rabago D, Nourani B. Prolotherapy for osteoarthritis and tendinopathy: a descriptive review. Curr Rheumatol Rep. 2017;19(6):34.

10. Ulasli A. Ultrasound imaging and guidance in the management of knee osteoarthritis in regenerative medicine field. J Clin Orthop Trauma. 2019;10(1):24–31.
11. Moraes VY, Lenza M, Tamaoki MJ, Faloppa F, Belloti JC. Platelet-rich therapies for musculoskeletal soft tissue injuries. Cochrane Database Syst Rev. 2014;4:CD010071.
12. Zhou Y, Wang JH-C. PRP treatment efficacy for tendinopathy: a review of basic science studies. Biomed Res Int. 2016;2016:9103792.
13. Dragoo JL, Wasterlain AS, Braun HJ, Nead KT. Platelet-rich plasma as a treatment for patellar tendinopathy: a double-blind, randomized controlled trial. Am J Sports Med. 2014;42(3):610–8.
14. Andia I, Maffulli N. Use of platelet-rich plasma for patellar tendon and medial collateral ligament injuries: best current clinical practice. J Knee Surg. 2015;28(1):11–8.
15. Kosaka M, Nakase J, Hayashi K, Tsuchiya H. Adipose-derived regenerative cells promote tendon-bone healing in a rabbit model. Arthrosc – J Arthrosc Relat Surg. 2016;32(5):851–9.
16. Hirzinger C, Tauber M, Korntner S, Quirchmayr M, Bauer HC, Traweger A, et al. ACL injuries and stem cell therapy. Arch Orthop Trauma Surg. 2014;134(11):1573–8.
17. Grote W, Delucia R, Waxman R, Zgierska A, Wilson J, Rabago D. Repair of a complete anterior cruciate tear using prolotherapy: a case report. Int Musculoskelet Med. 2009;31(4):159–65.

Chapter 13
Regenerative Medicine for the Foot and Ankle

Emily N. Fatakhov, Tina Bijlani, and Richard G. Chang

The foot is comprised of 28 bones, including 14 phalanges, 7 tarsal bones (talus, calcaneus, cuboid, navicular, and three cuneiforms), 5 metatarsals, and 2 sesamoids. Functionally, the foot is divided into three distinct sections. The hindfoot consists of the talus and calcaneus with the proximal ankle mortise connecting the tibia and fibula to the talus. The subtalar joint refers to the connection between the talus and calcaneus. The distal portion of the talus and calcaneus connects to the midfoot, known as the midtarsal or Chopart joint. The navicular, cuneiforms, and cuboid form the midfoot, a pyramid-like collection of bones, connecting the proximal metatarsals at the Lisfranc joint. Lastly, the forefoot contains everything distal to the Lisfranc joint, which includes the metatarsals, sesamoids, and phalanges. The hallux (big toe) contains two phalanx bones, distal and proximal. This articulates with the head of the first metatarsal forming the first metatarsophalangeal joint (MTPJ) [30]. Under the first metatarsal head lay two small round bones, the sesamoids.

The ankle (talocrural) joint is a synovial joint formed by the tibia, fibula, and talus. It is a hinge joint permitting dorsiflexion and plantar flexion, while eversion and inversion are produced by the subtalar joint. Multiple ligaments in the ankle provide support and resistance to specific movements including the tibiofibular, deltoid, and anterior and posterior talofibular and calcaneofibular ligaments. The Achilles tendon is the common tendon for the plantaris, gastrocnemius, and soleus with attachment to the calcaneus permitting plantar flexion of the foot. The peroneus (fibularis) longus and brevis tendons course posterior to the lateral malleolus and provide eversion and plantar flexion, while the peroneus tertius runs anterior to the lateral malleolus and provides eversion and dorsiflexion. Medially, the tarsal

E. N. Fatakhov · T. Bijlani
Rehabilitation Medicine, The Mount Sinai Hospital, Mount Sinai, New York, NY, USA

R. G. Chang (✉)
Department of Rehabilitation & Human Performance, Icahn School of Medicine at Mount Sinai, New York, NY, USA
e-mail: Richard.Chang@mountsinai.org

© Springer Nature Switzerland AG 2020
G. Cooper et al. (eds.), *Regenerative Medicine for Spine and Joint Pain*,
https://doi.org/10.1007/978-3-030-42771-9_13

225

tunnel contains the tibialis posterior, flexor digitorum longus and flexor hallucis longus tendons, posterior tibial artery, vein, and tibial nerve [30, 31].

Conventional treatment for musculoskeletal injury focuses on reducing inflammation and pain to provide symptomatic relief. However, it is now known that inflammation is an integral part of the healing process. These medications may impair the healing of damaged tissues, leading to chronic degenerative disruption and several adverse effects [28].

Plantar Fasciitis

The plantar fascia is a thick ligamentous connective tissue that originates from the heel at the calcaneus and runs out to attach to the ball of the foot at the bases of the five metatarsal heads. The aponeurosis consists of three bands: lateral, medial, and central. The central band originates from the medial tubercle of the calcaneus and travels to the five toes. At the metatarsal head, the central band divides into five slips, each of which inserts at the proximal phalanx of each toe. It has a static purpose, in which it supports the arch of the foot via tensioning and load bearing, as well as a dynamic purpose, in which it alternately elongates and contracts during the gait cycle, enabling the arch to flatten and elevate [25].

Plantar fasciitis (or plantar fasciosis/fasciopathy) is one of the most common causes of heel pain and is characterized by inflammation or degeneration of the plantar fascia [25]. In the United States, plantar fasciitis affects about two million people per year with an equal incidence between males and females. This results in approximately 1,000,000 patient visits per year and accounts for 10% of injuries in runners [25]. Plantar fasciitis results when increased load to the plantar fascia eventually leads to micro-tearing, inflammation, and pain. Scar tissue then damages the fascia, and with this increased force, heel spurs are prone to develop where the fascia attaches to the calcaneus. Rupture of the plantar fascia may sometimes occur. Pain usually begins when patients report a new repetitive activity, change in footwear, or walking on harder than usual surfaces [22]. Initially they may present with heel or midfoot pain, typically worse upon waking in the morning and again at the end of the day after increased activity. There are three different phases of pathology. The initial acute onset lasts up to 4 weeks, the subacute phase lasts up to 3 months, and afterward it is considered a chronic condition, at which point inflammation is replaced by degenerative changes, and tension enthesophytes often develop at the calcaneal insertion.

Per current evidence-based guidelines, treatment varies based on the timing of symptoms and clinical phase. In the acute phase, stretching of the plantar fascia and Achilles tendon, either manually or by rolling the foot over a tennis ball or a water bottle, is recommended [24]. Symptomatic relief may also be accomplished with the application of ice or by administering oral nonsteroidal anti-inflammatory drugs or acetaminophen [24]. Other options include heel cushions to act as shock absorbers, orthotic arch supports to alleviate stress of the plantar fascia, taping to decrease mobility of the joint, posterior night splints, and iontophoresis [25]. When symptoms progress to the subacute phase, ultrasound-guided corticosteroid injections, acupuncture, and manual therapy are recommended [23, 27]. Once it reaches the chronic phase, extracorporeal shock wave/sound therapy has yielded promising results [25, 27]. Botulinum toxin A is another, possible injectable treatment method that has shown some promise in some case series [20–22]. There are several instances in which conservative measures fail or patients do not opt for a surgical intervention. Alternatively, patient may not tolerate the side effects associated with medications. Nonsteroidal anti-inflammatory medications, via inhibition of the cyclooxygenase pathway, can potentiate damage to the gastrointestinal mucosa, resulting in peptic ulcer disease and gastrointestinal bleeding [28]. Glucocorticoids are associated with systemic increased risk for diabetes, glaucoma, and suppression of the hypothalamic-pituitary-adrenal axis, at the cellular level [26]. With these side effects and continued degenerative damage despite treatment, it is advantageous to find other treatment options for this common musculoskeletal disease. Regenerative medicine techniques can potentially help to promote remodeling of unhealthy tendinopathic tissue to healthy tendon but more importantly aid in decreasing the inflammatory environment [79, 80]. Several studies have shown improvement in pain and function with platelet-rich plasma injections utilized to treat plantar fasciitis. The injection of this centrifuged, autologous blood may provide cellular and humoral mediators to induce healing of degenerated tissues.

In a single-center, unblinded, prospective, preliminary study, Martinelli et al. demonstrated the safety of PRP injections when utilized for the treatment of chronic plantar fasciitis. Fourteen consecutive patients with chronic plantar fasciitis unresponsive to at least 3 months of icing, NSAIDs, and stretching received three once weekly, palpation-guided injections of PRP into the plantar fascia and were assessed 12 months after the procedure. The modified Roles and Maudsley (RM) score and a visual analogue scale (VAS) were used to evaluate the clinical results. At a year follow-up, results were rated as excellent in the majority of patients (9, 64.3%). The remaining 14.3% of patients rated results as good, acceptable in 14.3%, and poor in 7.1%. VAS for pain was found to be significantly decreased from 7.1 ± 1.1 before treatment to 1.9 ± 1.5 at 12 months follow-up with $p < 0.01$ [29].

In a prospective study by Kumar et al., 44 patients (50 heels) who had not responded to at least 1 year of standard conservative management were offered a one-time PRP injection. RM, VAS, and American Orthopedic Foot and Ankle Society (AOFAS) scores were collected prior to the procedure, at 3 months, and at 6 months. The PRP group was shown to have efficacy in these chronic cases. At 6-month review, RM scores improved from mean 4 to 2 ($p < 0.001$), VAS improved from 7.7 to 4.2, and AOFAS improved from 60.6 to 81.9. The study was without complication, and 28 patients (64%) were very satisfied, indicating they would opt for the injection again [6].

This was further demonstrated in a randomized controlled trial by Gill et al. with 179 patients who had greater than 6 months of pain due to plantar fasciitis (91 in treatment group and 88 in control group). For patients receiving the PRP, 10 ml of patient's blood was collected, mixed with 2 ml acid citrate dextrose (anticoagulant), and placed in Autologous Platelet Separator System, to yield PRP. Under sterile conditions, patients received 3 ml of PRP into the plantar fascia at site of maximum tenderness. Patients were followed at week 2, 4, 8, 12, and 52, during which VAS was utilized to assess pain relief. The mean VAS score in case group (PRP) decreased from baseline 6.6 to 0.54 at 52-week follow-up. This indicates that PRP may significantly improve pain in patients with chronic plantar fasciitis. Additionally, complication rates were minimal and symptom recurrence rate low [19].

A recent double-blinded, prospective randomized controlled trial (RCT) with 75 patients showed that PRP was as effective or more effective than corticosteroid injection when compared with normal saline injection control to reduce pain over 3 months of follow-up and improve functional scores for chronic plantar fasciitis [4]. Mahindra et al. found significant improvement in VAS and AOFAS in the PRP and corticosteroid group at 3-week and 3-month follow-up, while there was no improvement in the placebo group. PRP proves to have less side effects in comparison to traditional steroid injection, which may be unsafe for diabetics and those with multiple comorbidities. Glucocorticoids (GCs), the most important and frequently used class of anti-inflammatory drugs, are associated with diabetes, glaucoma, and suppression of the hypothalamic-pituitary-adrenal axis, at the cellular level [26]. Its potent anti-inflammatory and immunosuppressive actions allow it to remain the mainstay of treatment. However, with its multiple negative associations, it is vital to become equipped with alternate treatment strategies.

The effects of PRP not only showed improvements in pain but also showed a longer duration of benefit when compared to other current treatments. In a 2018, level I randomized controlled prospective study of 158 patients by Uğurlar et al., the therapeutic effects of four different treatment methods for chronic plantar fasciitis with a symptomatic heel spur not improved with 6 months of conservative treatment (including NSAIDs, orthotics, and gastrocnemius-soleus muscle stretching and confirmed on ultrasound imaging) were compared. Patients were randomized to one of four treatment modalities, which were given once a week for 3 weeks: extracorporeal shock wave therapy, platelet-rich plasma injection, local corticosteroid injection, and prolotherapy. Clinical outcomes were assessed using visual analogue scale and Revised Foot Function Index. While no significant improvements were noted in the Revised Foot Function Index, there was a discrepancy in the duration of pain relief. Corticosteroid injections were initially more effective in the first 3 months; extracorporeal shock wave therapy was found to be more effective in the first 6 months. Notably, the treatment groups with prolotherapy and platelet-rich plasma had the longest effect from 3 to 12 months [12].

Inflammation and degenerative changes were improved as evidenced by certain studies [11, 78]. In a prospective, unblinded, cohort study by Ragab et al., 25 patients with chronic plantar fasciitis were studied from Feb 2010 to June 2011. Ultrasound measurement of the medial, central, and lateral bands of the plantar fascia was done prior to injection of PRP in the affected foot and asymptomatic foot for comparison. Plantar fascial thickness greater than 4 mm was considered abnormal. Researchers injected 5 mL platelet concentrate into the most tender aspect of plantar fascia using a peppering technique and found a decrease in plantar fascial thickness, indicating improvement of tendinopathic changes [78].

PRP was directly compared to corticosteroids and found to be either equally or more effective with fewer side effects [3, 4, 5, 8, 15]. For example, Monto's 2014, single-blinded prospective randomized study of 40 patients found a single, 3 mL PRP injection under ultrasound guidance to be superior in terms of duration and effectiveness when compared to a single 40 mg methylprednisolone injection for treatment of chronic recalcitrant, plantar fasciitis. These patients did not respond to conservative management (NSAIDs, physical therapy, bracing). AOFAS hindfoot scores in the PRP group remained increased (indicating improved pain and function) at 3- and 6-month time periods, as well as at 1 and 2 years compared to the corticosteroid group [3]. In a comparative, single-blinded, randomized prospective study by Jain et al., they evaluated the result of single, palpation-guided injections of 3 mL PRP versus 40 mg triamcinolone and levobupivacaine hydrochloride injectate solution in 60 heels of patients with chronic plantar fasciitis of at least 1 year (not responsive to insoles, a full course of eccentric stretching exercises, and physical therapy). They found that both PRP and corticosteroid injection groups had significant improvement in VAS and modified Roles and Maudsley scores but were not statistically significant. PRP was as effective as a steroid injection at achieving symptom relief at 3 and 6 months; however, the PRP group's beneficial effects remained sustained and were statistically significant at the 12-month follow-up interval [5].

Stress Fracture: Metatarsal, Tarsal Navicular

Stress fractures in the foot are a type of chronic overuse injury, most often seen following periods of intense exercise without adequate rest and recovery. They are classified as low (calcaneus and cuboid) or high (navicular, fifth metatarsal, and sesamoids) risk, which has the potential to progress to nonunion or complete fracture. The second and third most common location out of all stress fractures are the tarsal navicular (17.6%) and metatarsal (16.2%), respectively, therefore accounting for a significant cause of foot injury.

Stress fractures account for 0.7–20% of all injuries at sports medicine clinics [18]. The pathophysiology results from damage secondary to repetitive and excessive microtrauma, leading to acceleration of normal bone remodeling with increased osteoblast activity, the production of microfractures (caused by insufficient time for repair of bone), the creation of a bone stress injury, and eventually a stress fracture. Simply put, chronic and persistent loading leads to a cortical break [17]. Certain risk factors for stress fracture include the consumption of greater than 10 alcoholic drinks per week, excessive physical activity with limited rest periods, female athlete triad, female sex, vitamin D deficiency, recreational running more than 25 miles per week, smoking, sudden increase in physical activity, and track (running sports) [13].

Patients will present with progressively worsening pain that is exacerbated by increased activity. They may have localized bony tenderness, swelling, or erythema on examination. The current standard of care for mild stress fractures is rest with progression to activity modification within 4–8 weeks. If the fracture is more critical, the rest period may extend up to 3 months, and the patient may require internal fixation surgery [1, 16]. Rest time may vary based on classification (grade 1–4) per the Arendt and Griffith's classification scale [7, 16].

During the bone healing process, cells of the periosteum in the proximal edge of the fracture and the fibroblasts in the granulation tissue convert into chondroblasts and form hyaline cartilage. Simultaneously, the periosteal cells in the distal edge of the fracture convert to osteoblasts. These two cell types mix over the fracture and form lamellar bone, known as early callus formation, which functions to provide stability of the fracture site. Lamellar bone then converts to trabecular bone and finally to compact bone, which restores full bone strength [9].

Biologics, such as growth factors, have shown benefit when applied to muscles, tendons, and ligaments. Bone marrow aspirate concentrate contains hematopoietic and mesenchymal stem cells and osteogenic growth factors, such as platelet-derived growth factor (PDGF), transforming growth factor-B (TGF-B), and vascular endothelial growth factor (VEGF), all of which have demonstrated efficacy in fracture nonunion treatment [13]. It has been shown that when these factors are utilized during surgical treatment of certain fractures, they may improve recovery. In a case report by Adams et al., a cannulated screw was utilized for delivery of bone marrow aspirate concentrate to a stress fracture nonunion, as previously studied intraosseous delivery via large bore needles and percutaneous delivery were not as effective. The patient was able to immediately bear weight despite postoperative instructions but without hardware failure. Postoperative radiographs and CT 10 weeks after the surgery confirmed union at the fracture site [2]. The use of orthopedic biologics to accelerate healing from fractures is still unknown.

Osteochondral Lesion of the Talus

Osteochondral lesion of the talus is a defect of the chondral surface and/or subchondral bone. Injuries are associated with pain, swelling, and negative impact on quality of life. The current standard of treatment for osteochondral lesions of the talus is isolated microfracture (BMS), which is a bone marrow stimulation procedure, in which subchondral bone plate is punctured into the bone marrow. This allows generation of a blood clot with precursor cells from the subchondral bone marrow, forming fibrocartilaginous repair tissue to fill the defect [14]. In short, the microfracture creates an inflammatory response. A prospective cohort study with 101 patients by Murphy et al. compared treatment of BMS alone (n = 52) to BMS augmented with bone marrow aspirate concentrate (n = 49) in the treatment of talus OCLs. BMAC consists of hematopoietic and mesenchymal stem cells with the potential to differentiate into platelets, chondrocytes, and osteoblasts, allowing for the proper environment for cartilage repair. It is generally harvested from the iliac crest and injected in layers into the surgical defect. In this study it was shown that patients with symptomatic osteochondral lesions who received combined treatment of microfracture plus bone marrow aspirate concentrate showed statistically significant improvement in terms of symptoms, pain, activities of daily living, sports, and quality of life [14].

In an RCT by Milano et al., the effects of autologous platelet-rich plasma combined with microfractures were evaluated in the treatment of chondral defects of 15 sheep. Macroscopic appearance was evaluated utilizing the International Cartilage Repair Society (ICRS) score. Cartilage stiffness was analyzed with electromechanical indenter, and histological appearance was scored according to modified O'Driscoll score. It was found that PRP enhanced cartilage repair after microfractures. It was found to be more effective when PRP was used as an intraoperative fibrin gel in comparison with liquid intra-articular injection. While this study included patients with chondral lesions of the medial femoral condyle, it would be interesting to study patients with osteochondral lesions of the talus.

Mei et al. took this a step further and compared the difference in short-term efficacy and safety in PRP versus hyaluronic acid for reducing pain and disability caused by osteochondral lesions. In this randomized controlled trial, 32 patients were allocated to treatment by intra-articular injections of either hyaluronic acid (HA) or PRP with efficacy being assessed via AOFAS Ankle-Hindfoot Scale (AHFS) and VAS scales. While the platelet-rich plasma treatment group led to a better outcome than the HA group indicated by better AHFS and VAS scores, both were found to have efficacy in decreasing pain and increasing function for at least 6 months [10].

Ankle Osteoarthritis

The pathophysiology of osteoarthritis includes progressive and irreversible cartilage degeneration due to the avascularity and thus inability of cartilage to heal and repair. Risk factors include mechanical, genetic, age, obesity, history of trauma, obesity, muscle weakness, component of the cartilage extracellular matrix, presence of pro-inflammatory mediators including free radicals and cytokines, and depleted local population of mesenchymal stem cells [32, 33]. The etiology of arthritis of the ankle joint most commonly occurs as post-traumatic osteoarthritis (PTOA) accounting for 20–78% of all cases of ankle OA. Within the subset of PTOA, 37% of cases are secondary to fractures, followed by recurrent ankle injuries and a history of ankle sprain [34]. Less commonly, ankle arthritis may also be secondary to degenerative OA, inflammatory arthropathies such as rheumatoid arthritis, as well as crystalloid deposition disease, mixed connective tissue disease, synovitis, and hemophilic arthropathy.

Ankle arthritis is a major cause of disability and chronic pain with resultant gait disturbance. In the foot and ankle, there is a weak correlation between abnormal imaging and patient symptoms. Physical exam reveals limited range of motion about the ankle joint, swelling, crepitus, and joint deformity [36]. Although no consensus or guideline statement exists for the treatment algorithm of ankle arthritis, the standard of care commonly involves physical therapy and symptomatic treatment including aspiration of effusion particularly if suspected with infection, crystalloid deposition disease, or Lyme arthritis [36]. Symptomatic management often includes corticosteroid injection. After failed conservative management, surgical interventions are considered including total ankle arthroplasty or arthrodesis [35]. Regardless of intensity and duration of the response following intra-articular anesthetic or corticosteroid injection, post-procedure pain relief is predictive of positive surgical outcomes [36].

Corticosteroid injections are often performed in the foot and ankle, preferably with imaging guidance to ensure accurate needle placement, as well as recognizing the possibility of inter-joint communications [36]. A retrospective review by Grice et al. showed that intra-articular steroid injections for midfoot and hindfoot osteoarthritis provided significant short-term pain relief for 82% of patients. However, only 32% showed sustained relief for 6 months and 12% at 2 years [37]. In a prospective cohort study including 289 subjects in whom 98 of 635 joints were ankles, Furtado et al. evaluated the impact of intra-articular steroid injection on VAS scores in rheumatoid arthritis patients. Overall, this study showed improvement in rest and movement VAS score in all joints from baseline to 4 weeks. The lowest statistically significant improvement was seen in the ankle and elbow arthritis. Additionally, there was no significant improvement for ankle pain at the longer-term (12 and 24 week) follow-up [38].

Hyaluronic acid (HA) injection for the management of ankle arthritis is promising particularly in the short term; however, the evidence is limited. Cohen et al. performed a double-blinded randomized control trial including 28 patients comparing injectate of Hyalgan to saline control in the tibiotalar joint. At 3-month follow-up, this study demonstrated a statistically significant improvement from baseline in the HA participants compared with control as measured by the Ankle Osteoarthritis Scale (AOS) and Western Ontario and McMaster Universities OA Index (WOMAC); at 6-month follow-up, the trend toward improvement at 6 months was not statistically significant [39]. In a randomized control trial by DeGroot et al. using the American Orthopedic Foot and Ankle Society (AOFAS) clinical rating score in 56 patients, there was a statistically significant improvement in the HA group at 6 weeks. At the 12-week follow-up, there was a substantial increase from baseline in both groups without a statistically significant difference [40]. Murphy et al. performed a prospective evaluation of 50 patients treated with a 3-injection protocol of HA injections comparing pre- and postinjection foot and ankle outcomes (FAOS) score which showed a statistically significant improvement (48 ± 6.3 to 78 ± 5.8) [41]. In order to evaluate the efficacy, safety, and dose dependency of Orthovisc injections, Witteveen et al. found that the weekly dosing (3x1mL) injection regimen showed the best results decreasing pain at rest and during walking [42]. In a prospective RCT, comparing HA injections with 6-week exercise therapy program, Karatosun et al. showed improvement without a statistically significant difference between the groups at 12-month follow-up [77].

Platelet-rich plasma may be a promising alternative in the management of ankle OA; however, there is limited evidence with low-powered studies currently available. Angthong et al. performed a retrospective case series of 12 chronic diseases of the hindfoot and ankle injected with PRP injection (3 mL) under fluoroscopic guidance. Eight out of the 12 patients showed satisfactory results [43]. In a retrospective case series of 20 patients with ankle OA, Repetto et al. performed four weekly PRP injections which demonstrated a positive effect on pain and function, with 80% of patients reporting feeling very satisfied or satisfied. In this study, 10% of patients required surgery due to early treatment failure [44]. Fukawa et al. performed a prospective case series of 20 patients with ankle OA administered with three ultrasound-guided PRP injections within a 2-week period. The results showed pain reduction on the VAS scale from 59.7 to 42.4 at 24 weeks. Statistically significant improvement in the Self-Administered Foot Evaluation Questionnaire (SAFE-Q) was seen at 12 weeks only [45].

Mesenchymal stem cells (MSCs) have the most limited data in ankle arthritis. Various preclinical and clinical trials of MSCs suggest it is a safe and therapeutically beneficial treatment (Freitag). Emadedin et al. performed autologous bone marrow (BM)-derived mesenchymal stem cell injections in 18 patients followed over a 30-month period, 6 of whom carried a diagnosis of ankle arthritis. In these patients, the mean walking distance measured at baseline was 1010 meters and increased to 1625 m and 2333 m at 6 and 30 months, respectively. Additionally, there was an improvement in WOMAC and FAOS scores and a decreased signal intensity related to subchondral edema in 4 of the 6 ankle OA patients at 6 months post-procedure [46].

As a sequela of osteoarthritis, patients often require arthrodesis. There is promising evidence for the use of bone morphogenetic protein (BMP) and platelet-derived growth factor (PDGF) in surgical management of arthritis and traumatic ankle nonunions requiring arthrodesis. Rearick et al., in a retrospective analysis studying 48 patients deemed high risk for nonunion, administered rhBMP-2 as augmentation for bone healing during ankle fusion. The results showed 92% per case union rate and 95.1% per site union rate with mean time to union of 111 days [47]. Similarly, Fourman et al. studied 82 patients undergoing complex ankle arthrodesis; half of the patients received intraoperative rhBMP-2. Those patients who received the BMP were more likely to obtain fusion after the initial surgery (93% vs 53%), required less time wearing the frame, and showed more bone bridging on CT scan [48]. Daniels et al., in a prospective randomized study, evaluated 217 patients undergoing standard internal fixation augmented with recombinant human platelet-derived growth factor BB homodimer (rhPDGF-BB) in 75 patients and 154 control subjects who underwent autograft supplementation. This study showed 84% fusion rate in PDGF compared with 65% in autograft-treated patient [49].

Overall, the data for regenerative medicine techniques for ankle osteoarthritis is promising but is limited. Most data is available for HA with good short-term results. PRP is an alternative approach also with limited evidence and low-powered studies; MSCs have the most limited data in ankle arthritis but show encouraging results. In the surgical model, the use of supplemental growth factors in the rat model is favorable, but limited data is available in humans.

Ankle Sprain

Ankle sprains are very common musculoskeletal conditions presenting to emergency departments and primary care providers and up to 10–30% of all sports-related injuries [51]. Intrinsic risk factors include limited balance, proprioception, and dorsiflexion. The main extrinsic risk factor is the type of sport played with indoor courts constituting the highest risk [50]. The most common mechanism of injury is an inversion injury causing a lateral ankle sprain with pathology involving first the anterior talofibular ligament, then the calcaneofibular ligament, and lastly the posterior talofibular ligament. Forced eversion injuries result in a medial ankle sprain, often resulting in an avulsion fracture of the medial malleolus. A syndesmotic injury (high ankle sprain) will result in significant ankle instability and a risk factor for recurrent ankle sprain.

Standard of care for ankle sprains commonly involves PRICE (protection, rest, ice, compression, and elevation) and limited weight-bearing, NSAIDs with consideration of immobilization and bracing depending on the severity of sprain. However, the mainstay of treatment involves functional rehabilitation and consideration of surgical intervention for patients with severe sprains and who participate in high-level sports.

PRP injections for ankle sprains show limited evidence for management of acute ankle sprain. In a prospective randomized double-blinded placebo-controlled trial by Rowden et al., 37 patients with acute ankle sprain evaluated in the emergency department underwent ultrasound-guided injection of leukocyte-rich PRP with local anesthetic compared with placebo at the point of maximal tenderness. The subjects were monitored on days 0, 3, 8, and 30. No statistical difference was found in pain score or lower-extremity functional scale [52]. Laver et al. studied 16 college elite athletes with grade 3 ankle sprain and syndesmotic instability who were randomized to treatment group (two leukocyte-poor PRP injections to the anterior-inferior tibiofibular ligament (AITFL) 7 days apart) followed by rehabilitation program and control group (only rehabilitation and return to play protocol). The treatment group demonstrated shorter return to play (40.8 vs 59.6 days) and less residual pain upon return to activity (12.5% vs 62.5%). Thus far, PRP does not appear to be efficacious in the setting of acute ankle sprain [53]. There is limited evidence suggesting PRP may be beneficial in a select group of high-level athletes with acute ankle sprain with syndesmotic instability.

Achilles Tendon Pathology

Chronic/Degenerative Achilles Tendinopathy

Overuse injury of the Achilles tendon is frequent in competitive and recreational athletes, as well as inactive middle-aged individuals. Achilles tendon injuries often lead to prolonged periods of sports cessation and interfere with ADLs. Acute

Achilles pain commonly develops with an abrupt increase in activity, whereas chronic pain (over 3 months) is due to cumulative microtrauma leading to degeneration and tendinopathy often exacerbated by improper footwear, poor running mechanics (lateral heel strike with pronation, gastrocnemius-soleus dysfunction), or sustained high-impact stress [56]. Pathology and concordant pain generally develop 2–6 cm proximal to the posterior calcaneus due to the relative hypovascularity of the tendon at this point.

Acute tendinitis care involves avoiding aggravating activities, ice, a short course of NSAIDs despite the lack of inflammation on histological evaluation, and support with taping or ACE. Chronic tendinopathy is managed with rehabilitation focusing on resistance training and either eccentric exercises or heavy slow resistance training program [54, 55]. Further management options include orthotics or bracing. Conservative treatment, often lasting more than 6 months, is disappointing with 25–45% of patients eventually requiring surgery with poor postoperative results and high failure rate [56].

Owing to the limited efficacy of conservative management, regenerative medicine treatments have primarily focused on PRP, with mixed results. A handful of recent trials on patients with chronic midportion Achilles tendinopathy are reviewed below. Boesen et al. followed 60 men with chronic midportion Achilles tendinopathy for 6 months. This RCT compared three arms: (1) high-volume injection (HVI) of steroid, saline, and local anesthetic versus (2) PRP (4 injections 14 days apart) versus (3) placebo (a few drops of saline under the skin). Each treatment was combined with an eccentric-based exercise program. The participants were followed at 6, 12, and 24 weeks. Although VISA-A initially only improved in the HVI group at 6 weeks, by the final time point, HVI (22 ± 4.5) and PRP (19.6 ± 4.5) showed significant improvement compared with placebo (8.8 ± 3.3). Objective parameters included ultrasound evaluation showing a significant decrease in the tendon thickness PRP group at 12 weeks and a larger decrease in PRP and HVI compared with placebo at 24 weeks [57]. A similar randomized, double-blinded placebo-controlled single-center trial performed by DeVos et al. randomized patients to an eccentric exercise program in combination with PRP or saline injection. VISA-A data was collected at 6, 12, and 24 weeks and in a second study at 1-year follow-up; the results showed an improvement but no statistically significant difference between the groups at any time points [58, 59]. There was no difference in secondary outcomes including patient satisfaction and return to sport. Using the same study group, DeVos et al. used ultrasound to identify echo-types suggestive of pathology or healing. In both the PRP and placebo groups, there was a decrease in echo-types suggesting tendinotic tissue and an increase in echo-types suggestive of organized tendon bundles. Additionally, there was no significant change in the neovascularization from baseline [60]. Similar results were demonstrated in a pilot study by Kearney et al. comparing PRP with eccentric loading program which found no difference in VISA-A and EuroQol-5D. Krogh et al. performed an RCT with 24 patients injected with PRP versus placebo (saline). At the 3-month follow-up, there was a statistically significant increase in the tendon thickness in the PRP group. However, there were no statistically significant differences in VISA-A score, pain at rest, pain when walking, pain when tendon was squeezed, and color Doppler activity [61].

More promising studies on PRP include Guelfi et al. who performed a retrospective study involving 83 tendons (73 patients) managed with a single PRP injection. Over follow-up duration at 3 weeks and 3 and 6 months (mean 50.1 months long term) showing significant improvement in VISA-A score, 92% of patients rated the result as satisfactory and would repeat the treatment; the remaining 8% were deemed unsatisfactory and underwent a repeat PRP injection at 6 months [62]. Monto performed a single PRP injection on 30 subjects monitoring AOFAS and evaluating tendon structure on MRI/ultrasound at 2-, 3-, 6-, 12-, and 24-month follow-up. In this study, 4 patients demonstrated intrasubstance tear, 8 showed insertional tendinopathy, and 22 showed non-insertional disease. The results showed improvement in AOFAS at 3 months and persisted through the 24-month follow-up. Pre-treatment imaging abnormalities resolved in 27/29 cases at the 6-month time point [63].

The data for mesenchymal stem cells in Achilles tendinopathy is extremely limited. A recent publication by Goldberg et al. designed a protocol for a phase IIa proof-of-concept study in which patients with chronic midportion Achilles tendinopathy will undergo MSC harvest and ultrasound-guided injection to measure safety, adverse events, as well as patient-reported and radiologic outcome measures [64].

Based on the current available literature, regenerative medicine is a promising tool for sure in chronic, degenerative Achilles tendinopathy, but routine use is not supported by the literature. The most beneficial results are seen in use of PRP and improvement in MRI/US parameters suggesting improved tendon healing. However, patient-reported subjective parameters including pain and function are not greatly improved with PRP.

Achilles Tendon Rupture

Achilles tendon rupture is the most common tendon rupture in the lower extremity. The incidence is approximately 18 per 100,000, most commonly occurring in adults in the third to fifth decade and affecting men 4–5× more frequently than women. Risk factors include underlying Achilles tendon pathology which has been reported in nearly 10% of ruptures, inflammatory arthritides, steroid injections, and fluoroquinolone use. Over 80% of ruptures occur during sporting activities often during sudden foot pivoting with forced plantar flexion or rapid acceleration during the push-off phase [67]. A pop or snap is often heard with a sensation of being kicked in the leg. However, it has been reported that up to $\frac{1}{3}$ of patients with tendon rupture do not report pain [65]. Physical exam findings are notable for inability to stand on toes and plantar flex the ankle with a positive Thompson test.

Initial management includes rest, pain control, and functional bracing with consideration of operative and nonoperative modalities providing similar healing rates but slightly longer return to work in patients managed nonoperatively. Additionally, the re-rupture rate in nonsurgical patients is nearly 40% compared with 0.5% in surgically managed patients [67]. Extensive rehabilitation is necessary to maintain ankle function.

PRP used in the nonoperative management of Achilles tendon rupture repair is limited. Kaniki et al. performed a retrospective comparative study of 145 patients including prospective (73 patients) and historical cohorts (72 patients) assessing PRP as adjunct to accelerated functional rehabilitation. This study showed no statistically significant difference between the PRP and control groups in regard to isokinetic plantar flexion strength, range of motion, calf circumference, or Leppilahti score at 1- and 2-year follow-up [66]. In a case report, Filardo et al. completed a series of PRP injections for a 34-year-old competitive basketball player with a partial Achilles tendon rupture. The first injection was performed at 6 days post-trauma, then 7 and 14 days later with slow progression to stretching and formal rehabilitation program. The patient was able to return to sport for 20 minutes 64 days after the injury and full game participation 75 days after injury. Eighteen months later, the player required no further treatment [68].

PRP has been suggested as surgical augmentation for acute tendon repair. Animal studies have shown optimistic results for augmentation with PRP in healing Achilles tendon ruptures; however the transition to the human model has not proved as efficacious. In a prospective trial by De Carli et al., 30 patients who underwent surgical tendon repair were evaluated: 15 control who underwent only surgery and 15 who underwent surgery with intraoperative administration of liquid and gelatinized PRP with repeat PRP injection 14 days post-op. Follow-up was measured at 1, 3, 6, and 24 months; there was no difference in VAS, FAOS and VISA-A scales, in isokinetic strength evaluation or ultrasound evaluation of tendon integrity. On MRI, there was a decrease in signal enhancement in the treatment group suggestive of better tendon remodeling [69]. Similarly, Zou et al. studied 36 patients with tendon rupture in a prospective RCT. In this study, the study group underwent surgical repair with PRP injected into the paratenon sheath and around ruptured tissue prior to skin suture and followed at 3, 6, 12, and 24 months. The treatment group showed better isokinetic calf strength at 3 months but not beyond. Patient-reported outcome measures showed higher SF-36 and Leppilahti scores at 6 and 12 months but no difference at 2 years [70]. In another RCT by Schepull et al., 30 patients were randomized with the treatment group receiving PRP intraoperatively; PRP had no significant effect on acute repair with regard to elasticity, heel raise index, or functional outcomes [71]. A prospective multicenter randomized placebo-controlled superiority trial is currently underway by Alsousou et al. to evaluate clinical efficacy of PRP in Achilles tendon rupture patients treated nonoperatively. The study will include 230 patients PRP vs placebo injection to the tendon rupture gap within 12 days of injury. Outcomes will include measurement of muscle-tendon function, quality of life, pain, and overall functional goals at 4, 7, 13, and 24 weeks and 24 months [72].

Although rat models using mesenchymal stem cells (MSC) for management of Achilles tendon rupture are promising, more research and data are required for humans. In the rat, Urdzikova et al. performed MSC injections during the post-op recovery period and showed increased collagen organization and improved vascularity with the injection [73]. Two additional rat studies involving MSC-coated sutures showed increased repair strength and lower failure load [74, 75]. In the human model, Stein et al. performed a retrospective review of a prospectively collected database of Achilles tendon rupture during recreational sports-related activity and during repair with BMAC augmentation. Twenty-seven subjects (28 tendons) were identified; in these patients, there was a 0.5 ± 1.3 cm difference in mean calf-circumference, 92% returned to sport at 6 ± 2 months, and there were no re-ruptures. However, there was no control group for comparison [75].

PRP does not appear to be beneficial to the operative or nonoperative management of acute Achilles tendinopathy or tendon rupture; more studies are needed. The rat models for MSC augmentation in operative repair are promising, but more human data is required.

Peroneal Tendinopathy

Peroneal tendinopathy involving the peroneus longus or brevis commonly occurs in runners and sports which involve frequent change of direction and lateral movements. Pain is located at lateral ankle and worse with standing or walking occasionally causing a limp. There is tenderness along the tendons just posterior to the lateral malleolus. Pain is reproduced with active-resisted ankle dorsiflexion and eversion. Standard of care includes activity modification, eccentric strength or heavy load exercises, and consideration of lateral heel wedge.

To date, in one retrospective descriptive study on chronic tendinopathies, Unlu et al. recruited 214 patients who received PRP injections for tendinopathy refractory to conventional treatment with follow-up at 6 weeks and 6 months. Of these participants, 12 underwent peroneal tendon PRP injections. In these patients, there was no statistically significant improvement in the VAS scores [76].

The literature for regenerative medicine in peroneal tendinopathy is extremely limited; more studies including high-quality RCTs will be needed to clarify its role in this overuse condition.

Summary

In conclusion, regenerative medicine is a promising field of nonoperative techniques that has shown benefit in certain musculoskeletal disorders. Evidence continues to grow to demonstrate its benefits in foot and ankle conditions; however, at present, there is limited evidence for its routine use (or as a recommended first-line therapeutic option) in the comprehensive treatment and management of foot and ankle injuries. Future studies will need to clarify what type of formulations are preferred (e.g., leukocyte rich/poor if PRP or mesenchymal stem cells are superior to corticosteroid injections, or alternatively if mesenchymal stem cell injections are superior to PRP), if their beneficial effects may be seen beyond 1 year, if such treatments may prevent and delay the need for surgical approaches, if image guidance when performing these injections are necessary and advantageous compared to palpation-guided approaches, and ultimately, if these procedures are cost-effective in the healthcare system.

References

1. Saxena A, Behan SA, Valerio DL, Frosch DL. Navicular stress fracture outcomes in athletes: analysis of 62 injuries. J Foot Ankle Surg. 2017;56(5):943–8.
2. Adams SB, Lewis JS, Gupta AK, Parekh SG, Miller SD, Schon LC. Cannulated screw delivery of bone marrow aspirate concentrate to a stress fracture nonunion. Foot Ankle Int. 2013;34(5):740–4.
3. Monto RR. Platelet-rich plasma efficacy versus corticosteroid injection treatment for chronic severe plantar fasciitis. Foot Ankle Int. 2014;35(4):313–8.
4. Mahindra P, Yamin M, Selhi HS, Singla S, Soni A. Chronic plantar fasciitis: effect of platelet-rich plasma, corticosteroid, and placebo. Orthopedics. 2016;39(2):e285–9.
5. Jain K, Murphy PN, Clough TM. Platelet rich plasma versus corticosteroid injection for plantar fasciitis: a comparative study. Foot. 2015;25(4):235–7.
6. Kumar V, Millar T, Murphy PN, Clough T. The treatment of intractable plantar fasciitis with platelet-rich plasma injection. Foot. 2013;23(2–3):74–7.
7. Mayer SW, Joyner PW, Almekinders LC, Parekh SG. Stress fractures of the foot and ankle in athletes. Sports Health. 2014;6(6):481–9.
8. Akşahin E, Doğruyol D, Yüksel HY, Hapa O, Doğan Ö, Çelebi L, Biçimoğlu A. The comparison of the effect of corticosteroids and platelet-rich plasma (PRP) for the treatment of plantar fasciitis. Arch Orthop Trauma Surg. 2012;132(6):781–5.
9. Jahagirdar R, Scammell BE. Principles of fracture healing and disorders of bone union. Surgery (Oxford). 2009;27(2):63–9.
10. Mei-Dan O, Carmont MR, Laver L, Mann G, Maffulli N, Nyska M. Platelet-rich plasma or hyaluronate in the management of osteochondral lesions of the talus. Am J Sports Med. 2012;40(3):534–41.
11. Baz AA, Gad AM, Waly MR. Ultrasound guided injection of platelet rich plasma in cases of chronic plantar fasciitis. Egypt J Radiol Nucl Med. 2017;48(1):125–32.
12. Uğurlar M, Sönmez MM, Uğurlar Özge Y, Adıyeke L, Yıldırım H, Eren OT. Effectiveness of four different treatment modalities in the treatment of chronic plantar fasciitis during a 36-month follow-up period: a randomized controlled trial. J Foot Ankle Surg. 2018;57(5):913–8.
13. Shakked RJ, Walters EE, O'Malley MJ. Tarsal navicular stress fractures. Curr Rev Musculoskelet Med. 2017;10(1):122–30.
14. Murphy EP, McGoldrick NP, Curtin M, Kearns SR. A prospective evaluation of bone marrow aspirate concentrate and microfracture in the treatment of osteochondral lesions of the talus. Foot Ankle Surg. 2018;25(4):441–8. pii: S1268-7731(18)30037-7.
15. Shetty VD, Dhillon M, Hegde C, Jagtap P, Shetty S. A study to compare the efficacy of corticosteroid therapy with platelet-rich plasma therapy in recalcitrant plantar fasciitis: a preliminary report. Foot Ankle Surg. 2014;20(1):10–3.
16. Astur DC, Zanatta F, Arliani GG, Moraes ER, de Castro Pochini A, Ejnisman B. Stress fractures: definition, diagnosis and treatment. Rev Bras Ortop. 2016;51(1):3–10. Available from: https://doi.org/10.1016/j.rboe.2015.12.008.
17. Patel D, Roth M, Kapil N. Stress fractures: diagnosis, treatment, and prevention. Am Fam Physician. 2011;83(1):39–6.

18. Wilder RP, Sethi S. Overuse injuries: tendinopathies, stress fractures, compartment syndrome, and shin splints. Clin Sports Med. 2004;23(1):55–1. Available from: https://doi.org/10.1016/s0278-5919(03)00085-1.
19. Gill S. A randomized control study to assess the efficacy of platelet rich plasma and local corticosteroid injection in treatment of chronic plantar fasciitis. IJOS. 2016;4(2):155–9.
20. Huang Y, Wei S, Wang H, Lieu F. Ultrasonographic guided botulinum toxin type A treatment for plantar fasciitis; an outcome-based investigation for treating pain and gait changes. J Rehabil Med. 2010;42(2):136–40. Available from: https://doi.org/10.2340/16501977-0491.
21. Babcock MS, Foster L, Pasquina P, Jabbari B. Treatment of pain attributed to plantar fasciitis with botulinum toxin A. Am J Phys Med Rehabil. 2019;84(9):649–54. Available from: https://doi.org/10.1097/01.phm.0000176339.73591.d7.
22. Placzek R. Treatment of chronic plantar fasciitis with botulinum toxin A: an open case series with a 1 year follow up. Ann Rheum Dis. 2005;64(11):1659–61. Available from: https://doi.org/10.1136/ard.2005.035840.
23. Renan-Ordine R, Alburquerque-Sendín F, Rodrigues De Souza DP, Cleland JA, Fernández-de-las-Peñas C. Effectiveness of myofascial trigger point manual therapy combined with a self-stretching protocol for the management of plantar heel pain: a randomized controlled trial. J Orthop Sports Phys Ther. 2011; 41(2):43–50. Available from: https://doi.org/10.2519/jospt.2011.3504.
24. Hillier S, Grimmer-Somers K, Merlin T, Middleton P, Salisbury J, Tooher R, Weston A. FORM: an Australian method for formulating and grading recommendations in evidence-based clinical guidelines. BMC Med Res Methodol. 2011;11(1). Available from: https://doi.org/10.1186/1471-2288-11-23.
25. Berbrayer D, Fredericson M. Update on evidence-based treatments for plantar fasciopathy. PM R. 2014;6(2):159–6. https://doi.org/10.1016/j.pmrj.2013.08.609.
26. Schacke H. Mechanisms involved in the side effects of glucocorticoids. Pharmacol Ther. 2002;96(1):23. https://doi.org/10.1016/s0163-7258(02)00297-8.
27. Porter MD, Shadbolt B. Intralesional corticosteroid injection versus extracorporeal shock wave therapy for plantar fasciopathy. Clin J Sport Med. 2005;15(3):119–24. Available from: https://doi.org/10.1097/01.jsm.0000164039.91787.dc.
28. Bhattacharyya T, Levin R, Vrahas MS, Solomon DH. Nonsteroidal antiinflammatory drugs and nonunion of humeral shaft fractures. Arthritis Rheum. 2005;53(3):364–7. Available from: https://doi.org/10.1002/art.21170.
29. Martinelli N, Marinozzi A, Carnì S, Trovato U, Bianchi A, Denaro V. Platelet-rich plasma injections for chronic plantar fasciitis. Int Orthop. 2013;37(5):839–42. Available from: https://doi.org/10.1007/s00264-012-1741-0.
30. Moore KL. Clinically oriented anatomy, 7th Ed. + Brs gross anatomy, 7th Ed. + Lww anatomy review, 7th Ed. Philadelphia: Lippincott Williams & Wilkins; 2013.
31. Harrast MA, Finnoff JT. Sports medicine 2E. 2nd ed: Springer Publishing Company; 2016.
32. Vannabouathong C, Del Fabbro G, Sales B, Smith C, Li CS, Yardley D, Bhandari M, Petrisor BA. Intra-articular injections in the treatment of symptoms from ankle arthritis: a systematic review. Foot Ankle Int. 2018;39(10):1141–50. Available from: https://doi.org/10.1177/1071100718779375.
33. Freitag J, Bates D, Boyd R, Shah K, Barnard A, Huguenin L, Tenen A. Mesenchymal stem cell therapy in the treatment of osteoarthritis: reparative pathways, safety and efficacy – a review. BMC Musculoskelet Disord. 2016;17(1). Available from: https://doi.org/10.1186/s12891-016-1085-9.
34. Thomas AC, Hubbard-Turner T, Wikstrom EA, Palmieri-Smith RM. Epidemiology of posttraumatic osteoarthritis. J Athl Train. 2017;52(6):491–6. Available from: https://doi.org/10.4085/1062-6050-51.5.08.
35. Martin RL, Stewart GW, Conti SF. Posttraumatic ankle arthritis: an update on conservative and surgical management. J Orthop Sports Phys Ther. 2007;37(5):253–9. Available from: https://doi.org/10.2519/jospt.2007.2404.

36. de Cesar Netto C, da Fonseca LF, Simeone Nascimento F, O'Daley AE, Tan EW, Dein EJ, Godoy-Santos AL, Schon LC. ☆ Diagnostic and therapeutic injections of the foot and ankle—an overview. Foot Ankle Surg. 2018;24(2):99–106. Available from: https://doi.org/10.1016/j.fas.2017.02.001.

37. Grice J, Marsland D, Smith G, Calder J. Efficacy of Foot and ankle corticosteroid injections. Foot Ankle Int. 2017;38(1):8–13. Available from: https://doi.org/10.1177/1071100716670160.

38. Furtado RNV, Machado FS, Luz KR da, Santos MF dos, Konai MS, Lopes RV, Natour J. Intra-articular injection with triamcinolone hexacetonide in patients with rheumatoid arthritis: prospective assessment of goniometry and joint inflammation parameters. Revista Brasileira de Reumatologia (English Edition). 2017;57(2):115–21. Available from: https://doi.org/10.1016/j.rbre.2016.08.001.

39. Cohen MM, Altman RD, Hollstrom R, Hollstrom C, Sun C, Gipson B. Safety and efficacy of intra-articular sodium hyaluronate (Hyalgan®) in a randomized, double-blind study for osteoarthritis of the ankle. Foot Ankle Int. 2008;29(7):657–63. Available from: https://doi.org/10.3113/fai.2008.0657.

40. DeGroot H, Uzunishvili S, Weir R, Al-omari A, Gomes B. Intra-articular injection of hyaluronic acid is not superior to saline solution injection for ankle arthritis. J Bone Joint Surg Am Volume. 2012;94(1):2–8. Available from: https://doi.org/10.2106/jbjs.j.01763.

41. Murphy EP, Curtin M, McGoldrick NP, Thong G, Kearns SR. Prospective evaluation of intra-articular sodium hyaluronate injection in the ankle. J Foot Ankle Surg. 2017;56(2):327–31. Available from: https://doi.org/10.1053/j.jfas.2016.09.017.

42. Witteveen AG, Sierevelt IN, Blankevoort L, Kerkhoffs GM, van Dijk CN. Intra-articular sodium hyaluronate injections in the osteoarthritic ankle joint: effects, safety and dose dependency. Foot Ankle Surg. 2010;16(4):159–63. Available from: https://doi.org/10.1016/j.fas.2009.10.003.

43. Angthong C, Khadsongkram A, Angthong W. Outcomes and quality of life after platelet-rich plasma therapy in patients with recalcitrant Hindfoot and ankle diseases: a preliminary report of 12 patients. J Foot Ankle Surg. 2013;2(4):475–80. Available from: https://doi.org/10.1053/j.jfas.2013.04.005.

44. Repetto I, Biti B, Cerruti P, Trentini R, Felli L. Conservative treatment of ankle osteoarthritis: can platelet-rich plasma effectively postpone surgery?. J Foot Ankle Surg. 2017;56(2):362–5. Available from: https://doi.org/10.1053/j.jfas.2016.11.015.

45. Fukawa T, Yamaguchi S, Akatsu Y, Yamamoto Y, Akagi R, Sasho T. Safety and efficacy of intra-articular injection of platelet-rich plasma in patients with ankle osteoarthritis. Foot Ankle Int. 2017;38(6):596–04. Available from: https://doi.org/10.1177/1071100717700377.

46. Emadedin M, Liastani M, Fazeli R, Mohseni F, Moghadasali R, Mardpour S, Hosseini S, Niknejadi M, Moeininia F, Fanni A. Long-term follow-up of intra-articular injection of autologous mesenchymal stem cells in patients with knee, ankle, or hip osteoarthritis. Arch Iran Med. 2015;18(6):336–44.

47. Rearick T, Charlton TP, Thordarson D. Effectiveness and complications associated with recombinant human bone morphogenetic protein-2 augmentation of foot and ankle fusions and fracture nonunions. Foot Ankle Int. 2014;35(8):783–8. Available from: https://doi.org/10.1177/1071100714536166.

48. Fourman MS, Borst EW, Bogner E, Rozbruch SR, Fragomen AT. Recombinant human BMP-2 increases the incidence and rate of healing in complex ankle arthrodesis. Clin Orthop Relat Res. 2014;472(2):732–9. Available from: https://doi.org/10.1007/s11999-013-3261-7.

49. Daniels TR, Younger ASE, Penner MJ, Wing KJ, Le ILD, Russell IS, Lalonde K-A, Evangelista PT, Quiton JD, Glazebrook M. Prospective randomized controlled trial of Hindfoot and ankle fusions treated with rhPDGF-BB in combination with a β-TCP-collagen matrix. Foot Ankle Int. 2015;36(7):739–48. Available from: https://doi.org/10.1177/1071100715576370.

50. Doherty C, Delahunt E, Caulfield B, Hertel J, Ryan J, Bleakley C. The incidence and prevalence of ankle sprain injury: a systematic review and meta-analysis of prospective epidemiological studies. Sports Med. 2014;44(1):123–40. Available from: https://doi.org/10.1007/s40279-013-0102-5.

51. Fong DT-P, Hong Y, Chan L-K, Yung PS-H, Chan K-M. A systematic review on ankle injury and ankle sprain in sports. Sports Med. 2007;37(1):73–4. Available from: https://doi.org/10.2165/00007256-200737010-00006.

52. Rowden A, Dominici P, D'Orazio J, Manur R, Deitch K, Simpson S, Kowalski MJ, Salzman M, Ngu D. Double-blind, randomized, placebo-controlled study evaluating the use of Platelet-rich Plasma Therapy (PRP) for acute ankle sprains in the emergency department. J Emerg Med. 2015;49(4):546–51. Available from: https://doi.org/10.1016/j.jemermed.2015.03.021.

53. Laver L, Carmont MR, McConkey MO, Palmanovich E, Yaacobi E, Mann G, Nyska M, Kots E, Mei-Dan O. Plasma rich in growth factors (PRGF) as a treatment for high ankle sprain in elite athletes: a randomized control trial. Knee Surg Sports Traumatol Arthrosc. 2015;23(11):3383–92. Available from: https://doi.org/10.1007/s00167-014-3119-x.

54. Malliaras P, Barton CJ, Reeves ND, Langberg H. Achilles and patellar tendinopathy loading programmes. Sports Med. 2013;43(4):267–86. Available from: https://doi.org/10.1007/s40279-013-0019-z.

55. Beyer R, Kongsgaard M, Hougs Kjær B, Øhlenschlæger T, Kjær M, Magnusson SP. Heavy slow resistance versus eccentric training as treatment for Achilles tendinopathy. Am J Sports Med. 2015;43(7):1704–11. Available from: https://doi.org/10.1177/0363546515584760.

56. Longo UG, Ronga M, Maffulli N. Achilles tendinopathy. Sports Med Arthrosc Rev. 2009;17(2):112–26. Available from: https://doi.org/10.1097/jsa.0b013e3181a3d625.

57. Boesen AP, Hansen R, Boesen MI, Malliaras P, Langberg H. Effect of high-volume injection, platelet-rich plasma, and sham treatment in chronic Midportion Achilles tendinopathy: a randomized double-blinded prospective study. Am J Sports Med. 2017;45(9):2034–43. Available from: https://doi.org/10.1177/0363546517702862.

58. de Vos RJ, Weir A, van Schie HTM, Bierma-Zeinstra SMA, Verhaar JAN, Weinans H, Tol JL. Platelet-rich plasma injection for chronic Achilles tendinopathy. JAMA. 2010;303(2):144. Available from: https://doi.org/10.1001/jama.2009.1986.

59. de Jonge S, de Vos RJ, Weir A, van Schie HTM, Bierma-Zeinstra SMA, Verhaar JAN, Weinans H, Tol JL. One-year follow-up of platelet-rich plasma treatment in chronic Achilles tendinopathy. Am J Sports Med. 2011;39(8):1623–30. Available from: https://doi.org/10.1177/0363546511404877.

60. de Vos RJ, Weir A, Tol JL, Verhaar JAN, Weinans H, van Schie HTM. No effects of PRP on ultrasonographic tendon structure and neovascularisation in chronic midportion Achilles tendinopathy. Br J Sports Med. 2011;45(5):387–92. Available from: https://doi.org/10.1136/bjsm.2010.076398.

61. Krogh TP, Ellingsen T, Christensen R, Jensen P, Fredberg U. Ultrasound-guided injection therapy of Achilles tendinopathy with platelet-rich plasma or saline. Am J Sports Med. 2016;44(8):1990–7. Available from: https://doi.org/10.1177/0363546516647958.

62. Guelfi M, Pantalone A, Vanni D, Abate M, Guelfi MG, Salini V. Long-term beneficial effects of platelet-rich plasma for non-insertional Achilles tendinopathy. Foot Ankle Surg. 2015;21(3):178–81. Available from: https://doi.org/10.1016/j.fas.2014.11.005.

63. Monto RR. Platelet rich plasma treatment for chronic Achilles tendinosis. Foot Ankle Int. 2012;33(5):379–85. Available from: https://doi.org/10.3113/fai.2012.0379.

64. Goldberg AJ, Zaidi R, Brooking D, Kim L, Korda M, Masci L, Green R, O'Donnell P, Smith R. Autologous Stem Cells in Achilles Tendinopathy (ASCAT): protocol for a phase IIA, single-centre, proof-of-concept study. BMJ Open. 2018;8(5):e021600.

65. Gravlee JR, Hatch RL, Galea AM. Achilles tendon rupture: a challenging diagnosis. J Am Board Fam Pract. 2000;13(5):371–3.

66. Kaniki N, Willits K, Mohtadi NG, Fung V, Bryant D. A retrospective comparative study with historical control to determine the effectiveness of platelet-rich plasma as part of nonoperative treatment of acute Achilles tendon rupture. Arthroscopy. 2014;30(9):1139–45. Available from: https://doi.org/10.1016/j.arthro.2014.04.086.

67. Gossman WG, Varacallo M. Achilles tendon rupture. StatPearls. 2019. Available from: https://www.ncbi.nlm.nih.gov/books/NBK430844/.

68. Filardo G, Presti ML, Kon E, Marcacci M. Nonoperative biological treatment approach for partial Achilles tendon lesion. Orthopedics. 2010;33(2):120–3. Available from: https://doi.org/10.3928/01477447-20100104-31.

69. De Carli A, Lanzetti RM, Ciompi A, Lupariello D, Vadalà A, Argento G, Ferretti A, Vulpiani MC, Vetrano M. Can platelet-rich plasma have a role in Achilles tendon surgical repair?. Knee Surg Sports Traumatol Arthrosc. 2016;24(7):2231–7. Available from: https://doi.org/10.1007/s00167-015-3580-1.

70. Zou J, Mo X, Shi Z, Li T, Xue J, Mei G, Li X. A prospective study of platelet-rich plasma as biological augmentation for acute Achilles tendon rupture repair. Biomed Res Int. 2016;2016:1–8. Available from: https://doi.org/10.1155/2016/9364170.

71. Schepull T, Kvist J, Norrman H, Trinks M, Berlin G, Aspenberg P. Autologous platelets have no effect on the healing of human Achilles tendon ruptures. Am J Sports Med. 2011;39(1):38–7. Available from: https://doi.org/10.1177/0363546510383515.

72. Alsousou J, Keene DJ, Hulley PA, Harrison P, Wagland S, Byrne C, Schlüssel MM, Dutton SJ, Lamb SE, Willett K. Platelet rich plasma in Achilles Tendon Healing 2 (PATH-2) trial: protocol for a multicentre, participant and assessor-blinded, parallel-group randomised clinical trial comparing platelet-rich plasma (PRP) injection versus placebo injection for Achilles tendon rupture. BMJ Open. 2017;7(11):e018135. Available from: https://doi.org/10.1136/bmjopen-2017-018135.

73. Machova Urdzikova L, Sedlacek R, Suchy T, Amemori T, Ruzicka J, Lesny P, Havlas V, Sykova E, Jendelova P. Human multipotent mesenchymal stem cells improve healing after collagenase tendon injury in the rat. Biomed Eng Online. 2014;13(1):42. Available from: https://doi.org/10.1186/1475-925x-13-42.

74. Yao J, Woon CY-L, Behn A, Korotkova T, Park D-Y, Gajendran V, Smith RL. The effect of suture coated with mesenchymal stem cells and bioactive substrate on tendon repair strength in a rat model. J Hand Surg Am. 2012;37(8):1639–45. Available from: https://doi.org/10.1016/j.jhsa.2012.04.038.

75. Adams SB, Thorpe MA, Parks BG, Aghazarian G, Allen E, Schon LC. Stem cell-bearing suture improves Achilles tendon healing in a rat model. Foot Ankle Int. 2014;35(3):293–9. Available from: https://doi.org/10.1177/1071100713519078.

76. Unlu MC, Kivrak A, Kayaalp ME, Birsel O, Akgun I. Peritendinous injection of platelet-rich plasma to treat tendinopathy: a retrospective review. Acta Orthop Traumatol Turc. 2017;51(6):482–7. Available from: https://doi.org/10.1016/j.aott.2017.10.003.

77. Karatosun V, Unver B, Gocen Z, Sen A, Gunal I. Intra-articular hyaluronic acid compared with progressive knee exercises in osteoarthritis of the knee: a prospective randomized trial with long-term follow-up. Rheumatol Int. 2006;26(4):277–84. Available from: https://doi.org/10.1007/s00296-005-0592-z.

78. Ragab EMS, Othman AMA. Platelets rich plasma for treatment of chronic plantar fasciitis. Arch Orthop Trauma Surg. 2012;132(8):1065–70. Available from: https://doi.org/10.1007/s00402-012-1505-8.

79. Henning PR, Grear BJ. Platelet-rich plasma in the foot and ankle. Curr Rev Musculoskelet Med. 2018;11(4):616–23. Available from: https://doi.org/10.1007/s12178-018-9522-z.

80. Le ADK, Enweze L, DeBaun MR, Dragoo JL. Current clinical recommendations for use of platelet-rich plasma. Curr Rev Musculoskelet Med. 2018;11(4):624–3. Available from: https://doi.org/10.1007/s12178-018-9527-7.

Chapter 14
The Future of Regenerative Medicine

Andrew Creighton and Jonathan S. Kirschner

Background on the Burden of MSK Conditions

Musculoskeletal diseases place a significant burden on the United States (US) healthcare system and contribute significantly to rising costs. In 2014, 66 million people sought medical care for a musculoskeletal injury [1, 2]. Current medical costs of musculoskeletal diseases are estimated at 873.8 billion US dollars (USD) annually. Osteoarthritis (OA), an example of a degenerative musculoskeletal disease with a significant impact on the US healthcare system, was responsible for raising aggregate annual medical care expenditures by 185.5 billion USD [3–5]. OA currently affects more than 27 million people in the United States and is forecasted to affect 25% of the adult US population or nearly 67 million people by the year 2030 [3, 5, 6]. At this time, there is no known cure for OA. With the potential to prevent or reverse disease progression, regenerative medicine provides an opportunity to reduce the financial burden of degenerative diseases like OA. This would significantly impact the overall financial burden of musculoskeletal diseases.

One model to describe regenerative medicine and the engineering of tissues divides the underlying component categories into three parts, analogous to a garden that requires seeds, dirt, and fertilizer: (1) cells or cellular components, (2) biomaterial scaffolds, and (3) chemical and physical growth factors including cytokines like those in PRP [7]. This triad involves cells which are cultured on either a natural or synthetic scaffold where attachment and differentiation or proliferation can take place.

A. Creighton · J. S. Kirschner (✉)
Physiatry, Hospital for Special Surgery, Rehabilitation Medicine, Weill Cornell Medicine, New York, NY, USA

© Springer Nature Switzerland AG 2020
G. Cooper et al. (eds.), *Regenerative Medicine for Spine and Joint Pain*,
https://doi.org/10.1007/978-3-030-42771-9_14

The future of regenerative medicine will focus on research and science on the efficacy and specific mechanisms of action of regenerative therapies (as broadly broken down into the above categories). A respect for Food and Drug Administration (FDA) regulations will be required. There will be an improved understanding of genetics pertaining to musculoskeletal diseases, and genetic targets involved with different degenerative diseases will be identified. Questions pertaining to the appropriate level of tissue loading and the appropriate post-procedure rehab protocols will need to be answered. Ultimately, controlled trials demonstrating efficacy, standardization in reporting, improved data collection processes, and improved outcome metrics will give merit to the field and allow physicians to feel confident recommending regenerative medicine treatments to patients.

Definitions/Nomenclature

Regenerative medicine and "stem cells" can be confusing and misleading terms, especially with regard to culture-expanded cells, cell products, and live or attenuated growth factors such as amniotic membrane-derived products. Names are used haphazardly, and nomenclature can be misleading and disconnected from the science and identity of cells in native tissues [3]. According to the National Institutes of Health (NIH), stem cells are defined by their ability to divide and renew themselves for long time periods, by their lack of specialization, and by their ability to give rise to specialized subtypes [8, 9]. Essentially, the current cell therapies offered in the United States involve transplanting adult cells obtained through harvest and minimal manipulation of native tissues (blood, bone marrow, and fat), which contain stem and progenitor cells [8]. While the concentration of these cells can be increased at the point of care [8, 10], stem and progenitor cells are the least plentiful cell type in these preparations. Specifically, only one in one thousand to one in one million cells harvested from healthy tissues is stem or progenitor cell capable of differentiating into one or more types of connective tissue [8, 11–13]. Another issue that contributes to confusion surrounding the nomenclature of stem cells is that both "mesenchymal stem cell" and "mesenchymal stromal cell" are abbreviated "MSC" and used to describe culture-expanded cells. Chu et al. suggested that the term "stem cell" has been overused to include uncharacterized minimally manipulated cell preparations as well as tissue-derived culture-expanded cell populations. It has been suggested, therefore, that these cell preparations and expanded cell populations be referred to as "cell therapy" [8]. While the term "stem cell" has become common, future work will need to clearly define what is meant when this term is used. The future of regenerative medicine will need to have a standardized and accurate nomenclature for descriptive, classification, and billing purposes but most importantly for the science and clinical applicability to move forward.

Regulations and Standardization

There have been two general approaches to cellular therapies within regenerative medicine [3]. The first approach involves specifically characterized cellular medical therapies provided by physicians who are diligent and committed to the scientific innovative process of first studying a product in animals and then through three phases of trials where appropriate informed consent is executed. Alternatively, the second approach utilizes unregulated cell- and tissue-based products and associated procedures that are unproven, offered without appropriate informed consent including an explanation of scientific limitations, and offered on a cash-only basis. It is estimated that these unproven therapies have a yearly financial impact of 2.4 billion USD [3, 14–19]. The demand of effective treatment for common diseases, hope from the public (and providers), poor and inaccurate marketing communications regarding the expectations, strengths and limitations of these therapies, availability of various technologies and systems for culturing, and patient ability and willingness to pay for care not covered by insurance companies have contributed to the hype around "stem cells" [3]. The surge of social media, gaps in regulation, and ethics and liability concerns of larger, more established companies have allowed small targeted clinics and manufacturers to bring forth lucrative business models without backing of controlled clinical studies [3]. This is concerning given reports of serious adverse events with treatments that at this point are not fully understood [20–22]. This second, unscrupulous approach highlights the need for regulations in the field of regenerative medicine to not only ensure patient safety but also allow potential strengths of these therapies to be demonstrated.

In response to these unregulated clinics, the FDA issued a guidance document on November 16, 2017, that had two directives: (1) identify and subsequently prosecute unscrupulous regenerative medicine clinics and (2) streamline the approval pathway for legitimate therapies [23]. The majority of regenerative medicine products is regulated under title 21 of the Code of Federal Regulations (21 CFR 1271), and there are two separate descriptions under part 1271: Section 361, which is reserved for tissues that are "minimally manipulated" and intended only for homologous use, and Section 351 used for a new drug or biologic product requiring FDA premarket review process that is more time intensive. If they originate from autologous bone marrow or adipose, stem cell preparations have traditionally been regulated under Section 361; however, recent guidance documents from the FDA caution that products from adipose, such as those created by mechanically processed lipoaspirate for orthopedic indications, are not considered minimally manipulated or homologously used and would therefore fall under Section 351 and have to undergo the rigors of an "investigational new drug." This would require appropriate regulatory submissions for the conduct of clinical trials and marketing [20].

While the FDA is targeting the unregulated practices of smaller clinics by necessitating approval standards, it demonstrated a sense of urgency by incorporating a mechanism for expediting the development of new therapies with an emphasis on those aimed at serious or life-threatening conditions [20]. For example, the 21st Century Cures Act enacted in December 2016 introduced an additional expedited program in which a product is designated as regenerative medicine advanced therapy (RMAT). This designation gives sponsors of a qualified regenerative medicine product intended for treating serious or life-threatening conditions an advantage in that it requires preliminary clinical evidence that the therapy addresses unmet medical needs as opposed to the requirement of preliminary clinical evidence of a substantial improvement over existing therapies [20]. In addition, RMAT-designated products that receive accelerated approval have potential eligibility for use of an expanded range of options, including the use of traditional studies along with submitting patient registries to fulfill post-approval commitments. Ultimately, the November 2017 policy from the FDA has given developers of lower-risk regenerative medicine products 36 months to determine if their products have undergone more than homologous use or minimal manipulation and if they need to submit an application for investigational new drug or marketing [20, 23]. Within the FDA's framework in thinking about musculoskeletal applications, if investigators are able to collaborate among different sites and agree on common manufacturing protocols and a common clinical trial protocol and the data along with the manufacturing information show a positive benefit-risk profile, there would be potential for receipt of biologics licenses at each of these sites by pooling the data [20]. This approach would be appropriate for developing products that, despite being more than minimally manipulated, would not be highly complex and would be able to be applied in simple trial designs.

The collaborative strategy outlined above highlights a need for standardization. There is an inconsistency in the literature with regard to reporting standards [3]. Direct-to-consumer marketing has allowed for erroneous claims. For example, aggregated claims of "stem cell" clinics suggested an average of 80% of patients experience "good results" or "symptomatic improvement," but published literature would suggest that there is a gap between what is reported and reality [3, 24]. Similarly, messages on social media about cell-based therapies are dominated by positive tone without discussing risks [3, 25]. Standardization is also needed from a research standpoint in terms of disease-specific clinical indications, reporting on how cells are sourced and characterized, the use of adjuvant therapies, the use of appropriate controls, trial methodology, and assessment of outcomes [3, 11, 12, 26, 27].

From a scientific standpoint, it is critical to develop a standardized and consistent approach to reporting in publications how cells are processed and characterized. Specifically, it is important to report the source of tissue, the selection or isolation method, expansion conditions, cell surface markers and their attributes, concentration, prevalence, gene expression profile and morphological features, and proteome profile. Publications vary widely with regard to relevant metrics of how the cells or components were processed and characterized [3]. When articles lack this information, it becomes difficult to communicate and repeat or compare one study to another. For example, Piuzzi et al. attempted to review the use of bone marrow aspirate concentrate in musculoskeletal disorders but, after reviewing 46 studies, found that no study gave enough details so that the methods could be repeated [3, 28]. Similarly, the composition of PRP can change depending on the time of day it is obtained or can vary when prepared using systems from different manufacturers [8, 29–31]. Demographic information is important to report as well because it has been noted that growth factor and cytokine concentrations vary by donor age, health status, and sex [8, 31, 32]. In a similar way, progenitor and MSC populations isolated from a given donor also differ widely from one preparation to another, along with being different in terms of age, sex, tissue source, harvest, and processing [8, 11–13, 28–30, 33–38]. Ultimately, the Delphi consensus approach describes a multidisciplinary group of investigators who defined minimum information for studies evaluating biologics in orthopedics (MIBO), specifically related to the use of PRP and MSCs, that serve as a checklist of the minimal requirements to guide study design and reporting [3, 39].

Registries

Registries can be a significant vehicle to direct the future of regenerative medicine toward standardization and facilitate outcomes-based research. There is a need for registries which include demographics (age, sex, medications, underlying medical conditions, and smoking status). Each patient who undergoes a procedure is very different. Would an older patient with multiple medical comorbidities respond to an injection of PRP, for example, the same way as a healthy patient with no comorbidities? A registry can be linked to a biorepository to capture and preserve clinical samples for future analysis and create cohorts that can help to power clinical trials [3, 8]. With cartilage, for example, one of the biggest barriers to establishing the safety and efficacy of these new therapies is the cost of clinical trials [3]. This is where the organization of multicenter registries for cartilage repair can be critical to reducing barriers to progress and allowing for multicenter trials to take place [3]. Overall, registries provide opportunities for collecting standardized data on both how the patient was doing clinically and what their outcome was for a variety of different interventions performed to treat the same disease [8].

The American Joint Replacement Registry [8, 40], the Kaiser Registries [8, 36], and the PRP registry at Veterans Hospital in Palo Alto, California, are model registries that have contributed important data on practice patterns, shown the potential issues from a particular treatment, or illustrated the potential for clinical evidence pertaining to PRP. The biorepository-linked PRP registry at the Veterans Hospital in Palo Alto, California, addressed the gap between the differing composition of PRP from patients and clinical outcomes [8]. Patients that received PRP injections for knee OA completed patient-reported outcomes (PROs) before treatment and at specific time points after treatment. At the same time, a sample of the PRP was stored for patients who consented to federally funded research and who additionally underwent functional and structural assessments of gait and quantitative MRI. In doing so, the registry supports correlating PRP proteomics with PRO and quantitative clinical outcome metrics in the interest of learning about potential mechanisms of action and clinical efficacy [8].

Effective registries require commitment and a team approach from physicians, clinics, and hospitals to recruit all qualifying patients, appropriate incentives for participation, and a process for financial support of the human resources required to accrue and report clinical and baseline outcomes data [8]. In addition, there will need to be a defined assessment of quality, technique of preparation, device used, and clinical laboratory data on the administered biologic [8]. Tissue specimens may also be collected to aid in stratifying the patient's disease state along with analyses of biomarkers, molecules, and genomes. These data could be required to help identify which patients would most likely respond to therapy and define the critical quality characteristics of a cell or biologic therapy.

Patient Access

Given the potential of these investigational therapies, there is a need to increase access to these treatments while still maintaining an environment committed to patient safety and respect. The acronym SMAC, which stands for science evidence, rigorous manufacturing process, accurate information for patients, and consistent product in terms of substance and how it is delivered, can be a guide [3]. The FDA, in its recent position paper, has demonstrated its commitment to both proper investigation and patient access to regenerative therapies by giving direction on ways to get an investigational drug into settings where there would be a potential for positively impacting a great number of patients [3, 41–43]. As previously mentioned, in the United States, the 21st Century Cures Act has provisions intended to expedite approvals of cell therapies and the recent "right-to-try" law to allow terminally ill patients access to products. An example from outside the United States can be seen by looking at Japan where a law passed emphasizing the utilization of conditional approvals for the purposes of stimulating the regenerative medicine industry.

Science

With an emphasis on patient registries and increasing patient access, scientists and clinicians need to maintain a sense of urgency in developing a better understanding of the mechanisms behind these regenerative therapies. Improved understanding of the science will allow the appropriate regenerative medicine therapy to be chosen for the appropriate patient. Rodeo (2016) noted that animal studies have been valuable in verifying "proof of principal" for cell-based therapies, PRP, cytokines, and tissue-engineered implants [44–48]. Despite the value of animal studies, there are limitations. In animals, it is challenging to stimulate chronic conditions like tendinopathy or slowly developing OA that is seen in humans [8]. In addition, there is an inability to control the mechanical loading environment or replicate the loading that takes place with humans. When thinking about humans, there is intrinsic variability in the soft tissues and joint spaces being treated that is poorly understood. The biologic targets need to be better identified [8]. For example, when looking at repair of the rotator cuff, primary targets are thought to be signaling molecules that drive cellular differentiation to reform the organized structure of the enthesis [8, 49]. Identifying biologic targets will necessitate a better understanding of the cellular mechanisms of tissue degeneration and repair for that disease state. Lastly, in terms of the three-part model, there is still much to be understood about the cells, biomaterial scaffolds, cytokines, and growth factors that are unique to the individual patient.

When analyzing stem cells, either marrow derived or adipose derived, there are numerous ways that these cells may work. They may function by way of their own inherent immunomodulatory and anti-inflammatory properties and by directly integrating into the healing tissue thereby directly participating in the healing response or have a local paracrine effect by stimulating and attracting intrinsic host cells [44]. The specific mechanisms by which they work are unknown at this time, however, and will need to be identified for regenerative medicine to progress.

One of the main goals of cell therapy is cartilage repair; however, there are a number of unknown factors involved with this process. Future research will need to work toward addressing current limitations including a lack of consensus regarding the optimal cell source, harvesting and processing techniques, and critical quality attributes (CQAs) that predict future performance [3, 50]. Specifically, when talking about the cell source, cells need to be selected that maintain an articular cartilage phenotype and do not undergo endochondral ossification, which can be a significant adverse effect [3, 50–53].

Scaffolds, as an important part of the tissue-engineering triad, interact with both cells and growth factors [54, 55]. Scaffolds can provide substrate for growth of cells and mechanical integrity for postsurgical implantation. They can also act as drug delivery systems for improved repair in vivo by being coated with bioactive molecules. One promising direction in scaffold production involves nanotechnology, specifically self-assembling peptides [54]. Natural and synthetic biomaterials have been investigated as scaffolds, but self-assembling peptide hydrogel (SAPH) scaffolds combine advantages of both natural and synthetic biomaterials because they are biocompatible and have easily modifiable properties [56]. For example, in a study looking at SAPH for intervertebral disc tissue engineering, after three-dimensional culture of nucleus pulposus cells (NPCs) in the SAPH, upregulation of nucleus pulposus-specific genes confirmed that the system could restore the nucleus pulposus (NP) phenotype in in vitro cultures [56]. The SAPH stimulated time-dependent increases in aggrecan and type II collagen deposition, which are two important NP extracellular matrix components. Overall, the suggestion from this study was that the SAPH could be used as a cell delivery system and scaffold in treating degenerative disc disease. Another promising application in the future of scaffolds will look to utilize 3D printing to achieve a clinically successful tissue-engineered product. 3D printing offers a way to control scaffold size, shape, pore size, geometry, and mechanical properties [54, 57]. Through the integration of computer-assisted design and modern medical imaging, scaffolds can be individualized to a specific patient and a specific defect [54, 58]. A new development has been biologically relevant bioinks, which are biomaterials that carry cells printed into 3D scaffolds and are an important component of the bioprinting effort [59, 60]. Faramarzi et al. incorporated PRP into an alginate hydrogel scaffold used in bioprinters and demonstrated that this bioink could positively affect the function of two important cell populations (mesenchymal stem cells and endothelial cells) involved in the tissue healing process in vitro [59].

PRP and the cytokines contained within it have played a large role in regenerative medicine and are relevant because they contain autologous growth factors that are easy to obtain and manipulate [3]. In a retrospective study by Mautner et al., in which PRP for chronic tendinopathy was evaluated, the majority of patients reported a moderate (>50%) improvement in pain symptoms [61]. However, despite showing an ability to contribute to symptom improvement, there are still many PRP-related questions that require clarification, many related to inconsistencies in published clinical trial results [3]. Due to variabilities in published studys' methods and results, the mechanism of action of PRP based on the various cell types it contains, optimal PRP formulation and system, dose number (single vs. serial), dose timing (intraoperative or delayed), and the impact of adding activating agents or anesthetics needs clarification in the future.

The optimal way of addressing the shortcomings in regenerative medicine is through controlled clinical trials [44]. In addition, it has also been suggested that clinicians carry out translational studies in conjunction with basic scientists to facilitate a thorough assessment of the biologic activity of these agents and then to compare and analyze this activity to clinical outcomes. A major limitation is that with general characteristics of the substance, such as platelet count or white blood cell count with PRP or cell number with stem cells, we do not know the biologic activity of the substance or how these general characteristics relate to that biologic activity. Extensive statistical analyses will be needed to study the interactions between intervention, time point after injury, and injury grade or severity [8]. There will also need to be stratification based on age, sex, and metabolic and systemic factors that may affect treatment response, like diabetes, rheumatologic conditions, and chronic use of anti-inflammatory or antifibrotic medications. At this point, given the amount of "unknowns" in regenerative medicine, has the usage of regenerative therapies outpaced the science supporting them?

Outcomes and Post-Procedure Rehabilitation

As with any treatment in medicine, the desired outcome for each regenerative medicine treatment needs to be clearly defined in controlled clinical trials. "Healed" versus "not healed" may not be the ideal outcome, and instead, the focus should be on the tissue quality at the site, the time it took to achieve tissue healing, pre- and post-procedure pain levels, and restoration of motion or strength [44]. The ultimate outcome may be to reduce pain or inflammation and not affect healing at all. For acute muscle injury, for example, the primary goal may be prevention of reinjury rather than faster return to sport [8]. Another example pertains to rotator cuff repair, where the goal may be to decrease the rate of retear of the repaired tendon. In addition, and maybe even more importantly, adverse outcomes need to be diligently reported. Given that many regenerative therapies are new, long-term adverse effects are unknown. The first priority is to do no harm to the patient. With a limited understanding of how these regenerative therapies work and limited long-term data available, the clinician is in a precarious position in offering these therapies to patients. Commitment to appropriate informed consent is imperative.

Posttreatment rehabilitation instructions have the potential to contribute to a positive outcome [8]. Mechanical loads are critical for healing tissue. There is a paucity of data on the appropriate timing and progression of rehabilitation after a regenerative medicine treatment. In addition, rehabilitation for shoulder osteoarthritis is very different than rehabilitation for Achilles tendinopathy. Therefore, rehabilitation protocols need to be identified for each location and regenerative treatment. Variables include when and how a tissue should be loaded, active vs. passive range of motion, medications and nutritional factors that may enhance or hinder healing, the role of hyperbaric oxygen, low-level laser therapies, and the types and frequencies of strength training exercises.

Genomics

Gene therapy administered through viral vectors can serve as a natural "drug store" for the body to help to regenerate tissues, slow aging, or modify disease processes. Improvement in the understanding of genetic and epigenetic factors related to the injury of tissues is needed to facilitate targets for therapy and more predictable results [44]. This improved understanding is also linked to the idea of a "personalized" patient-specific approach in which biological or gene expression markers are used to identify joints at risk and justify preemptive intervention with disease-modifying drugs that can preserve cartilage even before the osteoarthritic process ensues [3, 62]. For example, clustered regularly interspaced short palindromic repeats (CRISPR) genome-engineering technology enables strategies like Stem Cells Modified for Autonomous Regenerative Therapy (SMART), allowing for production of anti-inflammatory molecules that selectively reduce inflammation caused by chronic conditions [3]. With durable engraftment, these cells can then serve the role of vaccine – limiting the progression of OA.

Gene therapy has the potential to deliver proteins to specific tissues and cells for tissue-engineering purposes [1, 63]. Gene therapy involves transferring target genes into cells allowing for protein delivery, growth factors, or other therapeutic gene products to a specific anatomic site. The delivery process of transgenes can be through in vivo or ex vivo protocols with either viral (transduction) or nonviral (transfection) vectors [1]. Viral vectors can be integrating (retroviral and lentiviral) vectors which stably insert their genome into the DNA of infected cells and provide the best prospects for long-term gene expression as they are passed to both daughter cells during cell division. They also can be non-integrating (adenovirus and recombinant adeno-associated virus (AAV)) and stay in the nucleus as extrachromosomal episomes, which are not replicated during mitosis [1, 64]. The main issue with viral vectors is safety as they have demonstrated the potential to cause cell transformation and carcinogenesis [1, 65–67]. Given these concerns, nonviral vectors have been developed. They are associated with lower gene delivery efficiency compared to viral vector delivery systems [1, 68] but provide advantages with immunogenic response probability and cost-effective manufacturing [1, 69]. To improve the nonviral delivery efficiency problems, nonviral delivery systems have been engineered consisting of chemical or physical transfection systems [1].

There are two different ways of strategizing gene delivery: either in vivo or ex vivo strategies [1]. The vector is directly delivered to the host either systemically or locally with in vivo therapy. In ex vivo gene transfer, target cells are harvested, processed, and genetically manipulated outside the body prior to anatomic implantation. Ex vivo gene therapy is more technically challenging, more invasive, and less cost-effective. However, it is associated with higher transduction efficiency in allowing the delivery of potent cells and the gene product of interest to specific anatomic sites, a selective process of targeting the cell population of interest [1, 70–73]. Ex vivo gene therapy is also safer in only delivering transduced cells and not the actual vectors themselves, allowing for better control of the introduced factor. To overcome the limitations of ex vivo therapy, ex vivo strategies using either allogeneic cells or expedited single-step "same-day" approaches that eliminate the culture expansion step, decreasing the risk of contamination and gene mutations along with the increased cost, are being investigated [1, 74, 75]. Virk et al. evaluated this "same-day" approach using harvested bone marrow cells from a rat along with an osteoconductive scaffold assessing its effect on a critical-sized femoral defect on the rat [1, 75]. Radiographic, micro-CT, histologic, and biomechanical testing at 12 weeks post-implantation demonstrated that "same-day" ex vivo regional gene therapy was able to heal a rat's critical-sized femoral defect. In addition, for comparison to cultured bone marrow cells, "same-day" cells were associated with earlier radiographic healing and increased bone formation on micro-CT. Safety of this technique was assessed by Alaee et al., and the results indicated that viral vector copies were detected in the defect area following implantation of transduced cells but significantly decreased over time. There were no consistent findings of viral copies in the internal organs and no organ toxicity or histological abnormalities noted [1, 76]. The results suggested that ex vivo therapy, using a lentiviral vector, is safe but required further testing. Given the strengths of this expedited ex vivo approach along with safety, it is likely that this approach will be utilized in future studies.

When looking at possible indications for gene therapy in musculoskeletal diseases, such as articular cartilage repair or osteoarthritis, it is evident that gene therapy has the potential to make an impact on different disease processes. Unlike other therapeutic strategies that focus on alleviating the symptoms of OA, gene therapy focuses on cartilage growth factors and cytokines involved in inflammation and the pathogenesis of osteoarthritis like interleukin-1 (IL-1), IL-10, TNF-α, and TGF-β [1]. Usually, the process involves direct intra-articular administration of genetically manipulated cells or vectors alone. IL-1 is considered the most potent mediator of pain, inflammation, and cartilage loss in OA [1, 77]. IL-1 receptor antagonist (IL-1Ra), by blocking IL-1 and limiting inflammation and cartilage degradation, is a promising option for treatment of OA, and multiple studies in animal models of arthritis have shown efficacy of viral-mediated IL-1Ra gene transfer in inducing subsequent gene expression and biological response [1, 78–81]. Nonviral gene delivery into joints is also an approach that has shown promise. In a rabbit model, Fernandes et al. showed the ability to control progression of OA with intra-articular injection of a plasmid-lipid complex [1, 82]. In addition, using the cDNA of IL-1Ra in combination with TGF-β1 was more effective in cartilage repair than when each is used alone. Safety of in vivo intra-articular gene therapy was addressed by the Wang et al. group in a study that specifically evaluated the biodistribution and toxic effects of recombinant adeno-associated virus (AAV) carrying either rat or human IL-1Ra [1, 83]. In observational, body weight, and pathology studies, administration of this vector caused no local or systemic adverse effects. There was minimal vector leakage into the systemic circulation for the first 4–24 hours after injection, and the vector genome persisted for up to a year with only low levels of vector genomes detected outside the knee. This strategy needs further refinement but shows significant promise and requires future study.

OA is the only orthopedic-related disease being studied in clinical gene therapy trials [1, 84] in the United States and Korea. Phase I and II trials of "TissueGene-C" (TG-C), an ex vivo gene strategy utilizing retrovirally modified allograft chondrocytes in patients with knee OA, have been completed with phase III trials now underway. These patients had Cartilage Repair Society (ICRS) grade IV cartilage damage based on MRI and improved with pain, range of motion, and functional outcomes. Importantly, safety with TG-C has been demonstrated by analyzing peripheral blood in 12 patients treated with TG-C which showed normal levels of TGF-beta 1 and no circulating vector DNA for all patients at all dose levels at every time point [1, 85]. Recently in Korea, TG-C, named Invossa, became the first gene therapy to be approved for musculoskeletal applications and is indicated for moderate knee OA. In addition to Invossa, a single injection of sc-rAAV2.5IL-Ra is being assessed in a phase I clinical trial in patients with moderate knee OA [1, 86].

While there has been successful use of gene therapy in animal models treating difficult bone defects, cartilage defects, and osteoarthritis, there are still obstacles to clinical application [1]. We need to develop cost-effective, clinically relevant gene therapy strategies. Ideally, gene therapy should not require the clinician to develop a special skill set to prepare the product, and it will be off-the-shelf or easily extractable at the point of care. Safety is a special concern for the future application of gene therapy, and it is important that extensive biodistribution analysis of the transferred genes be consistently completed. The biology of gene therapy including the clinical indications, dose, cell source and scaffold, target gene, vector, and delivery system needs to be better defined.

Conclusion

The outlook on the future of regenerative medicine at this point is one of cautious optimism. Using the triad model framework, including cells, scaffolds, and PRP, along with an improving understanding of the human genome, it is evident that there is promising work being done that could lead to the future ability to modify degenerative diseases instead of simply managing symptoms. The challenge will be balancing patient demands and expectations with the limited evidence base for these therapies and an urgency from an increasing population of older patients. Given the regulations that are being enforced by the FDA, we are at a critical period of time where the onus to show data to support regenerative therapies has never been larger. This can be accomplished through collaboration and the development of registries along with standardization in methodology and outcome measures used in randomized controlled trials. For regenerative medicine to be successful we need an improved understanding of the science behind how stem cell therapy, scaffolds, and cytokines making up PRP work along with a better understanding of the human genome in the context of degenerative diseases like osteoarthritis. Given the immense potential of this field, will regenerative medicine be regarded as its own specialized area of medicine in the future?

References

1. Bougioukli S, Evans CH, Alluri RK, Ghivizzani SC, Lieberman JR. Gene therapy to enhance bone and cartilage repair in orthopaedic surgery. Curr Gene Ther. 2018;18(3):154–70. https://doi.org/10.2174/1566523218666180410152842.
2. United States Bone and Joint Initiative: the Burden of Musculoskeletal Diseases in the United States, Third Edition.
3. Piuzzi NS, Dominici M, Long M, Pascual-Garrido C, Rodeo S, Huard J, Guicheux J, McFarland R, Goodrich LR, Maddens S, Robey PG, Bauer TW, Barrett J, Barry F, Karli D, Chu CR, Weiss DJ, Martin I, Jorgensen C, Muschler GF. Proceedings of the signature series symposium "cellular therapies for orthopaedics and musculoskeletal disease proven and unproven therapies-promise, facts and fantasy," international society for cellular therapies, Montreal, Canada, May 2, 2018. Cytotherapy. 2018;20(11):1381–400. https://doi.org/10.1016/j.jcyt.2018.09.001.

4. Kotlarz H, Gunnarsson CL, Fang H, Rizzo JA. Insurer and out-of-pocket costs of osteoarthritis in the US: evidence from national survey data. Arthritis Rheum. 2009;60(12):3546–53. https://doi.org/10.1002/art.24984.
5. Lespasio MJ, Sultan AA, Piuzzi NS, Khlopas A, Husni ME, Muschler GF, Mont MA. Hip osteoarthritis: a primer. Perm J. 2018;22 https://doi.org/10.7812/tpp/17-084.
6. Jordan JM, Helmick CG, Renner JB, Luta G, Dragomir AD, Woodard J, Fang F, Schwartz TA, Nelson AE, Abbate LM, Callahan LF, Kalsbeek WD, Hochberg MC. Prevalence of hip symptoms and radiographic and symptomatic hip osteoarthritis in African Americans and Caucasians: the Johnston County Osteoarthritis Project. J Rheumatol. 2009;36(4):809–15. https://doi.org/10.3899/jrheum.080677.
7. Beldjilali-Labro M, Garcia Garcia A, Farhat F, Bedoui F, Grosset JF, Dufresne M, Legallais C. Biomaterials in tendon and skeletal muscle tissue engineering: current trends and challenges. Materials (Basel). 2018;11(7) https://doi.org/10.3390/ma11071116.
8. Chu CR, Rodeo S, Bhutani N, Goodrich LR, Huard J, Irrgang J, LaPrade RF, Lattermann C, Lu Y, Mandelbaum B, Mao J, McIntyre L, Mishra A, Muschler GF, Piuzzi NS, Potter H, Spindler K, Tokish JM, Tuan R, Zaslav K, Maloney W. Optimizing clinical use of biologics in orthopaedic surgery: consensus recommendations from the 2018 AAOS/NIH U-13 conference. J Am Acad Orthop Surg. 2019;27(2):e50–63. https://doi.org/10.5435/jaaos-d-18-00305.
9. NIH Stem Cell Information Home Page. National Institutes of Health, U.S., Department of Health and Human Services. 2016. https://stemcells.nih.gov/info/basics/1.htm. Accessed January 2, 2019.
10. Luangphakdy V, Boehm C, Pan H, Herrick J, Zaveri P, Muschler GF. Assessment of methods for rapid intraoperative concentration and selection of marrow-derived connective tissue progenitors for bone regeneration using the canine femoral multidefect model. Tissue Eng Part A. 2016;22(1–2):17–30. https://doi.org/10.1089/ten.TEA.2014.0663.
11. Chahla J, Piuzzi NS, Mitchell JJ, Dean CS, Pascual-Garrido C, LaPrade RF, Muschler GF. Intra-articular cellular therapy for osteoarthritis and focal cartilage defects of the knee: a systematic review of the literature and study quality analysis. J Bone Joint Surg Am. 2016;98(18):1511–21. https://doi.org/10.2106/jbjs.15.01495.
12. Piuzzi NS, Chahla J, Jiandong H, Chughtai M, LaPrade RF, Mont MA, Muschler GF, Pascual-Garrido C. Analysis of cell therapies used in clinical trials for the treatment of osteonecrosis of the femoral head: a systematic review of the literature. J Arthroplast. 2017;32(8):2612–8. https://doi.org/10.1016/j.arth.2017.02.075.
13. Muschler GF, Nakamoto C, Griffith LG. Engineering principles of clinical cell-based tissue engineering. J Bone Joint Surg Am. 2004;86-a(7):1541–58.
14. Srivastava A, Mason C, Wagena E, Cuende N, Weiss DJ, Horwitz EM, Dominici M. Part 1: defining unproven cellular therapies. Cytotherapy. 2016;18(1):117–9. https://doi.org/10.1016/j.jcyt.2015.11.004.
15. Weiss DJ, Rasko JE, Cuende N, Ruiz MA, Ho HN, Nordon R, Wilton S, Dominici M, Srivastava A. Part 2: making the "unproven" "proven". Cytotherapy. 2016;18(1):120–3. https://doi.org/10.1016/j.jcyt.2015.11.005.
16. Eldridge P, Griffin D, Janssen W, O'Donnell L. Part 3: understanding the manufacturing of unproven cellular therapy products. Cytotherapy. 2016;18(1):124–6. https://doi.org/10.1016/j.jcyt.2015.11.006.
17. O'Donnell L, Turner L, Levine AD. Part 6: the role of communication in better understanding unproven cellular therapies. Cytotherapy. 2016;18(1):143–8. https://doi.org/10.1016/j.jcyt.2015.11.002.
18. Nichols K, Janssen W, Wall D, Cuende N, Griffin D. Part 4: interaction between unproven cellular therapies and global medicinal product approval regulatory frameworks. Cytotherapy. 2016;18(1):127–37. https://doi.org/10.1016/j.jcyt.2015.11.003.
19. Deans RJ, Gunter KC, Dominici M, Forte M. Part 5: unproven cell therapies and the commercialization of cell-based products. Cytotherapy. 2016;18(1):138–42. https://doi.org/10.1016/j.jcyt.2015.11.001.

20. Marks P, Gottlieb S. Balancing safety and innovation for cell-based regenerative medicine. N Engl J Med. 2018;378(10):954–9. https://doi.org/10.1056/NEJMsr1715626.

21. Kuriyan AE, Albini TA, Townsend JH, Rodriguez M, Pandya HK, Leonard RE 2nd, Parrott MB, Rosenfeld PJ, Flynn HW Jr, Goldberg JL. Vision loss after intravitreal injection of autologous "stem cells" for AMD. N Engl J Med. 2017;376(11):1047–53. https://doi.org/10.1056/NEJMoa1609583.

22. Berkowitz AL, Miller MB, Mir SA, Cagney D, Chavakula V, Guleria I, Aizer A, Ligon KL, Chi JH. Glioproliferative lesion of the spinal cord as a complication of "stem-cell tourism". N Engl J Med. 2016;375(2):196–8. https://doi.org/10.1056/NEJMc1600188.

23. Rodeo SA. Moving toward responsible use of biologics in sports medicine. Am J Sports Med. 2018;46(8):1797–9. https://doi.org/10.1177/0363546518782182.

24. Piuzzi NS, Ng M, Chughtai M, Khlopas A, Ng K, Mont MA, Muschler GF. The stem-cell market for the treatment of knee osteoarthritis: a patient perspective. J Knee Surg. 2018;31(6):551–6. https://doi.org/10.1055/s-0037-1604443.

25. Piuzzi NS, Khlopas A, Newman JM, Ng M, Roche M, Husni ME, Spindler KP, Mont MA, Muschler G. Bone marrow cellular therapies: novel therapy for knee osteoarthritis. J Knee Surg. 2018;31(1):22–6. https://doi.org/10.1055/s-0037-1608844.

26. Piuzzi NS, Chahla J, Schrock JB, LaPrade RF, Pascual-Garrido C, Mont MA, Muschler GF. Evidence for the use of cell-based therapy for the treatment of osteonecrosis of the femoral head: a systematic review of the literature. J Arthroplast. 2017;32(5):1698–708. https://doi.org/10.1016/j.arth.2016.12.049.

27. Pas HI, Winters M, Haisma HJ, Koenis MJ, Tol JL, Moen MH. Stem cell injections in knee osteoarthritis: a systematic review of the literature. Br J Sports Med. 2017;51(15):1125–33. https://doi.org/10.1136/bjsports-2016-096793.

28. Piuzzi NS, Hussain ZB, Chahla J, Cinque ME, Moatshe G, Mantripragada VP, Muschler GF, LaPrade RF. Variability in the preparation, reporting, and use of bone marrow aspirate concentrate in musculoskeletal disorders: a systematic review of the clinical orthopaedic literature. J Bone Joint Surg Am. 2018;100(6):517–25. https://doi.org/10.2106/jbjs.17.00451.

29. Castillo TN, Pouliot MA, Kim HJ, Dragoo JL. Comparison of growth factor and platelet concentration from commercial platelet-rich plasma separation systems. Am J Sports Med. 2011;39(2):266–71. https://doi.org/10.1177/0363546510387517.

30. Mazzocca AD, McCarthy MB, Chowaniec DM, Cote MP, Romeo AA, Bradley JP, Arciero RA, Beitzel K. Platelet-rich plasma differs according to preparation method and human variability. J Bone Joint Surg Am. 2012;94(4):308–16. https://doi.org/10.2106/jbjs.k.00430.

31. Xiong G, Lingampalli N, Koltsov JCB, Leung LL, Bhutani N, Robinson WH, Chu CR. Men and women differ in the biochemical composition of platelet-rich plasma. Am J Sports Med. 2018;46(2):409–19. https://doi.org/10.1177/0363546517740845.

32. Weibrich G, Kleis WK, Hafner G, Hitzler WE. Growth factor levels in platelet-rich plasma and correlations with donor age, sex, and platelet count. J Craniomaxillofac Surg. 2002;30(2):97–102. https://doi.org/10.1054/jcms.2002.0285.

33. Crisan M, Yap S, Casteilla L, Chen CW, Corselli M, Park TS, Andriolo G, Sun B, Zheng B, Zhang L, Norotte C, Teng PN, Traas J, Schugar R, Deasy BM, Badylak S, Buhring HJ, Giacobino JP, Lazzari L, Huard J, Peault B. A perivascular origin for mesenchymal stem cells in multiple human organs. Cell Stem Cell. 2008;3(3):301–13. https://doi.org/10.1016/j.stem.2008.07.003.

34. Caplan AI. Mesenchymal stem cells. J Orthop Res. 1991;9(5):641–50. https://doi.org/10.1002/jor.1100090504.

35. Payne KA, Didiano DM, Chu CR. Donor sex and age influence the chondrogenic potential of human femoral bone marrow stem cells. Osteoarthr Cartil. 2010;18(5):705–13. https://doi.org/10.1016/j.joca.2010.01.011.

36. Maletis GB, Chen J, Inacio MC, Funahashi TT. Age-related risk factors for revision anterior cruciate ligament reconstruction: a cohort study of 21,304 patients from the Kaiser Permanente anterior cruciate ligament registry. Am J Sports Med. 2016;44(2):331–6. https://doi.org/10.1177/0363546515614813.

37. Baer PC, Geiger H. Adipose-derived mesenchymal stromal/stem cells: tissue localization, characterization, and heterogeneity. Stem Cells Int. 2012;2012:812693. https://doi.org/10.1155/2012/812693.

38. Trivanovic D, Jaukovic A, Popovic B, Krstic J, Mojsilovic S, Okic-Djordjevic I, Kukolj T, Obradovic H, Santibanez JF, Bugarski D. Mesenchymal stem cells of different origin: comparative evaluation of proliferative capacity, telomere length and pluripotency marker expression. Life Sci. 2015;141:61–73. https://doi.org/10.1016/j.lfs.2015.09.019.

39. Murray IR, Geeslin AG, Goudie EB, Petrigliano FA, LaPrade RF. Minimum Information for Studies Evaluating Biologics in Orthopaedics (MIBO): platelet-rich plasma and mesenchymal stem cells. J Bone Joint Surg Am. 2017;99(10):809–19. https://doi.org/10.2106/jbjs.16.00793.

40. Etkin CD, Springer BD. The American joint replacement registry-the first 5 years. Arthroplast Today. 2017;3(2):67–9. https://doi.org/10.1016/j.artd.2017.02.002.

41. HHS, FDA, CBER. Expedited programs for regenerative medicine therapies for serious conditions. 2017. https://www.fda.gov/downloads/biologicsbloodvaccines/guidancecompliance-regulatoryinformation/guidances/cellularandgenetherapy/ucm585414.pdf. Accessed January 2, 2019.

42. HHS, FDA, CBER, CDER. Regulatory considerations for human cells, tissues, and cellular and tissue-based products: minimal manipulation and homologous use. 2017. https://www.fda.gov/downloads/biologicsbloodvaccines/guidancecomplianceregulatoryinformation/guidances/cellularandgenetherapy/ucm585403.pdf. Accessed January 2, 2019.

43. HHS, FDA, CBER, CDER. Guidance for industry: expedited programs for serious conditions – drugs and biologics. 2017. https://www.fda.gov/downloads/Drugs/Guidances/UCM358301.pdf. Accessed January 2, 2019.

44. Rodeo SA. Biologic approaches in sports medicine: potential, perils, and paths forward. Am J Sports Med. 2016;44(7):1657–9. https://doi.org/10.1177/0363546516655130.

45. Dolkart O, Chechik O, Zarfati Y, Brosh T, Alhajajra F, Maman E. A single dose of platelet-rich plasma improves the organization and strength of a surgically repaired rotator cuff tendon in rats. Arch Orthop Trauma Surg. 2014;134(9):1271–7. https://doi.org/10.1007/s00402-014-2026-4.

46. Gulotta LV, Kovacevic D, Packer JD, Deng XH, Rodeo SA. Bone marrow-derived mesenchymal stem cells transduced with scleraxis improve rotator cuff healing in a rat model. Am J Sports Med. 2011;39(6):1282–9. https://doi.org/10.1177/0363546510395485.

47. Jo CH, Shin JS, Shin WH, Lee SY, Yoon KS, Shin S. Platelet-rich plasma for arthroscopic repair of medium to large rotator cuff tears: a randomized controlled trial. Am J Sports Med. 2015;43(9):2102–10. https://doi.org/10.1177/0363546515587081.

48. Patel JM, Merriam AR, Culp BM, Gatt CJ Jr, Dunn MG. One-year outcomes of total meniscus reconstruction using a novel fiber-reinforced scaffold in an ovine model. Am J Sports Med. 2016;44(4):898–907. https://doi.org/10.1177/0363546515624913.

49. Fitzpatrick J, Bulsara M, Zheng MH. The effectiveness of platelet-rich plasma in the treatment of tendinopathy: a meta-analysis of randomized controlled clinical trials. Am J Sports Med. 2017;45(1):226–33. https://doi.org/10.1177/0363546516643716.

50. Mantripragada VP, Bova WA, Boehm C, Piuzzi NS, Obuchowski NA, Midura RJ, Muschler GF. Progenitor cells from different zones of human cartilage and their correlation with histopathological osteoarthritis progression. J Orthop Res. 2018;36(6):1728–38. https://doi.org/10.1002/jor.23829.

51. Jiang Y, Cai Y, Zhang W, Yin Z, Hu C, Tong T, Lu P, Zhang S, Neculai D, Tuan RS, Ouyang HW. Human cartilage-derived progenitor cells from committed chondrocytes for efficient cartilage repair and regeneration. Stem Cells Transl Med. 2016;5(6):733–44. https://doi.org/10.5966/sctm.2015-0192.

52. Jiang Y, Tuan RS. Origin and function of cartilage stem/progenitor cells in osteoarthritis. Nat Rev Rheumatol. 2015;11(4):206–12. https://doi.org/10.1038/nrrheum.2014.200.

53. Caldwell KL, Wang J. Cell-based articular cartilage repair: the link between development and regeneration. Osteoarthr Cartil. 2015;23(3):351–62. https://doi.org/10.1016/j.joca.2014.11.004.

54. Smith BD, Grande DA. The current state of scaffolds for musculoskeletal regenerative applications. Nat Rev Rheumatol. 2015;11(4):213–22. https://doi.org/10.1038/nrrheum.2015.27.
55. Daher RJ, Chahine NO, Greenberg AS, Sgaglione NA, Grande DA. New methods to diagnose and treat cartilage degeneration. Nat Rev Rheumatol. 2009;5(11):599–607. https://doi.org/10.1038/nrrheum.2009.204.
56. Wan S, Borland S, Richardson SM, Merry CLR, Saiani A, Gough JE. Self-assembling peptide hydrogel for intervertebral disc tissue engineering. Acta Biomater. 2016;46:29–40. https://doi.org/10.1016/j.actbio.2016.09.033.
57. Hoque ME, Chuan YL, Pashby I. Extrusion based rapid prototyping technique: an advanced platform for tissue engineering scaffold fabrication. Biopolymers. 2012;97(2):83–93. https://doi.org/10.1002/bip.21701.
58. Rengier F, Mehndiratta A, von Tengg-Kobligk H, Zechmann CM, Unterhinninghofen R, Kauczor HU, Giesel FL. 3D printing based on imaging data: review of medical applications. Int J Comput Assist Radiol Surg. 2010;5(4):335–41. https://doi.org/10.1007/s11548-010-0476-x.
59. Faramarzi N, Yazdi IK, Nabavinia M, Gemma A, Fanelli A, Caizzone A, Ptaszek LM, Sinha I, Khademhosseini A, Ruskin JN, Tamayol A. Patient-specific bioinks for 3D bioprinting of tissue engineering scaffolds. Adv Healthc Mater. 2018;7(11):e1701347. https://doi.org/10.1002/adhm.201701347.
60. Zhu K, Shin SR, van Kempen T, Li YC, Ponraj V, Nasajpour A, Mandla S, Hu N, Liu X, Leijten J, Lin YD, Hussain MA, Zhang YS, Tamayol A, Khademhosseini A. Gold nanocomposite bioink for printing 3D cardiac constructs. Adv Funct Mater. 2017;27(12) https://doi.org/10.1002/adfm.201605352.
61. Mautner K, Colberg RE, Malanga G, Borg-Stein JP, Harmon KG, Dharamsi AS, Chu S, Homer P. Outcomes after ultrasound-guided platelet-rich plasma injections for chronic tendinopathy: a multicenter, retrospective review. PM R. 2013;5(3):169–75. https://doi.org/10.1016/j.pmrj.2012.12.010.
62. Rai MF, Sandell LJ, Zhang B, Wright RW, Brophy RH. RNA microarray analysis of macroscopically Normal articular cartilage from knees undergoing partial medial meniscectomy: potential prediction of the risk for developing osteoarthritis. PLoS One. 2016;11(5):e0155373. https://doi.org/10.1371/journal.pone.0155373.
63. Franceschi RT, Yang S, Rutherford RB, Krebsbach PH, Zhao M, Wang D. Gene therapy approaches for bone regeneration. Cells Tissues Organs. 2004;176(1–3):95–108. https://doi.org/10.1159/000075031.
64. Evans CH, Whalen JD, Evans CH, Ghivizzani SC, Robbins PD. Gene therapy in autoimmune diseases. Ann Rheum Dis. 1998;57(3):125–7.
65. Evans CH. Gene delivery to bone. Adv Drug Deliv Rev. 2012;64(12):1331–40. https://doi.org/10.1016/j.addr.2012.03.013.
66. Evans CH, Ghivizzani SC, Robbins PD. Getting arthritis gene therapy into the clinic. Nat Rev Rheumatol. 2011;7(4):244–9. https://doi.org/10.1038/nrrheum.2010.193.
67. Yi Y, Noh MJ, Lee KH. Current advances in retroviral gene therapy. Curr Gene Ther. 2011;11(3):218–28.
68. Yin H, Kanasty RL, Eltoukhy AA, Vegas AJ, Dorkin JR, Anderson DG. Non-viral vectors for gene-based therapy. Nat Rev Genet. 2014;15(8):541–55. https://doi.org/10.1038/nrg3763.
69. Thomas CE, Ehrhardt A, Kay MA. Progress and problems with the use of viral vectors for gene therapy. Nat Rev Genet. 2003;4(5):346–58. https://doi.org/10.1038/nrg1066.
70. Pensak MJ, Lieberman JR. Gene therapy for bone regeneration. Curr Pharm Des. 2013;19(19):3466–73.
71. Phillips JE, Gersbach CA, Garcia AJ. Virus-based gene therapy strategies for bone regeneration. Biomaterials. 2007;28(2):211–29. https://doi.org/10.1016/j.biomaterials.2006.07.032.
72. Evans CH, Ghivizzani SC, Herndon JH, Robbins PD. Gene therapy for the treatment of musculoskeletal diseases. J Am Acad Orthop Surg. 2005;13(4):230–42.
73. Carofino BC, Lieberman JR. Gene therapy applications for fracture-healing. J Bone Joint Surg Am. 2008;90(Suppl 1):99–110. https://doi.org/10.2106/jbjs.g.01546.

74. Zhang J, Huang X, Wang H, Liu X, Zhang T, Wang Y, Hu D. The challenges and promises of allogeneic mesenchymal stem cells for use as a cell-based therapy. Stem Cell Res Ther. 2015;6:234. https://doi.org/10.1186/s13287-015-0240-9.
75. Virk MS, Sugiyama O, Park SH, Gambhir SS, Adams DJ, Drissi H, Lieberman JR. "Same day" ex-vivo regional gene therapy: a novel strategy to enhance bone repair. Mol Ther. 2011;19(5):960–8. https://doi.org/10.1038/mt.2011.2.
76. Alaee F, Bartholomae C, Sugiyama O, Virk MS, Drissi H, Wu Q, Schmidt M, Lieberman JR. Biodistribution of LV-TSTA transduced rat bone marrow cells used for "ex-vivo" regional gene therapy for bone repair. Curr Gene Ther. 2015;15(5):481–91.
77. Evans CH, Gouze JN, Gouze E, Robbins PD, Ghivizzani SC. Osteoarthritis gene therapy. Gene Ther. 2004;11(4):379–89. https://doi.org/10.1038/sj.gt.3302196.
78. Pelletier JP, Caron JP, Evans C, Robbins PD, Georgescu HI, Jovanovic D, Fernandes JC, Martel-Pelletier J. In vivo suppression of early experimental osteoarthritis by interleukin-1 receptor antagonist using gene therapy. Arthritis Rheum. 1997;40(6):1012–9. https://doi.org/10.1002/art.1780400604.
79. Frisbie DD, Ghivizzani SC, Robbins PD, Evans CH, McIlwraith CW. Treatment of experimental equine osteoarthritis by in vivo delivery of the equine interleukin-1 receptor antagonist gene. Gene Ther. 2002;9(1):12–20. https://doi.org/10.1038/sj.gt.3301608.
80. Goodrich LR, Grieger JC, Phillips JN, Khan N, Gray SJ, McIlwraith CW, Samulski RJ. scAAVIL-1ra dosing trial in a large animal model and validation of long-term expression with repeat administration for osteoarthritis therapy. Gene Ther. 2015;22(7):536–45. https://doi.org/10.1038/gt.2015.21.
81. Kay JD, Gouze E, Oligino TJ, Gouze JN, Watson RS, Levings PP, Bush ML, Dacanay A, Nickerson DM, Robbins PD, Evans CH, Ghivizzani SC. Intra-articular gene delivery and expression of interleukin-1Ra mediated by self-complementary adeno-associated virus. J Gene Med. 2009;11(7):605–14. https://doi.org/10.1002/jgm.1334.
82. Fernandes J, Tardif G, Martel-Pelletier J, Lascau-Coman V, Dupuis M, Moldovan F, Sheppard M, Krishnan BR, Pelletier JP. In vivo transfer of interleukin-1 receptor antagonist gene in osteoarthritic rabbit knee joints: prevention of osteoarthritis progression. Am J Pathol. 1999;154(4):1159–69. https://doi.org/10.1016/s0002-9440(10)65368-0.
83. Wang G, Evans CH, Benson JM, Hutt JA, Seagrave J, Wilder JA, Grieger JC, Samulski RJ, Terse PS. Safety and biodistribution assessment of sc-rAAV2.5IL-1Ra administered via intra-articular injection in a mono-iodoacetate-induced osteoarthritis rat model. Mol Ther Methods Clin Dev. 2016;3:15052. https://doi.org/10.1038/mtm.2015.52.
84. https://clinicaltrials.gov/ct2/results?term=TGC+joint&Search=Search.   Cited: 3rd January 2019.
85. Ha CW, Noh MJ, Choi KB, Lee KH. Initial phase I safety of retrovirally transduced human chondrocytes expressing transforming growth factor-beta-1 in degenerative arthritis patients. Cytotherapy. 2012;14(2):247–56. https://doi.org/10.3109/14653249.2011.629645.
86. Safety of Intra-Articular Sc-rAAV2.5IL-1Ra in Subjects With Moderate Knee OA. https://ClinicalTrials.gov/show/NCT02790723.

Index

© Springer Nature Switzerland AG 2020
G. Cooper et al. (eds.), *Regenerative Medicine for Spine and Joint Pain*,
https://doi.org/10.1007/978-3-030-42771-9

Printed in the United States
by Baker & Taylor Publisher Services